Management of Spinal Cord Injuries
A Guide for Physiotherapists

For Elsevier:

Publisher: Heidi Harrison
Associate Editor: Siobhan Campbell
Production Manager: Anne Dickie
Design: Charles Gray
Illustration Buyer: Merlyn Harvey
Illustrator: Cactus
Original illustrations from www.physiotherapyexercises.com: Paul Pattie

Management of Spinal Cord Injuries
A Guide for Physiotherapists

Lisa Harvey BAppSc, GradDipAppSc(ExSpSc), MAppSc, PhD
Senior Lecturer, Rehabilitation Studies Unit, Northern Clinical School,
University of Sydney, Sydney, Australia

Clinical Consultant, Moorong Spinal Unit, Royal Rehabilitation Centre Sydney, Australia

Foreword by
William H. Donovan MD
Clinical Professor and Chair, Physical Medicine and Rehabilitation,
University of Texas Health Science Centre at Houston, Houston, Texas, USA

Medical Director, Memorial Hermann/The Institute for Rehabilitation and Research (TIRR),
Houston, Texas, USA

Principal Investigator, Model Systems SCI Centre, Houston, Texas, USA

President, International Spinal Cord Society

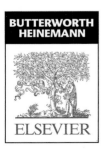

BUTTERWORTH
HEINEMANN

ELSEVIER

EDINBURGH LONDON NEW YORK OXFORD PHILADELPHIA ST LOUIS SYDNEY TORONTO 2008

BUTTERWORTH
HEINEMANN
ELSEVIER

Butterworth-Heinemann
An imprint of Elsevier Limited

First published 2008
© 2008, Elsevier Ltd

The following figures and tables are adapted with permission from www.
physiotherapyexercises.com: Tables 3.1–3.9, 6.1, 6.2 and Figures 3.4–3.13, 3.15,
4.2–4.10, 6.1–6.3, 6.5–6.7, 6.11, 7.1–7.7, 8.1, 8.2, 8.4–8.6, 8.8, 9.3–9.9, 9.11–9.14,
12.1, 13.4.

ISBN: 978 0 443 06858 4

British Library Cataloguing in Publication Data
A catalogue record for this book is available from the British Library.

Library of Congress Cataloging in Publication Data
A catalog record for this book is available from the Library of Congress.

Note
Neither the Publisher nor the Authors assume any responsibility for any loss or
injury and/or damage to persons or property arising out of or related to any use
of the material contained in this book. It is the responsibility of the treating prac-
titioner, relying on independent expertise and knowledge of the patient, to determine the best treatment and method of application for the patient.

Contents

Foreword by *William H. Donovan*   vii
Preface   ix
Acknowledgements   xi
Reviewers   xiii
Abbreviations   xvii

SECTION 1: The bare essentials

Chapter 1:   Background information   3
Chapter 2:   A framework for physiotherapy management   35

SECTION 2: Understanding how people with paralysis perform motor tasks

Chapter 3:   Transfers and bed mobility of people with lower limb paralysis   57
Chapter 4:   Wheelchair mobility   79
Chapter 5:   Hand function of people with tetraplegia   93
Chapter 6:   Standing and walking with lower limb paralysis   107

SECTION 3: Management of impairments

Chapter 7:   Training motor tasks   137
Chapter 8:   Strength training   155
Chapter 9:   Contracture management   177
Chapter 10:   Pain management   193
Chapter 11:   Respiratory management   205
Chapter 12:   Cardiovascular fitness training   227

SECTION 4: Environmental factors

Chapter 13:   Wheelchair seating   245

SECTION 5: The way forward

Chapter 14:   Evidence-based physiotherapy   275

Appendix   283
Index   287

Foreword

William H. Donovan

It is indeed a privilege to be asked to write a foreword to a book that has been definitely needed for a long time. Departing from formats of other physiotherapy texts, Dr Lisa Harvey has centred all pertinent therapeutic approaches around spinal cord injury (SCI) and explains how they should be applied to this unique population, considering all aspects of the post-impairment physiological changes.

Dr Harvey's impressive research and contributions to the literature, as well as her accomplishments as a teacher in the dissemination of knowledge, have prepared her well to write this text. Clear and concise explanations are augmented with numerous illustrations, making the learning of physiotherapy principles, as applied to SCI, easy for students and therapists new to SCI alike.

While relating all sections back to the basic concepts of the World Health Organization's international classification of function, disability and health (ICF), Dr Harvey continually reminds the reader of the importance of relating all mobility tasks to functions that are attainable and relevant to each person within his/her environmental and personal circumstances.

The students, as well as trained therapists, seeking to refresh or expand their knowledge of SCI, will especially benefit from the chapters on learning of motor tasks, since so much of SCI rehab relies on the learning capacity of the patient/consumer. Likewise, Dr Harvey's clear explanations on gait, the contribution of the key muscle groups during normal gait and the orthoses which substitute for their functions when those muscles are weakened, contain information that must be mastered. Similarly, her treatment of the concepts involved in strength training and wheelchair prescription are as easy to read as they are illuminating.

Chapters on pain, and the respiratory and cardiac aspects that pertain to the SCI population, provide therapists with knowledge that will allow them to contribute to patient management in these challenging areas, while also imparting sufficient information about how the more medically-oriented issues are addressed by the physicians.

I must say I have enjoyed reading this opus which provides ample evidence of Dr Harvey's teaching skills, dedication to the scientific approach aimed at evidence-based treatment and leads me to say she is a role model for all therapists, particularly those inclined towards an academic career.

William H. Donovan, MD

Clinical Professor and Chair, Physical Medicine and Rehabilitation

The University of Texas Health Science Centre at Houston

Medical Director, Memorial Hermann/The Institute for Rehabilitation and Research (TIRR)

President, the International Spinal Cord Society

Preface

The aim of this book is to equip readers with a theoretical framework to manage people with spinal cord injury. It is intended for students and junior physiotherapists with little or no experience in the area of spinal cord injury but with a general understanding of the principles of physiotherapy. There are also sections which will be of interest to senior clinicians, especially those keen to explore the evidence base of different interventions.

When writing this book, I tried to take myself back to my early career. I tried to remember the feeling of inadequacy when I was first expected to train a person with C6 tetraplegia to transfer and the anxiety I felt when late one night I was asked to manage a critically ill person with tetraplegia who was unable to clear his own chest secretions. I have considered the challenge for physiotherapists faced with the management of these patients and why it is difficult to transfer general principles of physiotherapy to this specific group. I have also tried to remember all those questions that came to my mind as a junior physiotherapist, to many of which there are still no clear answers. Then, as now, I had questions about the relative effectiveness of different interventions and about long-held assumptions of what physiotherapists should and should not do.

There are three important influences on this book. The first is evidence-based practice. The move towards evidence-based practice has changed physiotherapy. We can no longer accept as fact all beliefs about physiotherapy management of people with spinal cord injury which have been passed down through the years. The demand for high quality evidence to support our work is appropriate because good evidence optimizes patient outcomes and reduces the costs of rehabilitation. Good evidence also heightens job satisfaction for physiotherapists because it provides unequivocal evidence that their work is important and effective and their interventions make a clear difference to their patients' quality of life. However, the push for evidence-based practice raises practical problems of what to do in the face of clinical scenarios where there is little or no evidence to guide us. It also introduces ambiguity and uncertainty. Ours is still a young profession and in many areas we are yet to clearly distinguish between effective and non-effective interventions. This is a challenge but it also makes the profession a dynamic and exciting one to belong to.

A second major influence on this book is the International Classification of Functioning, Disability and Health (ICF). The ICF was adopted by the World Health Organization as a universally accepted language. It is also useful for providing a framework for the physiotherapy management of people with spinal cord injury and it underpins the problem-solving approach advocated in this book. Goals of treatment are identified in terms of 'activity limitations' and 'participation restrictions' after taking into account 'contextual' and 'environmental' factors. Physiotherapy-specific goals are largely directed at patients' ability to perform functional motor tasks so they are classified within the mobility domain of ICF. Difficulties performing motor tasks are analysed in terms of impairments and impairments are largely defined within the neuromusculoskeletal and movement-related domains of ICF. The key impairments are lack of strength, skill, fitness and joint mobility, as well as pain and compromised respiratory function. Patient outcomes can be measured at the activity limitation and participation restriction level or at the impairment level. The ICF encourages physiotherapists to ensure that treatments are driven by the contribution of impairments to activity limitations and participation restrictions, not by impairments alone.

The third influence on this book is theories about motor learning and motor control. Often patients with spinal cord injury have difficulties mastering important mobility tasks because they lack skill. That is, they do not know how to transfer, roll, walk or manoeuvre a wheelchair with their newly acquired patterns of paralysis. They need to learn to appropriately activate non-paralysed muscles for purposeful movement. The motor tasks are novel and need to be learnt. The physiotherapist's role is to facilitate the learning process and act as 'coach'. To do this effectively, physiotherapists need to understand how patients learn motor tasks and how the environment can be structured to optimize learning. These and other issues related to the effective teaching of motor tasks are emphasized throughout the book.

When writing this book, I needed to make decisions about what to include and exclude. Medical, surgical, psychosocial and nursing issues have only been covered briefly in one chapter, in enough detail for a junior physiotherapist.

Hopefully this strategy will enable readers to appreciate issues related to the broader management of people with spinal cord injury but not at the risk of diverting attention to issues which are not the prime focus of physiotherapy. There are many good books on these topics which interested readers are encouraged to consult.

Initially when writing the book I tried to avoid the term 'patient' and instead refer to 'people' or 'individuals' with spinal cord injury. The term 'patient' implies illness, passivity and dependence, so it is less than ideal. However, the alternate terminology was so clumsy and confusing I relented and used the word 'patient' through most of the book, except in titles and the beginning sections of chapters.

My hope is that this book will be of practical use to readers and will help them develop the problem-solving skills necessary to manage patients with all types of spinal cord injury. I also hope that it will inspire young and junior physiotherapists working in the area of spinal cord injuries to embrace evidence-based physiotherapy within an ICF and motor learning framework. Hopefully, this next generation of physiotherapists will critically reflect on their practice to further develop the physiotherapy care of people with spinal cord injury.

Acknowledgements

This book would not have been possible without the ongoing support of the Motor Accidents Authority of New South Wales. The Motor Accidents Authority has provided me with financial support over the last 10 years in the form of scholarships and project grants, and it currently funds my academic position within the Faculty of Medicine at the University of Sydney. I would not be in a position to write a book without the Motor Accidents Authority's ongoing support.

I also wish to thank my fellow clinicians and students with whom I have had the privilege of working over the years. They have encouraged and challenged my thinking, and helped me in innumerable ways. Many have contributed to the research and other projects mentioned in this book. I am particularly grateful to Julia Batty.

In the early days of writing this book, Joanne Glinsky provided the critical encouragement and, once the book started to take shape, she read and edited large sections and provided sensible advice and guidance. Other colleagues who provided assistance are Jill Eyles, Donna Ristev, Craig Drury, Nicola Shelton, Damien Barratt, Adrian Byak, Sophie Denis, Jenni Barker, Sean Hogan, Ann Thompson, Bronwyn Thomas, Emilie Myers, Lyndall Katte, Greg Ungerer, Paula Cunningham, Ross Chafetz, Merrick Smith, Alicon Bennie, Mary Schmidt and Courtney Fiebig. Academics who generously provided feedback include Professor Andre De Troyer, Dr Jane Butler, Dr Anne Moseley, Ms Carolyn Gates, Professor Bruce Dobkin and Professor Ian Cameron.

I am especially grateful for the valuable advice and feedback I received from my reviewers, some of whom I have never met (see p. xiii). Despite their busy workloads and high profiles, they all responded enthusiastically to my written requests for help. They graciously and generously corrected mistakes and steered the book in the right direction. Any remaining errors are, of course, entirely my responsibility.

I acknowledge with gratitude the assistance I received from staff and volunteers of the Rehabilitation Studies Unit and the Royal Rehabilitation Centre Sydney. Chris Lin, a research assistant, helped review the literature and checked over 1500 references. Librarians Michelle Lee and Judith Allan endlessly and enthusiastically retrieved books and articles. Ms Penny Lye, a volunteer with a long background in publication, proofread the entire manuscript. Professor Ian Cameron, the director of the Rehabilitation Studies Unit, saw worth in the project and provided support over an extended period of time.

I wish to make special mention of my physiotherapy colleagues from India, Pakistan, South Africa and Vietnam. Over recent years I have had the privilege of visiting and teaching physiotherapists from these countries. They have provided me with an international perspective for which I am grateful. I salute the good work they do. I have tried to ensure that this book caters for their needs and is equally relevant to their circumstances.

Most of the illustrations in this book are drawn by Paul Pattie, originally for the website www.physiotherapyexercises. com. My colleagues and I established this website. It is a not-for-profit initiative funded by various organizations including the Motor Accidents Authority of New South Wales, Royal Rehabilitation Centre Sydney and New South Wales State Spinal Service. It was made possible by the generous volunteer work of Peter Messenger. Owen Katalinic and Joanne Glinsky took all the photographs which the website is based upon and laboured behind the scenes. I am grateful to Peter, Owen, Joanne and all involved who made the creation of the website possible.

Lastly, thanks to my family, Rob, Dan and Jemma Herbert, as well as my parents, Pat and Frank Harvey. Special thanks to Pat and Rob who both proofread and edited the entire book.

Reviewers

Chapter 1

Dr James Middleton MD, PhD
NSW State Spinal Cord Injury Services, Australia

Associate Professor Ralph Marino MD, PhD
Department of Rehabilitation Medicine, Jefferson Medical College, Thomas Jefferson University, Philadelphia, USA

Dr Paul Kennedy PhD
Department of Clinical Psychology, University of Oxford, Warneford Hospital, England

Chapter 2

Associate Professor Louise Ada PhD
Discipline of Physiotherapy, University of Sydney, Australia

Ms Joanne Glinsky MAppSc
Physiotherapy Department, Moorong Spinal Unit, Royal Rehabilitation Centre Sydney, Australia

Dr Paul Kennedy PhD
Department of Clinical Psychology, University of Oxford, Warneford Hospital, England

Chapter 3

Associate Professor Robert Herbert PhD
Discipline of Physiotherapy and Centre for Evidence-Based Physiotherapy, Faculty of Health Science, University of Sydney, Australia

Associate Professor Garry Alison PhD
The Centre for Musculoskeletal Studies, The University of Western Australia, Australia

Dr Colleen Canning PhD
Discipline of Physiotherapy, University of Sydney, Australia

Ms Joanne Glinsky MAppSc
Physiotherapy Department, Moorong Spinal Unit, Royal Rehabilitation Centre Sydney, Australia

Chapter 4

Professor Lee Kirby MD, FRCPC
Division of Physical Medicine and Rehabilitation, Department of Medicine, Dalhousie University, Halifax, Nova Scotia, Canada

Mr Craig Jarvis AssDip (Recreation)
Spinal Injury Unit, Prince of Wales Hospital, Sydney, Australia

Chapter 5

Ms Helga Lechner MSc
Swiss Paraplegic Research, Nottwil, Switzerland

Ms Cathy Cooper BAppSc
Upper Limb Program, Victorian Spinal Cord Service, Royal Talbot Campus, Melbourne, Australia

Chapter 6

Associate Professor Jack Crosbie PhD
Discipline of Physiotherapy, University of Sydney, Australia

Mr Kevin Brigden Cert(Orthotics)
Department of Orthotics, Royal North Shore Hospital, Sydney, Australia

Chapter 7

Associate Professor Louise Ada PhD
Discipline of Physiotherapy, University of Sydney, Australia

Professor Lee Kirby MD, FRCPC
Division of Physical Medicine and Rehabilitation, Dalhousie University, Halifax, Nova Scotia, Canada

Mr Karl Schurr MAppSc
Department of Physiotherapy, Bankstown Hospital, Sydney, Australia

Associate Professor Karim Fouad PhD
University of Alberta, Faculty of Rehabilitation Medicine, Edmonton, Canada

Chapter 8

Mr Tom Gwinn MAppSc
Department of Exercise and Sports Science, University of Sydney, Australia

Professor Karen Dodd PhD
School of Physiotherapy, La Trobe University, Melbourne, Australia

Associate Professor Robert Herbert PhD
Discipline of Physiotherapy and Centre for Evidence-Based Physiotherapy, University of Sydney, Australia

Chapter 9

Mr Karl Schurr MAppSc
Department of Physiotherapy, Bankstown Hospital, Sydney, Australia

Mr Tom Gwinn MAppSc
Department of Exercise and Sports Science, University of Sydney, Australia

Associate Professor Robert Herbert PhD
Discipline of Physiotherapy and Centre for Evidence-Based Physiotherapy, University of Sydney, Australia

Chapter 10

Clinical Associate Professor Philip Siddall PhD
Pain Management Research Institute, University of Sydney, Royal North Shore Hospital, Sydney, Australia

Dr Karen Ginn PhD
School of Biomedical Sciences, University of Sydney, Australia

Chapter 11

Associate Professor Jenny Alison PhD
Discipline of Physiotherapy, University of Sydney, Australia

Dr Jane Butler PhD
Prince of Wales Medical Research Institute, Australia

Professor Marc Estenne PhD
Chest Service, Erasme University Hospital, Brussels, Belgium

Chapter 12

Dr Jackie Raymond PhD
Department of Exercise and Sports Science, University of Sydney, Australia

Associate Professor Norman Morris PhD
School of Physiotherapy and Exercise Science, Griffith University, Queensland, Australia

Chapter 13

Mr Craig Jarvis AssDip (Recreation)
Physiotherapy Department, Prince of Wales Hospital, Sydney, Australia

Dr Bill Fisher PhD
Department of Biomedical Engineering, Royal North Shore Hospital, Sydney, Australia

Chapter 14

Associate Professor Robert Herbert PhD
Discipline of Physiotherapy and Centre for Evidence-Based Physiotherapy,
University of Sydney, Australia

Abbreviations

1 RM	one repetition maximum
AFO	ankle–foot orthosis
ASIA	American Spinal Injury Association
CPAP	continuous positive airways pressure
DIP	distal interphalangeal joint
ER	expiratory reserve
FEV_1	forced expiratory volume in 1 second
FRC	functional residual capacity
HGO	hip guidance orthosis
ICF	International Classification of Functioning, Disability and Health
IP	interphalangeal joint
IRV	inspiratory reserve volume
MCP	metacarpophalangeal joint
MLO	medial-linkage orthosis
PIP	proximal interphalangeal joint
RGO	reciprocating gait orthosis
RM	repetition maximum
RV	residual volume
SMART	Specific, Measurable, Attainable, Realistic and Timebound
TLC	total lung capacity
T_v	tidal volume
VC	vital capacity
WB	wheelbase

"

The bare essentials

CHAPTER 1
Background
information
3

CHAPTER 2
A framework for
physiotherapy
management
35

"

Contents

Motor, sensory and
autonomic pathways 4

The ASIA assessment of
neurological deficit 6

Common patterns of
neurological loss with
incomplete lesions 11

Upper and lower motor
neuron lesions 12

Prognosis 12

Impairments associated
with spinal cord injury 13

Skin management 22

Psychological well-being 24

Spinal cord injury and
traumatic brain injury 25

Aging with spinal cord injury . .26

Background information

The spinal cord travels within the vertebral canal of the spine and is vital for conveying and integrating sensory and motor information between the brain and somatic and visceral structures. A spinal cord injury impairs motor, sensory and autonomic functions, the implications of which are profound and lead to an array of secondary impairments.

The term 'spinal cord injury' is used to refer to neurological damage of the spinal cord following trauma. In most developed countries, the incidence of spinal cord injury is between 10 and 80 cases per million per year.[1,2] Approximately half of all spinal cord injuries occur in people aged under 30 years.[3-6] The typical person with spinal cord injury is male, aged between 15 and 25 years; only about 15% of spinal cord injuries affect females and only 18% affect people over 45 years.[3] Obvious exceptions to these demographics occur in natural disasters. For example, in the Pakistan earthquakes of 2005 the majority of spinal cord injuries (estimated to be over 1500) were in young women and children.

The most common causes of spinal cord injury are motor vehicle and motor-bike accidents, followed by falls.[3,7] Work-related injuries are also common, as are injuries from sport and water-based activities. In some countries the incidence of spinal cord injury from gun, stab or war-related injuries is high. Spinal cord lesions can also be due to disease, infection and congenital defect.

Over 55% of all spinal cord injuries are cervical; the remainder are approximately equally divided between thoracic, lumbar and sacral levels.[8,9] The most common level of injury is C5, followed by C4, C6 and T12, in that order.[10] A spinal cord injury in the cervical region affects all four limbs, resulting in *tetraplegia* (also called quadriplegia). Spinal cord injuries in the thoracic, lumbar or sacral region affect the lower limbs and result in *paraplegia*. Most spinal cord injuries do not involve transection or severing of the spinal cord.[11,12] Rather, the cord remains intact and the neurological damage is due to secondary vascular and pathogenic events, including oedema, inflammation and changes to the blood–spinal cord barrier.[13,14]

The extent of damage to the spinal cord is highly variable and, consequently, a spinal cord injury can prevent the transmission of all or just some neural messages across the site of the lesion.[9] In some patients the only sign that part of the spinal cord

Figure 1.1 Prevalence of different types of spinal cord injuries in developed countries. Prevalence refers to the number of people living with SCI. Reproduced from Martin Ginis KA, Hicks AL: Exercise research issues in the spinal cord injured population. Exerc Sport Sci Rev 2005; 33: 49–53, with permission of Lippincott Williams & Wilkins.

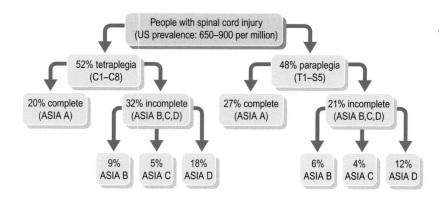

has been preserved is very slight movement or sensation below the level of the injury. For other patients there may be extensive preservation of motor and sensory pathways enabling them to walk almost normally. Partial preservation of the spinal cord is more common following cervical, lumbar and sacral injuries than thoracic injuries. It is also more common today than 20 years ago because of advances in retrieval, emergency and acute management reducing secondary neural damage (see Figure 1.1).[15]

Motor, sensory and autonomic pathways

The vertebral column consists of seven cervical, 12 thoracic, five lumbar, five sacral and four coccygeal vertebrae, although the sacral and coccygeal vertebrae are fused. Emerging from the spinal cord are 31 pairs of anterior and posterior nerve roots: eight cervical, 12 thoracic, five lumbar, five sacral and one coccygeal. At each level an anterior (ventral) pair of nerve roots carries motor nerves and a posterior (dorsal) pair of nerve roots carries sensory nerves. The anterior and posterior roots join to form two spinal nerves, one on either side of the spine, which then exit the vertebral canal through the intervertebral foramina. Once outside the intervertebral foramina they form peripheral nerves.[16]

While there are eight pairs of cervical spinal nerves there are only seven cervical vertebrae. This disparity occurs because the first pair of cervical spinal nerves exits *above* the first cervical vertebra just below the skull. However, the eighth pair of cervical spinal nerves exits *below* the last cervical vertebra (see Figure 1.2).[17]

Motor pathways

Upper and lower motor neurons connect the motor cortex and muscles. The upper motor neurons originate within the motor cortex and then travel down the spinal cord within the corticospinal tracts. These tracts are also called pyramidal tracts. Approximately 85% of upper motor neurons cross over to the contralateral side in the brainstem and then travel within the lateral corticospinal tract. The other 15% cross within the spinal cord at the level they terminate and are carried within the medial corticospinal tract. The cervical upper motor neurons are centrally located within the corticospinal tract and the lumbar and sacral neurons are peripherally located (see Figure 1.3). This explains patterns of neurological loss seen with certain types of incomplete spinal cord injuries where the peripheral rim of the spinal cord

Figure 1.2 The spinal cord, illustrating relationship between vertebrae and nerve roots. Reproduced from Parent A: Carpenter's Human Neuroanatomy, 9th edn. Baltimore, Williams & Wilkins, 1996, with permission of Lippincott Williams & Wilkins.

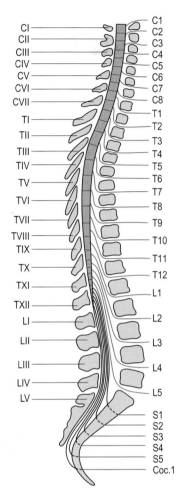

Figure 1.3 Cross-section of the spinal cord illustrating the corticospinal and spinothalamic tracts, and the posterior (or dorsal) columns.

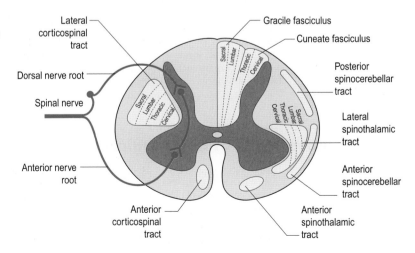

is undamaged (see p. 11). There are also other complex motor pathways contained within the extrapyramidal system.

The upper motor neurons synapse in the spinal cord with anterior horn cells of lower motor neurons, usually via interneurons. The anterior horn cells are the cell bodies of the lower motor neurons and are located in the grey matter of the spinal cord. Axons project from the cell bodies of lower motor neurons to form the anterior nerve roots before mixing with the posterior sensory nerve roots to form spinal nerves.

In the cervical region the spinal nerves are short and exit the vertebral canal almost immediately after forming. However, this is not the case further down the spine where the spinal nerves travel progressively longer distances within the vertebral canal before exiting. This is particularly apparent in the cauda equina which consists solely of lumbar, sacral and coccygeal spinal nerves. That is, it consists solely of lower motor neurons. The cell bodies of the lower motor neurons of the cauda equina are positioned within the conus, located at approximately the L1 vertebral body. However, even above the conus, spinal nerves travel down within the vertebral canal before exiting. Consequently, the anterior horn cells of lower motor neurons are often positioned at a higher level in the vertebral canal than where they exit.

Sensory pathways

There are many sensory tracts and pathways carrying different types of sensory information from the periphery to the cerebral cortex. The key ones are the lateral and anterior spinothalamic tracts and the gracile and cuneate tracts within the posterior columns. The spinothalamic tracts sit within the dorsal horn of the spinal cord. Most of the fibres cross at or near the level they enter the spinal cord. The lateral spinothalamic tract carries information about pain and temperature, and the anterior spinothalamic tract carries information about crude touch. The gracile and cuneate tracts carry information about proprioception and light touch. The *gracile tract* is positioned medially and predominantly carries sensory fibres from the lower body while the *cuneate tract* is positioned laterally and predominantly carries fibres from the upper body. The fibres within the gracile and cuneate tracts cross in the brainstem.

Autonomic pathways

The spinal cord not only carries motor and sensory nerves but also autonomic nerves (see Figure 1.4). Sympathetic nerves exit the vertebral canal via thoraco-lumbar spinal nerves, and parasympathetic nerves exit via sacral spinal nerves. Consequently, patients with cervical lesions lose supraspinal control of the entire sympathetic nervous system[18] and of the sacral part of the parasympathetic nervous system. Patients with thoracic, lumbar or sacral lesions lose varying amounts of supraspinal control of the sympathetic and parasympathetic nervous system as determined by the level of the lesion. Some parasympathetic fibres are carried within cranial nerves and are unaffected by spinal cord injury.

The ASIA assessment of neurological deficit

Spinal cord injuries are classified according to The American Spinal Injury Association (ASIA) classification system.[19] The classification is based on a standardized motor and sensory assessment (see Figure 1.5). It is used to define two motor, two sensory and one neurological level. It is also used to classify injuries as either complete (ASIA A) or incomplete (ASIA B, C, D or E).

Figure 1.4 Schematic representation of the autonomic nervous system. Reproduced from Parent A: Carpenter's Human Neuroanatomy, 9th edn. Baltimore, Williams & Wilkins, 1996, with permission of Lippincott Williams & Wilkins.

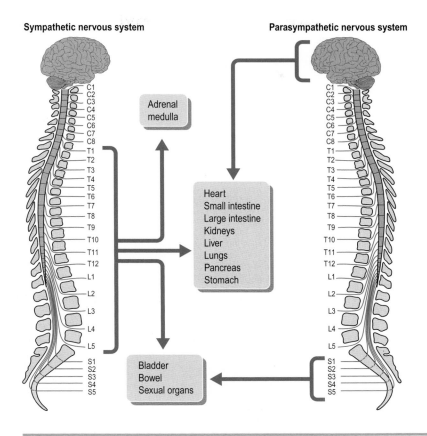

The ASIA motor level

A motor assessment is used to define two motor levels: one for the right and one for the left side of the body. An ASIA motor assessment involves testing the strength of ten key muscles. Each key muscle group represents one myotome between C5 and T1, and between L2 and S1 (see Table 1.1).

Each muscle is tested for strength on the original six-point manual muscle testing scale where:

0 = no muscle contraction
1 = a flicker of muscle contraction
2 = full range of motion with gravity eliminated
3 = full range of motion against gravity
4 = full range of motion with added resistance
5 = normal strength

The main difference between an ASIA motor assessment and a standard manual muscle test[20] (see Chapter 8) is that the ASIA test is performed with patients in the supine position. This position is used because it is important to standardize the testing position and often recently injured patients cannot be moved from the supine position. Limb positions are manipulated to vary the effects of gravity (e.g. testing the iliopsoas muscle for a grade 2/5 involves asking the patient to flex the hip from

Figure 1.5 ASIA assessment form. (From American Spinal Injury Association: International Standards for Neurological Classification of Spinal Cord Injury, revised 2006,[19] with permission of American Spinal Cord Injury Association, Chicago, IL.)

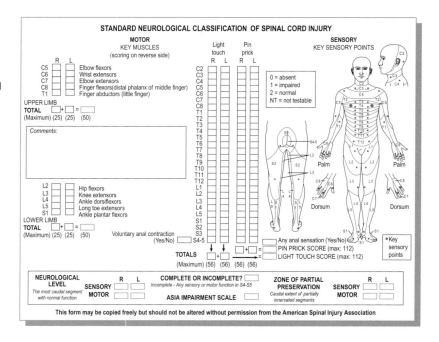

TABLE 1.1 ASIA muscles

C5	Elbow flexors	L2	Hip flexors
C6	Wrist extensors	L3	Knee extensors
C7	Elbow extensors	L4	Ankle dorsiflexors
C8	Finger flexors (middle finger)	L5	Long toe extensors
T1	Little finger abductors	S1	Ankle plantarflexors

an externally rotated position; see Table 1.2 for some general rules about ASIA motor testing). In addition, there are a few complexities in the ASIA motor assessment. For example, grade 1/5 strength in the upper limbs is tested in the gravity-eliminated position whereas in the lower limbs it is tested in the anti-gravity position, except in the case of the plantarflexor muscles (see Table 1.2).

The ASIA *motor level* for each side of the body is determined by the most caudal (distal) key muscle that has at least grade 3/5 (anti-gravity) strength provided all key muscles above have grade 5/5 (normal) strength. The motor level for the right side of the body may be different from the left. There are no specified ASIA muscles for the thoracic segments of the spinal cord. Consequently, the motor level of patients with thoracic paraplegia (lower limb paralysis but no upper limb weakness) is assumed to correspond with their ASIA sensory level.

It is possible to sum the motor scores of the five key ASIA upper limb muscles on both sides of the body and express the total with respect to a maximum possible score of 50. The same can be done for the lower limbs.[21]

TABLE 1.2 **Ten rules for ASIA motor testing**	
1	Test for a grade 3/5 first, then test up or down depending on findings
2	Only downgrade strength if due to neurological deficit. Patients unable to fully cooperate due to pain should not be downgraded
3	Do not test if the patient has a serious contracture (50% or more loss of joint mobility), severe pain or severe spasticity (mark as not testable)
4	Test for a grade 1/5 in the upper limbs with the body segment in its gravity-eliminated position
5	Test for a grade 1/5 in the lower limbs with the body segment in its anti-gravity position (except when testing the plantarflexor muscles)
6	Test for a grade 4/5 in the upper and lower limbs with the body segment in the anti-gravity position (except when testing T1 and S1 muscles)
7	Do not use half marks, pluses or minuses
8	Test for grade 2/5, 3/5, 4/5 or 5/5 by asking the patient to move all the way through range. Grade 4/5 and 5/5 should be tested with resistance applied throughout range
9	Ensure that the patient is not performing trick movements (e.g. ensure grade 3/5 elbow extension occurs without the shoulder dropping into extension)
10	Modify testing positions if the patient has loss of extensibility in underlying muscles that span two or more joints (e.g. finger flexion can be tested with the wrist flexed if the patient has shortening of the extrinsic finger flexor muscles)

The ASIA sensory level

A sensory assessment is used to define two sensory levels: one for the right and one for the left side of the body. An ASIA sensory assessment involves testing light touch and pinprick sensation in 28 key points on each side of the body. Each point represents one dermatome (see Figure 1.5). For example, a precise spot over the back of the hand and just distal to the metacarpophalangeal (MCP) joint of the third digit represents the C7 dermatome. A three-point scale is used for light touch and pinprick where normal sensation is given a score of 2, abnormal (i.e. heightened or reduced) sensation is given a score of 1, and absent sensation is given a score of 0 (see Table 1.3).

The ASIA *sensory level* for each side of the body is determined by the most caudal (distal) key point that has grade 2/2 for pinprick and light touch, provided all key points above are also grade 2/2. Like the motor assessment, the sensory level for the right side of the body may be different from the left. It is also possible to sum the scores for light touch and pinprick of all 28 dermatomes on each side of the body. The total possible score is 224.

The ASIA neurological level

The ASIA motor and sensory assessment is also used to depict one overall *neurological level*.[19] This is relatively straightforward in patients who have the same motor and

TABLE 1.3 Definitions of ASIA sensory scores for pinprick and light touch	
Grade 0	
Light touch	the patient *cannot consistently distinguish* between being touched and not touched with a light cotton bud
Pinprick	the patient *cannot consistently distinguish* between being touched with the sharp end of a safety pin and touched with the blunt end of a safety pin
Grade 1	
Light touch	the patient *can consistently distinguish* between being touched and not touched with a light cotton bud but light touch *feels different* from light touch on the face (this comparison is tested at each dermatome)
Pinprick	the patient *can consistently distinguish* between being touched with the sharp end of a safety pin and touched with the blunt end of a safety pin BUT the sharp side of the pin *feels different* from the sharp side of the pin on the face (this comparison is tested at each dermatome)
Grade 2	
Light touch	the patient *can consistently distinguish* between being touched and not touched with a light cotton bud AND light touch *feels the same as* light touch on the face (this comparison is tested at each dermatome)
Pinprick	the patient *can consistently distinguish* between being touched with the sharp end of a safety pin and touched with the blunt end of a safety pin and the sharp side of the pin *feels the same as* the sharp side of the pin on the face (this comparison is tested at each dermatome)

sensory levels on both sides of the body. In this situation, the neurological level corresponds with the motor and sensory levels. However, in patients who have asymmetrical lesions, the highest motor or sensory level on either side of the body is used to define the neurological level of the lesion. For instance, a patient with a right sensory level of C5 but bilateral motor and left sensory levels of C6 has an overall neurological level of C5.

The ASIA Impairment Scale

Spinal cord injuries are classified as complete (ASIA A) or incomplete (ASIA B, C, D and E). The distinction between different ASIA impairments is made on the basis of:

1. Motor function in S4–S5. This is reflected by the ability to voluntarily contract the anal sphincter.
2. Sensory function in S4–S5. This is reflected by appreciation of deep anal pressure or preservation of either light touch or pinprick sensation in the perianal area.
3. Strength in muscles below the motor and neurological level.

The importance of the S4–S5 segments is linked to prognosis. Its preservation is a strong predictor of neurological recovery.[22] Likewise preservation of pinprick sensation anywhere on the body helps predict motor recovery (this is thought to be due to the proximity of the spinothalamic and corticospinal tracts).[23]

The definition of each ASIA impairment is:

ASIA A: no motor or sensory function in S4–S5.
ASIA B: preservation of sensory function in S4–S5.

ASIA C: preservation of sensory function in S4–S5 provided there is also motor function more than three levels below the *motor* level OR just preservation of motor function in S4–S5. In addition, less than grade 3/5 strength (i.e. grades 0/5–2/5) in more than half the key muscles below the *neurological level*.

ASIA D: preservation of sensory function in S4–S5 provided there is also motor function more than three levels below the *motor* level OR preservation of motor function in S4–S5. In addition, grade 3/5 or more strength (i.e. grades 3/5–5/5) in at least half the key muscles below the *neurological level*.

ASIA E: normal motor and sensory function.

ASIA A lesions can also have *zones of partial preservation* reflecting some preservation of motor or sensory function below the neurological level. This is recorded by noting the lowest segment with some sensory or motor function. Importantly, however, if there is motor or sensory function in S4–S5 the lesion is no longer complete but rather incomplete.

Common patterns of neurological loss with incomplete lesions

There are some common patterns of neurological loss with incomplete spinal cord injury. These are:

Sacral sparing. Sacral sparing occurs when the peripheral rim of the spinal cord is preserved. This can happen in vascular injuries when the small radicular arteries supplying the outer rim of the spinal cord are preserved. Consequently, motor and sensory pathways to the sacral segments remain intact and the patient retains sacral sensation, voluntary anal control and, possibly, toe movement (see Figure 1.3).

Brown-Sequard lesion. Brown-Sequard lesions occur when one side of the spinal cord is damaged (i.e. lateral hemi-section). They are usually due to penetrating injuries such as gunshot or knife injuries and account for only 2–4% of all spinal cord injuries. The consequence of damage to half the spinal cord is loss of proprioception and motor function on the same side as the injury and loss of pain and temperature sensation on the opposite side. The pattern of neurological loss is due to the crossing of different motor and sensory pathways within the spinal cord (see p. 4–6). For example, most fibres carrying pain and sensation cross at or near the level they enter the spinal cord. In contrast, fibres carrying motor and proprioception cross in the brainstem.

Central cord lesion. Central cord lesions commonly occur following hyperextension injuries of the cervical spine in older people with cervical spondylosis. The hyperextension injury causes compression, hypoxia and haemorrhage of the central grey matter of the cord, although the peripheral rim of the spinal cord remains intact. Typically, a patient with a cervical central cord lesion has more severe paralysis of the upper limbs than of the lower limbs. This is because the cervical motor tracts are centrally located while the lumbar and sacral tracts are more peripheral (see Figure 1.3). Quite often a mixed lesion occurs combining features of central cord and Brown-Sequard lesions.

Anterior cervical cord syndrome. This syndrome is usually associated with a flexion injury that damages the anterior two-thirds of the spinal cord. Most often it is caused by vascular insult to the anterior vertebral artery, leaving the two posterior vertebral arteries intact. Consequently, the posterior columns are undamaged. Typically, a patient with anterior cervical cord syndrome has preservation of light touch and proprioception but not motor function, pain or temperature sensation below the level of the lesion.

Upper and lower motor neuron lesions

Injuries above the conus are predominantly upper motor neuron lesions. Spinal cord-mediated reflexes remain intact and consequently the lesion results in a spastic paralysis. The exceptions are spinal cord injuries which are associated with extensive ischaemic damage. In these types of injuries the anterior horn cells of lower motor neurons are damaged over many segments and sometimes down the entire length of the spinal cord. Similarly, it is common for the anterior horn cells of lower motor neurons to be damaged at the site of the injury.[24,25] In this latter scenario, the patient has quite specific and isolated damage of the lower motor neurons associated with the level of the injury although the spinal cord injury is predominantly an upper motor neuron lesion. For example, a patient with a motor C6 level may have lower motor neuron damage of the C7 and/or C8 myotomes but upper motor neuron damage of all other myotomes below the level of the lesion. The lesion is largely an upper motor neuron lesion although the patient has a flaccid paralysis of one or two myotomes.

Injuries involving the cauda equina are lower motor neuron lesions. The main implication of lower motor neuron lesions is the loss of spinal cord-mediated reflexes. Damage to lower motor neurons results in a flaccid paralysis. Injuries at the conus can involve both upper and lower motor neurons and result in a 'mixed' lesion.

The type of motor neuron lesion (upper or lower) has implications for spasticity and bladder, bowel and sexual functions (each discussed later in this chapter). It also has implications for the potential use of therapeutic electrical stimulation because effective electrical stimulation requires intact lower motor neurons. Electrical simulation cannot be easily used to stimulate the leg muscles of patients with cauda equina injuries.

Prognosis

Most neurological recovery occurs within the first 2 months after injury although recovery may continue for up to 1 year and occasionally after this.[26-29] In patients with complete lesions (i.e. ASIA A), the probability of extensive neurological recovery is low.[30] One study indicated that only 6% of patients initially diagnosed with a complete lesion had a motor incomplete lesion 1 year later.[31] However, patients with complete lesions often regain one neurological level in the months after injury. For example, an individual presenting with C5 tetraplegia at the time of injury may present with C6 tetraplegia 3 months later. Motor recovery following an incomplete lesion is more common. Approximately 50% of patients initially diagnosed with ASIA B or C lesions improve over the first few months by one ASIA level (i.e. from ASIA B to ASIA C, or from ASIA C to ASIA D). It is less common for patients with ASIA D to fully recover (i.e. to ASIA E).[29,32]

It is difficult to predict patients' ability to walk at the time of injury but the best estimates indicate that very few patients with ASIA A lesions at the time of injury ultimately ambulate with or without assistance, 30–45% of patients with ASIA B lesion ambulate for at least short distances and most patients with ASIA C and D lesions become community ambulators.[33-35] Patients with Brown-Sequard or cervical central cord syndrome have a reasonably good prognosis for walking but not if they are elderly (see Chapter 6).[33,36]

Impairments associated with spinal cord injury

Vertebral damage and instability

Traumatic spinal cord injuries may or may not be associated with structural damage and instability of the vertebral column. At the time of injury, all effort is directed at minimizing further spinal cord injury, managing associated impairments and optimizing neurological recovery. If there is no vertebral instability or damage (as can occur following ischaemic injuries) patients are generally mobilized within a few days of injury provided they are medically stable. However, when there is instability of the vertebral column, the management is quite different.

Instability of the vertebral column is generally managed in one of two ways. The first approach is conservative and involves immobilizing the spine for a period of 6–12 weeks. Sometimes this is done with extensive bracing such as can be provided with a halo-thoracic jacket and patients are mobilized in a wheelchair relatively soon after injury. More commonly, patients are confined to bed for 6–12 weeks. During this period the spine is immobilized with skeletal traction (for cervical lesions) or with some type of pillow wedge (for thoracic, lumbar and sacral lesions). There are tight restrictions placed on therapies which may cause movement at the injury site, and patients are turned and moved only under strict medical supervision. The precise limitations on therapies, such as passive movements and stretches, vary from hospital to hospital depending on medical protocols.[37] For example, some hospitals limit hamstring stretches for 2 weeks, and others for 3 months. Similarly, some hospitals place tight restrictions on shoulder movements in people with cervical lesions and others encourage movement from the time of injury. The prolonged bedrest associated with conservative management can cause respiratory complications (see Chapter 11) and pressure ulcers, promote disuse weakness (see Chapter 8) and encourage contractures (see Chapter 9).

Once the spine is deemed stable, the patient is mobilized in a wheelchair, often with a spinal orthosis[38] which is worn for a further few months (see Figure 1.6).

The second and more common approach to the management of vertebral damage and instability is surgical. Typically, vertebrae are realigned and fixated with or without spinal decompression. There are many different surgical options.[39,40] Patients managed surgically are often permitted to mobilize much more rapidly than those managed conservatively, sometimes within a week or so of surgery. They may or may not require some type of bracing once mobilized (see Figure 1.7). The main implication of this approach for physiotherapy management is that patients are confined to bed for a shorter period, and so experience fewer complications associated with immobilization. On the other hand, anaesthesia depresses respiratory function, increasing risk of respiratory compromise in the days after surgery (see Chapter 11).

Spinal shock

Immediately after the onset of a spinal cord injury, patients develop a condition called spinal shock.[13,41] As the name implies, the spinal cord has an acute reaction to the injury and there is a temporary loss of spinal cord-mediated reflexes below the level of the lesion.[13] The extent of disruption to reflexes is variable. The precise definition and duration of spinal shock is debated because different reflexes are lost for varying lengths of time and there is not one reflex used to define spinal shock. For

Figure 1.6 Typical brace used for thoracic injury.

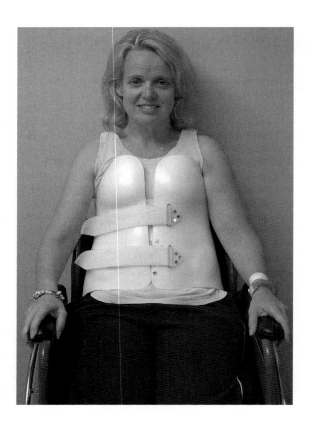

Figure 1.7 Typical brace used to mobilize a patient with tetraplegia following surgical stabilization of the cervical spine.

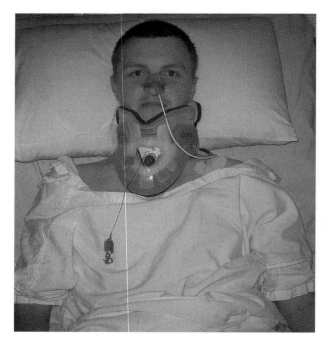

instance, reflexes around the ankle, such as the delayed plantar response, are often only lost for 1–6 hours after injury, while those associated with bladder and bowel function can be lost for many months.[41] Some clinicians define spinal shock solely by the absence of deep tendon reflexes[42] (typically lost for several weeks) while others define it by the loss of the bulbocavernosus reflex (a reflex associated with anal function which is typically lost for 1–3 days).[43] For a long time it was believed that caudal reflexes returned before cephalad ones, with the bulbocavernosus reflex (S4 to S5) being one of the first to return.[13] However, this has been disputed.[44] It is now generally agreed that spinal shock gradually resolves in a series of stages lasting from a few days to a few months.[41]

As spinal shock resolves patients with upper motor neuron lesions gradually develop spasticity. The development of spasticity is not solely due to the resolution of spinal shock but may also be due to associated neurophysiological and physical changes.[13,41] The development of spasticity has important implications for physiotherapy management and especially for the management of contractures (see Chapter 9).

Paralytic ileus

The development of a paralytic ileus is associated with spinal shock. Like spinal shock, this condition presents immediately after injury and can last from a few days to a few weeks. The main consequence of a paralytic ileus is that food cannot be digested and, if untreated, patients develop abdominal distension and may vomit. The distended abdomen increases the work of breathing, and vomiting heightens the risk of aspiration pneumonia (see Chapter 11). Typical management includes 'nil by mouth'. A nasogastric tube is inserted to regularly aspirate stomach contents (the tube is not for feeding). Nutrition and fluids are provided intravenously.

Deep venous thrombosis and pulmonary embolus

Patients are particularly vulnerable to deep venous thromboses during the first 2 weeks after injury. During this period the dislodgement of deep venous thromboses is one of the leading causes of death.[45–50] Deep venous thromboses are caused by stasis of blood within the venous system that results from paralysis and lack of movement. The stasis is exacerbated by bedrest and lack of vasomotor control in people with lesions involving the sympathetic nervous system.[47,51] Deep venous thromboses are particularly common in the veins of the calf but potentially more dangerous in the veins of the thigh and groin. The signs of deep venous thromboses are low grade fever and localized swelling, warmth and discolouration.[46] Pain may be present in patients with intact sensation. Definitive diagnoses are based on the results of impedance plethysmography, ultrasound or venography.[46]

The dislodgement of deep venous thromboses can result in pulmonary emboli, which are life-threatening. The presence of emboli is characterized by any number of the following symptoms: loss of consciousness, shortness of breath, hypoxia, sweating, haemoptysis, tachycardia, confusion or chest pain. Sometimes the first sign of an embolus is respiratory or cardiac arrest.[46] Deep venous thromboses are particularly likely to be dislodged when patients are moved for routine care or when patients' limbs are moved during passive movements. Therefore, if deep venous thromboses are suspected or diagnosed, movement of the patient should be kept to a minimum and passive movements of the legs should cease.[52]

To prevent deep venous thromboses during the period immediately after injury, patients are routinely placed on anticoagulation medication,[47,53,54] provided with tight-fitting stockings, regularly screened for deep venous thromboses, and mobilized as soon as feasible. External pneumatic compression devices[46,54-56] and electrical stimulation have also been advocated.[47] For a long time it was believed that passive movements prevented deep venous thromboses, although this is now disputed[46] (see Ref. 57 for clinical guidelines on prevention of thromboembolism). Deep venous thromboses and pulmonary emboli are treated with thrombolytic agents or low molecular weight heparin, e.g. enoxaparin.[58]

Spasticity

Spasticity is present in up to 80% of patients with spinal cord injury.[59] It is only present in patients with intact lower motor neurons so is not present in patients with cauda equina injuries. Spasticity is more troublesome for patients with incomplete rather than complete lesions,[60] and tends to gradually increase over the first year before it plateaus. The increase may be due to neural sprouting or changes in the sensitivity of neural receptors. Spasticity can be elicited with many stimuli but stretch and touch are the most common.[61] Sudden increases in spasticity are usually indicative of illness or injury, or an over-distended bladder or bowel.[59] Many tests[62,63] are used to quantify spasticity but the two most widely used are the Tardieu Scale[64] and the Modified Ashworth Scale[65-67] (see Table 1.4). The usefulness of these and other tests of spasticity is widely debated.[68,69]

The neurophysiology of spasticity is complex and not fully understood (see Refs 59, 68, 70, 71 for comprehensive overviews). It can have many different features but the two key ones are an abnormal and velocity-dependent increase in resistance to stretch.[70] Spinal cord injury changes the excitability of the tonic and phasic stretch reflexes, which are controlled by the balance of excitatory and inhibitory inputs onto alpha motor neurons. These inputs arise from a large number of segmental and descending neural circuits. There are many theories about precisely how and to what extent these circuits are disrupted, and which disruption is most important.[72] Until

TABLE 1.4 Modified Ashworth Scale	
0	No increase in muscle tone
1	Slight increase in muscle tone, manifested by a catch and release or by minimal resistance at the end of range of motion when the affected part(s) is moved in flexion or extension
1+	Slight increase in muscle tone, manifested by a catch, followed by minimal resistance throughout the remainder (less than half) of the range of motion
2	More marked increase in muscle tone through most of the range of motion but affected part(s) easily moved
3	Considerable increase in muscle tone, passive movement difficult
4	Affected part(s) rigid in flexion or extension

Reproduced from Bohannon RW, Andrews AW: Interrater reliability of hand-held dynamometry. Phys Ther 1987; 67:931–933, with permission of the American Physical Therapy Association.

recently it was believed that spasticity primarily resulted from unchecked hyperactivity of gamma motor neurons, driving intrafusal muscle fibres and increasing reflex facilitation of alpha motor neurons. However, the importance of gamma motor activity has been disputed,[61] and spasticity is now believed to be due primarily to a direct increase in the excitability of the alpha motor neurons. This may be related to enhanced sensitivity of the alpha motor neurons.[13,61] The increased excitability of the alpha motor neurons is also thought to be due to a loss in the normal dampening effects of the descending fibres of the corticospinal tract. With less dampening, the alpha motor neurons are more excitable and responsive to sensory inputs. The alpha motor neurons of antagonistic muscles are also easily excited because there is a loss of activity in the cells which are responsible for reciprocal inhibition (i.e. Renshaw cells).

Spasticity is primarily managed with pharmacological agents.[73] There are two main categories of drugs, some acting predominantly within the central nervous system (e.g. baclofen, diazepam, gabapentin, clonidine, tizanidine) and others acting peripherally, either within the muscle or at the neuromuscular junction (e.g. dantrolene and Botulinum toxin). Severe spasticity is sometimes managed by administering drugs directly to the spinal cord (i.e. intrathecally).

The main implications of spasticity are that it predisposes patients to pain, contractures and pressure ulcers, and makes movement and hygiene difficult.[59,61,68] For some patients, spasticity limits function and quality of life.[74] Physiotherapy interventions such as hydrotherapy, stretch, heat, TENS, cold, electrical stimulation, therapeutic exercise techniques, passive movements, standing and vibration may provide transient relief from spasticity, but there is no evidence that any of these interventions produce lasting reductions in spasticity.[73,75] In addition, the application of heat can cause burns and therefore should only be used with extreme caution in patients who lack sensation.

Autonomic dysreflexia

Autonomic dysreflexia is an exaggerated reflex response of the sympathetic nervous system to noxious stimuli. It is seen in patients with total or profound loss of supraspinal sympathetic control (see p. 6). Typically, patients with lesions above T6 are most vulnerable. It can occur at any time throughout patients' lives but not before spinal shock has resolved.[52,76–79]

Stimuli which typically precipitate autonomic dysreflexia include blocked catheters, over-distended bladders or bowels, fractures, pressure ulcers or ingrown toenails. However, any stimulus normally associated with pain or discomfort can cause autonomic dysreflexia. Sometimes even something as mild as a stretch of the hamstring muscles can aggravate symptoms in already vulnerable patients. These stimuli directly excite neurons in the isolated sympathetic chain. Without supraspinal control to dampen the reflex sympathetic response, the sympathetic nervous system makes an exaggerated and unchecked reflex response. This causes widespread vasoconstriction below the level of the lesion with associated increases in blood pressure, headache, sweating, flushing and, initially, tachycardia. The increased blood pressure is sensed by the carotid and aortic baroreceptors. This information is transmitted to the brain via cranial nerves IX and X.[52] Homeostatic mechanisms act to combat the increase in blood pressure by increasing cranial nerve X activity (i.e. parasympathetic activity). Heart rate response is variable as it is determined by the balance between the accelerating effect of the sympathetic nervous system and the dampening effect of the vagal nerve.[76] However, patients consistently become flushed in the face and neck but white below the lesion level, and complain of nausea, anxiety, blurred vision and headache.[77] All these responses can occur rapidly (i.e. in minutes), although in some patients they can develop over a few days.

Patients with lesions above T6 are most susceptible to autonomic dysreflexia because the large splanchnic blood vessels are supplied by sympathetic fibres carried within T6 to T10 nerve roots. Unchecked vasoconstriction of the splanchnic blood vessels in response to noxious stimuli can cause a marked increase in blood pressure. The primary concern with autonomic dysreflexia is the associated sudden increase in intracerebral blood pressure. If sufficiently high and untreated it can cause cerebrovascular accident or death.

Patients who present with any symptoms of autonomic dysreflexia need to be immediately assessed. Initially, blood pressure needs to be taken, remembering that systolic blood pressure for patients with spinal cord injury is typically 90–110 mm Hg. A sudden increase in systolic blood pressure of more than 20 mm Hg is usually indicative of autonomic dysreflexia. Treatment involves identifying and removing the source of noxious stimuli, loosening tight stockings and abdominal binders, lowering the legs and elevating the head. The supine position should be avoided if possible because it increases intracerebral blood pressure. Medical assistance must be immediately sought so blood pressure-relieving medication can be administered if necessary. Typically, nifedipine and nitrates are used.[52,80] Further information about management of autonomic dysreflexia is available in clinical guidelines.[79,81]

Postural hypotension

Postural hypotension is typically a problem for patients with lesions above T6. It is due to a loss of supraspinal control of the sympathetic nervous system and the resultant inability to regulate blood pressure. It is exacerbated by poor venous return secondary to lower limb paralysis and the loss of the lower limb 'muscle pump' (see Chapter 12).[18,52,82,83]

Postural hypotension predominantly occurs when patients move from lying to sitting. Without leg movement or a capacity to increase sympathetic activity, blood remains pooled in the legs and abdomen, and blood pressure drops. This causes the patient to feel faint and to lose consciousness. The immediate treatment is to lie the patient down and raise the feet or tilt the wheelchair backwards. Graduated compression stockings and abdominal binders may help maintain blood pressure although evidence of their effectiveness is conflicting.[84]

Postural hypotension is particularly pronounced when patients first mobilize after injury, especially if there has been an extended period of prior bedrest. For this reason mobilization needs to be implemented slowly. For the first few days the patient may just tolerate sitting up in bed. Subsequently, the patient may then be sat out of bed in a reclined wheelchair with the legs elevated. Over time patients 'acclimatize' and better tolerate the transition from lying to sitting; this is thought to be due to an increased tolerance to feelings of lightheadedness with lower blood pressure. Alternatively, blood pressure may be better maintained because of the additional release of circulating catecholamines and hormones (i.e. antidiuretic hormones and hormones associated with the renin–angiotensin–aldosterone system),[85–88] or because of increases in sensitivity to these hormones.

Bladder, bowel and sexual function

Spinal cord injury commonly affects bladder, bowel and sexual function. One of the most comprehensive studies in this area found that 81% of people with spinal cord injury had impaired bladder function and 63% had impaired bowel function 1 year post injury.[3] While the control of these three bodily functions is complex, they all rely on coordinated activity between the sympathetic and parasympathetic nervous system as well as skeletal muscle control via the S2–S4 nerve roots. Injuries below the conus result in a flaccid paralysis of skeletal muscles associated with bladder, bowel and sexual function, and loss of the sacral part of parasympathetic spinal cord-mediated reflexes. In contrast, injuries above the conus result in a spastic paralysis of the bladder, bowel and sexual skeletal muscles with retention of sacral reflexes. The site of the lesion therefore has important implications for management and function.[89]

Bladder management

Bladder drainage can be managed in several different ways. Most patients with some hand function perform intermittent catheterization. This requires the patient (or the patient's carer) to temporarily introduce a catheter into the bladder every 3–6 hours. The catheter is removed once the bladder is drained. Intermittent catheterization is preferred over other options because it is associated with lower rates of infection[90] and is aesthetically more acceptable (i.e. it does not require use of external leg bags to collect urine).[91] In males, external drainage sheaths can be used to ensure continence. These are like condoms that cover the penis and are attached to leg bags. There is no equivalent device for females so sanitary pads are often used.[91] Patients who are unable to intermittently catheterize typically have an indwelling catheter. The catheter is initially inserted via the urethra but ultimately is often inserted surgically through the suprapubic abdominal wall.[92] Some patients rely on reflex emptying of the bladder: voiding is elicited by either tapping over the bladder or manually stimulating the perineal region. This technique can be assisted by manual overpressure on the bladder provided there is no risk of urine tracking up to the kidneys.[93]

Patients with spinal cord injury have an increased susceptibility to bladder stones, kidney stones and urinary tract infections, all contributing to an increased risk of late-life kidney failure.[93,94] All these potential problems are managed and monitored by controlling fluid intake, optimizing medication and by regularly reviewing kidney and bladder function. Urinary incontinence can be an ongoing problem for some patients.[93,95]

Bowel management

Bowel management is an important and often time-consuming issue for people with spinal cord injury. Patients with lower motor neuron lesions tend to have more problems with incontinence because they have flaccid paralysis of the anal sphincter[96] and loss of associated spinal cord-mediated reflexes.[97–99] In contrast, patients with upper motor neuron lesions can take advantage of remaining bowel reflexes.

Bowels can be managed in a variety of ways, but key strategies include a high-fibre diet, adequate fluid intake and a regular routine for bowel emptying. Other options include oral and/or anal medication, digital stimulation or manual evacuation.[98,100] Often bowel regimes are initially difficult to establish and faecal incontinence or constipation can be a problem.[101–104] It is not unusual for bowel accidents to be precipitated by exercise.

Sexuality

When people think of spinal cord injuries and sexuality, they most commonly think of the physical aspects of sex. Spinal cord injury clearly affects sexual intercourse and

Figure 1.8 The physiological responses associated with sexual intercourse and sexual arousal are determined by sensory and psychogenic inputs onto the sympathetic and parasympathetic nervous pathways.

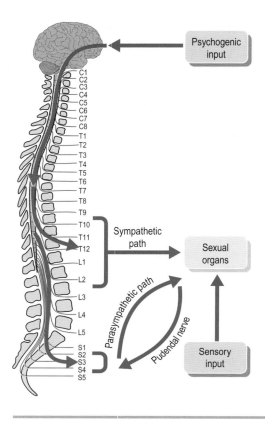

the associated physical sexual responses in both males and females.[105,106] Patients with upper motor neuron lesions retain reflexive but not psychogenic responses, patients with lower motor neuron lesions lose reflexive but may retain psychogenic responses, and all retain the ability for non-genital sexual arousal (see Figure 1.8).[69,106–109]

Spinal cord injury can affect male fertility by impairing ejaculation and reducing semen quality. However semen, if required, can often be obtained with vibration and electro-ejaculation techniques. More sophisticated techniques are being increasingly used for fertilization. Female fertility and menstruation are largely unchanged by spinal cord injury but pregnancies are associated with increased risks.[110] Females generally cease menstruating for 1–3 months following injury. Studies of men with spinal cord injury have found that genital sensation, erectile function and capacity for orgasm are not strong predictors of sexual satisfaction nor behaviour.[111] The stronger predictors are perceptions of partners' satisfaction with the sexual relationship,[111] intimacy of relationships and willingness for sexual experimentation.[112]

Spinal cord injuries have implications not only for patients' experiences of sexual intercourse but also for males' and females' sexuality. That is, spinal cord injury affects how people perceive their own maleness or femaleness.[113] For example, a spinal cord injury may affect a male's ability to earn money for the family, play sport with the kids, drink beer with the mates or pump iron at the gym. Some men perceive that the inability to readily engage in these types of activities undermines their maleness. In the same way, a female may perceive that her femininity has been adversely affected by her difficulty wearing fashion shoes, making up her face, looking after her children or going to nightclubs. The issues are complex and management often involves reappraisal of preconceived ideas about the expression of both sex and sexuality.

Most rehabilitation teams have psychologists, social workers, nurses or medical personnel specifically trained to counsel patients on sex and sexuality. Ongoing sexual support and education post-discharge are particularly important.[112,114] Physiotherapists need a general understanding of these issues so they can be appropriately supportive and knowledgeable when these issues are raised during therapy sessions. However, it is not normally the physiotherapist's role to provide counselling or detailed information on these issues.

Osteoporosis

Osteoporosis is a common long-term complication of spinal cord injury which predisposes individuals to fractures.[115–117] Over a lifetime patients may experience a 25–50% reduction in bone mineral content of the lower limbs with most bone mineral loss occurring in the first year following injury.[115–124] It has been assumed that bone mineral loss is primarily due to the lack of weight bearing and axial loading.[125,126] However, it is now believed that bone mineral loss is due to multiple factors involving metabolic, endocrine, neural and vascular changes associated with spinal cord injury.[116,120–122,127–129]

Bone loss is primarily managed with pharmacological agents (i.e. bisphosphonates). Early standing[130,131] and electrical stimulation programmes[132–134] are also advocated, although their effectiveness is yet to be clearly demonstrated.[122,135,136]

Heterotopic ossification

Heterotopic ossification, also called ectopic ossification and myositis ossificans, refers to the formation of bone outside the skeletal system, and occurs below the level of the injury, typically around the hips, knees, elbows and shoulders.[137–140] It occurs in up to 50% of adults with spinal cord injury.[140] Presentation is usually within the first few months after injury but can be many years later.[137,138,140–142] If severe, it restricts joint mobility and impedes function.[137]

The first clinical signs of heterotopic ossification are swelling and reduced range of motion, with or without fever, spasticity and pain.[138–140] A number of these clinical signs are similar to those of fracture and deep venous thrombosis.[139] A definitive diagnosis of heterotopic ossification is usually made on the basis of ultrasound, CT scan or bone scan, although blood tests may also give some indication.[138–140]

The cause of heterotopic ossification is not known[139,140] but it has been observed after repeated and aggressive passive movements of immobilized joints in animals.[143,144] Partly for this reason it is often attributed to excessively enthusiastic physiotherapy,[145] although a causal relationship between physiotherapy and heterotopic ossification has not been demonstrated. While doubt remains, it would be prudent to avoid aggressive manual therapy interventions.[146] It is unclear whether stretches and passive movements should cease altogether during the acute inflammatory stage of heterotopic ossification, although some low quality evidence suggests that gentle passive movements maintain range of motion during this stage.[146,147]

Heterotopic ossification is managed with varying degrees of success through drug therapy.[138–140] Occasionally, surgery is used to remove excessive bone but this is not without risk and can exacerbate the condition.[138] For these reasons, surgery is only performed once heterotopic ossification has stabilized (typically 1–2 years after onset) and primarily in situations where function and quality of life are adversely affected[138] or where there is resulting nerve compression.[140]

Skin management

Pressure ulcers are one of the commonest and most troubling complications of spinal cord injury.[148–150] They can occur at any time and are a source of frustration and disruption to patients' lives and rehabilitation.[151] In the long term, they can prevent individuals from successfully holding jobs and they can adversely affect quality of life. They can also increase spasticity and pain, and predispose to autonomic dysreflexia and contracture. In severe cases, pressure ulcers develop into large wounds which become infected, leading to osteomyelitis and other serious medical complications which may be fatal. In some developing countries with limited resources, life-threatening pressure ulcers are a constant threat.

Causes of pressure ulcers

Pressure ulcers are due to necrosis of soft tissues. The necrosis occurs when blood supply is compromised by the compression of small arteries and capillaries between internal bony prominences and external hard surfaces.[152] For example, the tissues overlying the ischial tuberosities are compressed when sitting on a wooden stool. Prolonged compression disrupts blood supply, causing necrosis.[151] Normally, in able-bodied individuals, destructive pressures are associated with discomfort and pain which precipitates a voluntary change of posture. This relieves and redistributes pressure. However, with absent or impaired sensation, people with spinal cord injury have no warning mechanism to indicate a need for change of posture so pressure can continue unrelieved.

Constant unrelieved pressure and excessive frictional or shearing forces are particularly problematic.[153] The tissues most vulnerable are those overlying the heel, head of fibula, greater trocanter of femur, ischial tuberosity, sacrum, inferior tip of scapula, olecranon and the back of the head.[154] Other factors contributing to the development of pressure ulcers include spasticity, bladder or bowel incontinence, age, loss of supraspinal sympathetic control, poor circulation, tight clothing, oedema, infection and poor nutrition.[151,152,155]

The first sign of excessive pressure is not skin breakdown, but redness that does not blanch with localized pressure.[156] This indicates damage to underlying tissues, which are more vulnerable to pressure than skin. Consequently, underlying tissues are the first to be damaged and the last to be repaired. Skin breakdown is a later sign of a pressure ulcer and usually indicates more sinister underlying soft tissue destruction. During recovery from a pressure ulcer the skin repairs first. It is important not to assume that because an open wound has covered with new skin, the underlying tissues have healed.[151]

Prevention of pressure ulcers

The key to pressure management is prevention.[151] Prevention requires a multi-faceted and interdisciplinary approach involving education, good nutrition, anti-spasticity medication and strategies to ensure regular changes in position. Perhaps more importantly, prevention involves the appropriate prescription of pressure-relieving equipment such as bed mattresses, wheelchair cushions and wheelchairs.

Regular change in position

Recently-injured patients confined to bed are initially turned every 2 hours.[151] The frequency of turning is gradually decreased but depends on many factors, including the type of mattress upon which the patient is lying and susceptibility to skin problems. Once patients start to sit in their wheelchairs, they need to relieve pressure from under the ischial tuberosities at least once every 15–30 minutes.[152,157] Some evidence indicates that the lift should be sustained for approximately 2 minutes.[158] The frequency and length of pressure relief can often be decreased over time, but only in conjunction with careful monitoring. There are many different ways pressure can be relieved when sitting. A vertical lift that clears the buttocks from the seat is the most commonly used method by those with sufficient upper limb strength (see Chapter 3, Figures 3.8 and 3.9). Patients unable to perform a vertical lift can relieve pressure by regularly leaning forwards or sidewards, or, if necessary, by resting forwards with their arms on a table.[159] Patients with high levels of tetraplegia sitting in power wheelchairs can redistribute pressure by regularly changing the tilt of their wheelchairs and elevating the feet (see Chapter 13).[153,157,160,161]

Patient, staff and family education

Education of patients, staff and families is an important aspect of pressure care management.[151,152] All must be made aware of the appropriate use and maintenance of pressure-relieving equipment. A common mistake is to place a wheelchair cushion upside down or around the wrong way. This usually reduces the pressure-relieving qualities of the cushion.

Skin needs to be checked daily and, initially, more regularly if trialling new equipment.[151] Patients need to be aware of the first signs of skin damage. They also should know how to appropriately manage problems when they arise. Adequate pressure relief is particularly important when sitting in cars or on commodes or other hard surfaces. Similarly, pressure from orthoses, splints, straps or casts can be a problem and these need careful monitoring. Medical sheepskin overlays can be used to relieve shearing forces although they should not be used on top of most pressure-relieving cushions or mattresses.

Pressure-relieving equipment

Pressure-relieving equipment is important for effective skin management. Its prescription is sometimes the responsibility of physiotherapists but more often occupational therapists. A brief outline of some of the key issues is provided below and in Chapter 13, but therapists prescribing this type of equipment would be well advised to seek additional information and training.[162–165] Prescription of pressure-relieving equipment is something which requires careful consideration with deleterious consequences for patients if it is done poorly.

Equipment that has provided adequate pressure protection during hospitalization may prove to be insufficient when patients return home. This is partly because patients regularly change position as part of therapy and nursing care programmes when in hospital but may not change position as frequently on discharge. Skin problems at home can be avoided by trialling pressure-relieving equipment under conditions that closely mimic the home situation. For example, patients unlikely to turn at night when home need to trial bed mattresses under the same conditions while in hospital. If in doubt, it is better to err on the side of caution and prescribe overprotective equipment.

Bed mattresses. There are many different varieties of pressure-relieving mattresses. Mattresses may be either foam-, air- or water-based. The more expensive ones use power to cycle air through different chambers, systematically alternating pressure. A recent Cochrane systematic review concluded that in people at high risk of developing pressure ulcers, foam mattresses designed for relieving pressure are superior to standard hospital mattresses.[156] The merits of more elaborate and expensive mattresses have not been scientifically validated, although most clinicians consider them superior to foam mattresses.

Wheelchair seating. Poor seating is a common cause of pressure. Soft tissues that are weight bearing or in contact with the wheelchair, especially those overlying the ischial tuberosities, are most vulnerable to the destructive pressures associated with prolonged sitting. These pressures are influenced by factors such as height of the footplates, tilt of the pelvis, tilt of the wheelchair and length of the seat. For example, footplates which are too high shift weight posteriorly, concentrating pressure over the ischial tuberosities. A posteriorly rotated pelvis turns the sacrum into a weight-bearing area, increasing susceptibility to sacral pressure ulcers.[166] A seat which is too short distributes the weight of the thighs over a smaller surface area, increasing pressure. All these issues need to be considered when prescribing wheelchairs[159,161,162,167] (see Chapter 13 for more details).

Patients with deformities present complex seating problems because correction of deformities invariably requires the application of pressure. Most solutions involve dissipating pressure over wide areas, preferably through soft tissues that do not overlie bony prominences.

Wheelchair cushions. There has been growing commercialization of wheelchair cushions and there are now hundreds of different types on the market.[168] Most are air-, foam- or gel-based, and designed for specific purposes (see Chapter 13). The most important pressure-relieving quality of a cushion is its ability to minimize pressures in the soft tissues overlying the ischial tuberosities. These pressures can be measured with either simple or sophisticated equipment designed to measure skin interface pressures.[153,168–170] However, there is not one critical pressure, below which patients are safe from skin damage and above which they are not. It depends on many factors, including the length of time that pressure remains unrelieved.[171] As a general rule, however, peak pressures over vulnerable sites should be kept well below 60 mm Hg.[153,168,172,173]

Treatment of pressure ulcers

Not surprisingly, the treatment of pressure ulcers includes strategies to minimize pressure.[151,152] These must be instigated with the first signs of destructive pressure, and may include confinement to bed, adjustment of a wheelchair or cushion, remoulding of a hand splint, realignment of an orthosis, or education. If a severe pressure ulcer develops, hospitalization may be required for many months, with or without accompanying surgery. For further details, interested readers are directed to clinical practice guidelines on the treatment and prevention of pressure ulcers.[151,152,157]

Psychological well-being

The psychological implications of spinal cord injury are profound.[174–179] Some of the common emotions experienced immediately after injury include anger, grief, despondency, denial, depression and apathy.[180,181] Factors found to be associated with patients' psychological reactions include coping skills, pre-morbid personality, family support, substance abuse, extent of permanent paralysis and home situation.[174,179,180,182] Some studies put the rate of depression in the first 2 years following spinal cord injury as high as 38%,[83] although most place it between 15% and 23%.[184–186] The incidence of ongoing depression appears to be strongly linked to restrictions in participation.[180,187] Suicide rates are higher amongst people with spinal cord injury than in the general population.[188–190] However, these statistics mask the proportion of people with spinal cord injury who go on to live happy and fulfilling lives. Health care workers often underestimate the long-term satisfaction with life following spinal cord injury.[191,192]

Psychological distress impacts on patients' ability to cooperate with physiotherapy programmes, especially when the distress is associated with poor sleep, appetite and energy. In particular, psychological distress can lead to passivity, self-neglect, poor drive and motivation, and low adherence. Not surprisingly, patients with depressive symptoms achieve poorer outcomes than their non-depressed counterparts. However, psychological distress is not always associated with poor adherence. It can present as unbridled determination and drive for success in physiotherapy. Sometimes this is expressed by unrealistic goals, especially those that are gait-orientated (e.g. "I am going to walk at any cost"). Alternatively, it can be expressed by preoccupation with physiotherapy and unrealistic demands for intensive attention from therapists. These issues are best managed through a coordinated team response under the leadership of a clinical psychologist (see Refs 179, 193, 194 for more details on management of depression following spinal cord injury).

Family and friends

Families and friends of people with spinal cord injury are often overlooked by health professionals.[195] However, the practical and psychological implications for parents, siblings, children or friends can be multifaceted.[195] Family members, particularly spouses, are often the primary providers of physical and emotional support.[196] The marital status of a patient with spinal cord injury is the strongest predictor of long-term psychological adjustment and quality of life,[197,198] although divorce is common.[176] Family members often become responsible for providing a range of care services. This can cause them considerable stress, burnout, resentment and depression.[195,196]

In the early days after injury physiotherapists can assist members of the family and friends by involving them as much as possible in patients' programmes. Family and friends often welcome the opportunity to assist in real and tangible ways. This can be achieved by requesting them to help patients with practice activities, positioning and stretching programmes, and helping monitor skin integrity, either within or outside formal therapy sessions. Of course, patients must be happy to have family and friends involved in this way; patient consent for family involvement should not be assumed.

Spinal cord injury and traumatic brain injury

It is estimated that up to 40–50% of people with spinal cord injury have a co-morbid traumatic brain injury.[199–201] Although traumatic brain injury is often mild, more serious injuries can be associated with cognitive impairments such as poor insight, problem-solving, attention and memory. Not surprisingly, patients with a dual diagnosis of spinal cord injury and traumatic brain injury often achieve lower levels of independence than those with spinal cord injury alone.[202] Physiotherapists need to ensure their treatment programmes are appropriately designed to cater for patients with co-morbid traumatic brain injuries. They also need to be aware that often the effects of mild traumatic brain injury are overlooked due to the more obvious deficits of the spinal cord injury.

Aging with spinal cord injury

Only 50 years ago 80% of people died within 3 years of sustaining a spinal cord injury. Today, the life expectancy of people with paraplegia is similar to that of their able-bodied counterparts, although the life expectancy of people with tetraplegia is reduced by 10%. In addition, a larger number of people incurring spinal cord injury later in life are surviving.[203] The implications are that for the first time there is a growing prevalence of people aging with spinal cord injury.[203,204]

The 'normal' aging process combined with the long-term deleterious implications of spinal cord injury compromises general health and increases disability.[52,205,206] Painful musculoskeletal conditions are particularly problematic. If severe, these problems compromise independence and necessitate greater assistance from others, modification of existing home and work environments, and revision of equipment, aids and orthoses.

Elderly people with long-standing spinal cord injury are particularly vulnerable to health problems. These may be related to skin problems, decreased mobility and poor nutrition. Chronic renal failure from a lifetime of compromised bladder function and cardiovascular disease are also common (see Chapter 12).[18,52,203,205,207] The most obvious implication is the increased need for physical assistance and care.[206,208,209] In all, an aging population of people with spinal cord injury presents substantial challenges to health care systems trying to meet this population's increasing physical, social and psychological needs.

References

1. Wyndaele M, Wyndaele J-J: Incidence, prevalence and epidemiology of spinal cord injury: what learns a worldwide literature survey? Spinal Cord 2006; 44:523–508.
2. Sekhon LH, Fehlings MG: Epidemiology, demographics, and pathophysiology of acute spinal cord injury. Spine 2001; 26:S2–S12.
3. Go BK, De Vivo NJ, Richards JS: The epidemiology of spinal cord injury. In Stover SL, DeLisa JA, Whiteneck GG (eds): Spinal Cord Injury: Clinical Outcomes from the Model Systems. Gaithersburg, MD, Aspen Publications, 1995:21–54.
4. Shingu H, Ohama M, Ikata T et al: A nationwide epidemiological survey of spinal cord injuries in Japan from January 1990 to December 1992. Paraplegia 1995; 33:183–188.
5. Silberstein B, Rabinovich S: Epidemiology of spinal cord injuries in Novosibirsk, Russia. Paraplegia 1995; 33:322–325.
6. O'Connor P: Spinal cord injury, Australia 2000–01. Injury Research and Statistics Series Number 16. Adelaide, Australian Institute of Health and Welfare (AIHW cat no. INJCAT 50), 2003.
7. Cripps RA: Spinal cord injury, Australia, 2003–04. Injuries Research and Statistics Series Number 25. Adelaide, Australian Institute of Health and Welfare, 2006.
8. De Vivo MJ, Richards JS, Stover SL et al: Spinal cord injury. Rehabilitation adds life to years. West J Med 1991; 154:602–606.
9. De Vivo MJ, Krause JS, Lammertse DP: Recent trends in mortality and causes of death among persons with spinal cord injury. Arch Phys Med Rehabil 1999; 80:1411–1419.
10. Stover SL, DeLisa JA, Whiteneck GG (eds): Spinal Cord Injury: Clinical Outcomes from the Model Systems. Gaithersburg MD, Aspen Publications, 1995.
11. Hansebout RR: The neurosurgical management of cord injuries. In Bloch RF, Basbaum M (eds): Management of Spinal Cord Injuries. Baltimore, Williams & Wilkins, 1986:1–27.
12. Kakulas BA: A review of the neuropathology of human spinal cord injury with emphasis on special features. J Spinal Cord Med 1999; 22:119–124.
13. Atkinson PP, Atkinson JL: Spinal shock. Mayo Clin Proc 1996; 71:384–389.
14. Mautes AE, Weinzierl MR, Donovan F et al: Vascular events after spinal cord injury: contribution to secondary pathogenesis. Phys Ther 2000; 80:673–687.
15. Martin Ginis KA, Hicks AL: Exercise research issues in the spinal cord injured population. Exerc Sport Sci Rev 2005; 33:49–53.
16. Williams PL, Bannister LH, Berry MM et al: Gray's Anatomy, 38th edn. New York, Churchill Livingstone, 1995.

17. Parent A: Carpenter's Human Neuroanatomy, 9th edn. Baltimore, Williams & Wilkins, 1996.
18. Ragnarsson KT: The cardiovascular system. In Whiteneck GG, Charlifue SW, Gerhart KA (eds): Aging With Spinal Cord Injury. New York, Demos Publications, 1993.
19. American Spinal Injury Association: Reference Manual for the International Standards for Neurological Classification of Spinal Cord Injury. Chicago, ASIA, 2003.
20. Hislop HJ, Montgomery J: Daniels and Worthingham's muscle testing: techniques of manual examination, 8th edition. St Louis, Saunders, 2007.
21. Graves DE: The construct validity and explanatory power of the AISA Motor Score and the FIM: implications for theoretical models of spinal cord injury. Top Spinal Cord Inj Rehabil 2005; 10:65–74.
22. Waters RL, Adkins RH, Yakura JS: Definition of complete spinal cord injury. Paraplegia 1991; 29:573–581.
23. Crozier KS, Graziani V, Ditunno JF et al: Spinal cord injury: prognosis for ambulation based on sensory examination in patients who are initially motor complete. Arch Phys Med Rehabil 1991; 72:119–121.
24. Peckham PH, Mortimer JT, Marsolais EB: Upper and lower motor neuron lesions in the upper extremity muscles of tetraplegics. Paraplegia 1976; 14:115–121.
25. Bryden AM, Sinnott KA, Mulcahey MJ: Innovative strategies for improving upper extremity function in tetraplegia and considerations in measuring functional outcomes. Top Spinal Cord Inj Rehabil 2005; 10:75–93.
26. Waters RL, Adkins RH, Yakura JS et al: Motor and sensory recovery following incomplete tetraplegia. Arch Phys Med Rehabil 1994; 75:306–311.
27. Waters RL, Adkins RH, Yakura JS et al: Motor and sensory recovery following incomplete paraplegia. Arch Phys Med Rehabil 1994; 75:67–72.
28. Waters RL, Adkins R, Yakura J et al: Prediction of ambulatory performance based on motor scores derived from standards of the American Spinal Injury Association. Arch Phys Med Rehabil 1994; 75:756–760.
29. Wolfe DL, Hsieh JTC: Rehabilitation practice and associated outcomes following spinal cord injuries. In Eng JJ, Teasell RW, Miller WC et al (eds): Spinal Cord Injury Rehabilitation Evidence. Vancouver, 2006:3.1–3.44.
30. Marino RJ: Neurological and functional outcomes in spinal cord injury: review and recommendations. Top Spinal Cord Inj Rehabil 2005; 10:51–64.
31. Burns AS, Lee BS, Ditunno JF et al: Patient selection for clinical trials: the reliability of the early spinal cord injury examination. J Neurotrauma 2003; 20:477–482.
32. Consortium for Spinal Cord Medicine: Outcomes Following Traumatic Spinal Cord Injury: Clinical Practice Guidelines for Health Care Professionals. Washington, DC, Paralyzed Veterans of America, 1999.
33. Burns SP, Golding DG, Rolle WA et al: Recovery of ambulation in motor incomplete tetraplegia. Arch Phys Med Rehabil 1997; 78:1169–1172.
34. Tattersall R, Turner B: Brown-Sequard and his syndrome. Lancet 2000; 356:61–63.
35. Gittler MS, McKinley WO, Stiens SA et al: Spinal cord injury medicine. 3. Rehabilitation outcomes. Arch Phys Med Rehabil 2002; 83:S65–71, S90–8.
36. Merriam WF, Taylor TK, Ruff SJ et al: A reappraisal of acute traumatic central cord syndrome. J Bone Joint Surg (Br) 1986; 68B:708–713.
37. Schmitz TJ: Traumatic spinal cord injury. In O'Sullivan SB, Schmitz TJ (eds): Physical Rehabilitation: Assessment and Treatment. Philadelphia, FA Davis Company, 2000.
38. Bussell M, Merritt J, Fenwick L: Spinal orthoses. In Redford JB, Basmajian JV, Trautman P (eds): Orthotics: Clinical Practice and Rehabilitation Technology. New York, Churchill Livingstone, 1995:71–101.
39. Daffner SD, Vaccaro AR, Katsos MS et al: Advances in operative stabilization for unstable cervical spine injuries: implications for early mobilization and rehabilitation. Top Spinal Cord Inj Rehabil 2003; 9:1–13.
40. Nolden M, Mirkovic S: Operative treatment of cervical spine injuries: an update. Top Spinal Cord Inj Rehabil 2004; 9:39–59.
41. Ditunno JF, Little JW, Tessler A et al: Spinal shock revisited: a four-phase model. Spinal Cord 2004; 42:383–395.
42. Wolpaw JR, Tennissen AM: Activity-dependent spinal cord plasticity in health and disease. Annu Rev Neurosci 2001; 24:807–843.
43. Stauffer ES: Diagnosis and prognosis of acute cervical spinal cord injury. Clin Orthop Relat Res 1975; 112:9–15.
44. Ditunno JF, Flanders AE, Kirchblum SC et al: Predicting outcome in traumatic spinal cord injury. In Kirshblum S, Campagnolo DI, DeLisa JA (eds): Spinal Cord Medicine. Philadelphia, Lippincott Williams & Wilkins, 2002:108–122.
45. Chen D, Apple DA, Hudson LM et al: Medical complications during acute rehabilitation following spinal cord injury — current experience of the model systems. Arch Phys Med Rehabil 1999; 80:1397–1401.

46. Chen D: Treatment and prevention of thromboembolism after spinal cord injury. Top Spinal Cord Inj Rehabil 2003; 9:14–25.

47. Merli GJ, Herbison GJ, Ditunno JF et al: Deep vein thrombosis: prophylaxis in acute spinal cord injured patients. Arch Phys Med Rehabil 1988; 69:661–664.

48. Gunduz S, Ogur E, Mohur H et al: Deep vein thrombosis in spinal injured patients. Paraplegia 1993; 31:606–610.

49. Ragnarsson KT, Hall KM, Wilmot CB et al: Management of pulmonary, cardiovascular and metabolic conditions after spinal cord injury. In Stover S, DeLisa JA, Whiteneck GG (eds): Spinal Cord Injury: Clinical Outcomes from the Model Systems. Gaithersburg, MD, Aspen Publishers, 1995:79–99.

50. Lamb GC, Tomski MA, Kaufman J et al: Is chronic spinal cord injury associated with increased risk of venous thromboembolism? J Am Paraplegia Soc 1993; 16:153–156.

51. Myllynen P, Kammonen M, Rokkanen P et al: Deep venous thrombosis and pulmonary embolism in patients with acute spinal cord injury: a comparison with nonparalyzed patients immobilized due to spinal fractures. J Trauma 1985; 25:541–543.

52. Phillips WT, Kiratli BJ, Sarkarati M et al: Effect of spinal cord injury on the heart and cardiovascular fitness. Curr Probl Cardiol 1998; 23:649–716.

53. Gruber UF, Thoni F: Prevention of thrombo-embolic complications in paraplegics. Paraplegia 1985; 23:124.

54. Anonymous: Prevention of venous thrombosis and pulmonary embolism. NIH Consensus Development. JAMA 1986; 256:744–749.

55. Green D, Rossi EC, Yao JST et al: Deep vein thrombosis in spinal cord injury: effect of prophylaxis with calf compression, aspirin, and dipyridamole. Paraplegia 1982; 20:227–234.

56. Merli GJ, Crabbe S, Doyle L et al: Mechanical plus pharmacological prophylaxis for deep vein thrombosis in acute spinal cord injury. Paraplegia 1992; 30:558–562.

57. Consortium for Spinal Cord Medicine: Prevention of Thromboembolism in Spinal Cord Injury. Washington, DC, Paralyzed Veterans of America, 1999.

58. Dong B, Jirong Y, Liu G et al: Thrombolytic therapy for pulmonary embolism. The Cochrane Database of Systematic Reviews. 2006: Issue 2. Art. No.: CD004437. DOI: 10.1002/14651858.CD004437.pub2.

59. Priebe MM, Goetz LL, Wuermser LA: Spasticity following spinal cord injury. In Kirshblum S, Campagnolo DI, DeLisa JA (eds): Spinal Cord Medicine. Philadelphia, Lippincott Williams & Wilkins, 2002:221–233.

60. Maynard FM, Karunas RS, Waring WP: Epidemiology of spasticity following traumatic spinal cord injury. Arch Phys Med Rehabil 1990; 71:566–569.

61. Young RR: Physiology and pharmacology of spasticity. In Gelber DA, Jeffery DR (eds): Clinical Evaluation and Management of Spasticity. Totowa, NJ, Humana Press, 2002:3–12.

62. Platz T, Eickhof C, Nuyens G et al: Clinical scales for the assessment of spasticity, associated phenomena, and function: a systematic review of the literature. Disabil Rehabil 2005; 27:7–21.

63. Skold C: Spasticity in spinal cord injury: self- and clinically rated intrinsic fluctuations and intervention-induced changes. Arch Phys Med Rehabil 2000; 81:144–149.

64. Patrick E, Ada L: The Tardieu Scale differentiates contracture from spasticity whereas the Ashworth Scale is confounded by it. Clin Rehabil 2006; 20:173–182.

65. Gregson JM, Leathley M, Moore AP et al: Reliability of the Tone Assessment Scale and the modified Ashworth scale as clinical tools for assessing poststroke spasticity. Arch Phys Med Rehabil 1999; 80:1013–1016.

66. Haas BM, Bergstrom E, Jamous A et al: The inter rater reliability of the original and of the modified Ashworth scale for the assessment of spasticity in patients with spinal cord injury. Spinal Cord 1996; 34:560–564.

67. Bohannon RW, Andrews AW: Interrater reliability of hand-held dynamometry. Phys Ther 1987; 67:931–933.

68. Priebe MM: Assessment of spinal cord injury spasticity in clinical trials. Top Spinal Cord Inj Rehabil 2006; 11:69–77.

69. Sipski ML, Richards JS: Spinal cord injury rehabilitation: State of the science. Am J Phys Med Rehabil 2006; 85:310–342.

70. Burchiel KJ, Hsu FP: Pain and spasticity after spinal cord injury: mechanisms and treatment. Spine 2001; 26:S146–S160.

71. Pandyan AD, Gregoric M, Barnes MP et al: Spasticity: Clinical perceptions, neurological realities and meaningful measurement. Disabil Rehabil 2005; 27:2–6.

72. Pierrot-Deseilligny E, Mazieres L: Spinal mechanisms underlying spasticity: contribution to assessment and pathophysiology. In Delwaide PJ, Young RR (eds): Clinical Neurophysiology in Spasticity. Amsterdam, Elsevier, 1985.

73. Hsieh JTC, Wolfe DL, Connolly S et al: Spasticity following spinal cord injury. In Eng JJ, Teasell RW, Miller WC et al (eds): Spinal Cord Injury Rehabilitation Evidence. Vancouver, 2006:21.1–21.56.

74. Levi R, Hultling C, Seiger A: The Stockholm Spinal Cord Injury Study: 2. Associations between clinical patient characteristics and post-acute medical problems. Paraplegia 1995; 33:585–594.

75. Pierson SH: Physical and occupational approaches. In Gelber DA, Jeffery DR (eds): Clinical Evaluation and Management of Spasticity. Totowa, Humana Press, 2002:47–66.

76. Gao SA, Ambring A, Lambert G et al: Autonomic control of the heart and renal vascular bed during autonomic dysreflexia in high spinal cord injury. Clin Auton Res 2002; 12:457–464.

77. Blackmer J: Rehabilitation medicine: 1. Autonomic dysreflexia. Can Med Assoc J 2003; 169:931–935.

78. Karlsson AK: Autonomic dysreflexia. Spinal Cord 1999; 37:383–391.

79. Krassioukov A, Warburton DER, Teasell RW et al: Autonomic dysreflexia. In Eng JJ, Teasell RW, Miller WC et al (eds): Spinal Cord Injury Rehabilitation Evidence. Vancouver, 2006:17.1–17.27.

80. Campagnolo DI, Merli GJ: Autonomic and cardiovascular complications of spinal cord injury. In Kirshblum S, Campagnolo DI, DeLisa JA (eds): Spinal Cord Medicine. Philadelphia, Lippincott Williams & Wilkins, 2002:123–134.

81. Consortium for Spinal Cord Medicine: Acute Management of Autonomic Dysreflexia: Individuals with Spinal Cord Injury Presenting to Health-Care Facilities. Washington, DC, Paralyzed Veterans of America, 2001.

82. Mathias CJ, Fankel HL: Autonomic disturbances in spinal cord lesions. In Mathias CJ, Bannister R (eds): Autonomic Failure. A Textbook of Clinical Disorders of the Autonomic Nervous System. Oxford, Oxford University Press, 1999:494–513.

83. Mathias CJ, Kimber JR: Postural hypotension: causes, clinical features, investigation and management. Annu Rev Med 1999; 50:317–336.

84. Krassioukov A, Warburton DER, Teasell RW et al: Orthostatic hypotension following spinal cord injury. In Eng JJ, Teasell RW, Miller WC et al (eds): Spinal Cord Injury Rehabilitation Evidence. Vancouver, 2006:16.1–16.7.

85. Sved AF, McDowell FH, Blessing WW: Release of antidiuretic hormone in quadriplegic subjects in response to head-up tilt. Neurology 1985; 35:78–82.

86. Senard JM, Arias A, Berlan M et al: Pharmacological evidence of alpha 1- and alpha 2-adrenergic supersensitivity in orthostatic hypotension due to spinal cord injury: a case report. Eur J Clin Pharmacol 1991; 41:593–596.

87. Mathias CJ, Christensen NJ, Corbett JL et al: Plasma catecholamines, plasma renin activity and plasma aldosterone in tetraplegic man, horizontal and tilted. Clin Sci Mol Med 1975; 49:291–299.

88. Teasell RW, Arnold JM, Krassioukov A et al: Cardiovascular consequences of loss of supraspinal control of the sympathetic nervous system after spinal cord injury. Arch Phys Med Rehabil 2000; 81:506–516.

89. Benevento BT, Sipski ML: Neurogenic bladder, neurogenic bowel, and sexual dysfunction in people with spinal cord injury. Phys Ther 2002; 82:601–612.

90. Weld KJ, Cmochowski RR: Effect of bladder management on urological complications in spinal cord injured patients. J Urol 2000; 163:768–772.

91. Singh G, Thomas DG: The female tetraplegic: an admission of urological failure. Br J Urol 1997; 79:708–712.

92. Ersoz M, Akyuk M: Bladder-filling sensation in patients with spinal cord injury and the potential for sensation-dependent bladder emptying. Spinal Cord 2004; 42:110–116.

93. Horton JA, Chancellor MB, Labatia I: Bladder management for the evolving spinal cord injury: options and considerations. Top Spinal Cord Inj Rehabil 2003; 9:36–52.

94. Drake MJ, Cortina-Borja M, Savic G et al: Prospective evaluation of urological effects of aging in chronic spinal cord injury by method of bladder management. Neurourol Urodyn 2005; 24:111–116.

95. Hicken BL, Putzke JD, Richards JS: Bladder management and quality of life after spinal cord injury. Am J Phys Med Rehabil 2001; 80:916–922.

96. Korsten MA, Rosman AS, Ng A et al: Infusion of neostigmine-glycopyrrolate for bowel evacuation in persons with spinal cord injury. Am J Gastroenterol 2005; 100:1560–1565.

97. Krogh K, Olsen N, Christensen P et al: Colorectal transport during defecation in patients with lesions of the sacral spinal cord. Neurogastroenterol Motil 2003; 15:25–31.

98. Stiens SA, Bergman SB, Goetz LL: Neurogenic bowel dysfunction after spinal cord injury: Clinical evaluation and rehabilitative management. Arch Phys Med Rehabil 1997; 78:S86–102.

99. Yim SY, Yoon SH, Lee IY et al: A comparison of bowel care patterns in patients with spinal cord injury. Upper motor neuron bowel vs lower motor neuron bowel. Spinal Cord 2001; 39:204–207.

100. House JG, Stiens SA: Pharmacologically initiated defecation for persons with spinal cord injury: effectiveness of three agents. Arch Phys Med Rehabil 1997; 78:1062–1065.

101. Banwell JG, Creasey GH, Aggarwal AM et al: Management of the neurogenic bowel in patients with spinal cord injury. Urol Clin North Am 1993; 20:517–526.

102. Stone JM, Nino-Murcia M, Wold VA et al: Chronic gastrointestinal problems in spinal cord injury patients: a prospective analysis. Am J Gastroenterol 1990; 85:114–119.

103. Glickman S, Kamm MA: Bowel dysfunction in spinal-cord-injury patients. Lancet 1996; 347:1651–1653.

104. Menter R, Weitzenkamp D, Cooper D et al: Bowel management outcomes in individuals with long-term spinal cord injuries. Spinal Cord 1997; 35:608–612.

105. Kreuter M, Sullivan M, Siosteen A: Sexual adjustment and quality of relationship in spinal paraplegia: a controlled study. Arch Phys Med Rehabil 1996; 77:541–548.

106. Sipski ML, Alexander CJ, Rosen RC: Physiological parameters associated with psychogenic sexual arousal in women with complete spinal cord injuries. Arch Phys Med Rehabil 1995; 76:811–818.

107. Sipski ML, Alexander CJ, Rosen RC: Physiologic parameters associated with sexual arousal in women with incomplete spinal cord injuries. Arch Phys Med Rehabil 1997; 78:305–313.

108. Martinez-Arizala A, Brackett NL: Sexual dysfunction in spinal cord injury. In Singer C, Weiner WJ (eds): Sexual Dysfunction: A Neuro-medical Approach. Armonk, NY, Futura Publishing, 1994:135–153.

109. Brackett NL, Nash MS, Lynne CM: Male fertility following spinal cord injury: facts and fiction. Phys Ther 1996; 76:1221–1231.

110. Deforge D, Blackmer J, Garritty C et al: Fertility following spinal cord injury: a systematic review. Spinal Cord 2005; 43:693–703.

111. Phelps J, Albo M, Dunn K et al: Spinal cord injury and sexuality in married or partnered men: activities, function, needs, and predictors of sexual adjustment. Arch Sex Behav 2001; 30:591–602.

112. Fisher TL, Laud PW, Byfield MG et al: Sexual health after spinal cord injury: a longitudinal study. Arch Phys Med Rehabil 2002; 83:1043–1051.

113. Gittler MS: Acute rehabilitation in cervical spinal cord injuries. Top Spinal Cord Inj Rehabil 2004; 9:60–73.

114. Johnson KMM, Lanig IS: Promotion and maintenance of sexual health in individuals with spinal cord injury. In Chase TM, Butt LM, Hulse KL et al (eds): A Practical Guide to Health Promotion after Spinal Cord Injury. Gaithersburg, MD, Aspen Publications, 1996:171–202.

115. Lazo MG, Shirazi P, Sam M et al: Osteoporosis and risk of fracture in men with spinal cord injury. Spinal Cord 2001; 39:208–214.

116. Ott SM: Osteoporosis in women with spinal cord injuries. Phys Med Rehabil Clin N Am 2001; 12:111–131.

117. Ingram RR, Suman RK, Freeman PA: Lower limb fractures in the chronic spinal cord injured patient. Paraplegia 1989; 27:133–139.

118. Chantraine A, Nusgens B, Lapiere CM: Bone remodeling during the development of osteoporosis in paraplegia. Calcif Tissue Int 1986; 38:323–327.

119. Garland DR, Stewart CA, Adkins RH et al: Osteoporosis after spinal cord injury. J Orthop Res 1992; 10:371–378.

120. Uebelhart D, Demiaux-Domenech B, Roth M et al: Bone metabolism in spinal cord injured individuals and in others who have prolonged immobilisation. A review. Paraplegia 1995; 33:669–673.

121. Chen B, Stein A: Osteoporosis in acute spinal cord injury. Top Spinal Cord Inj Rehabil 2003; 9:26–35.

122. Needham-Shropshire BM, Broton JG, Klose K et al: Evaluation of a training programme for persons with SCI paraplegia using the Parastep 1 Ambulation System: part 3. Lack of effect on bone mineral density. Arch Phys Med Rehabil 1997; 78:799–803.

123. Freehafer AA, Hazel CM, Becker CL: Lower extremity fractures in patients with spinal cord injury. Paraplegia 1981; 19:367–372.

124. Ragnarsson KT, Sell GH: Lower extremity fractures after spinal cord injury: a retrospective study. Arch Phys Med Rehabil 1981; 62:418–423.

125. Guttman L: Spinal Cord Injuries: Comprehensive Management and Research, 2nd edn. Oxford, Blackwell Scientific Publications, 1976.

126. Kaplan PE, Gannhavadi B, Richards L et al: Calcium balance in paraplegic patients: influence of injury duration and ambulation. Arch Phys Med Rehabil 1978; 59:447–450.

127. Chantraine A: Actual concept of osteoporosis in paraplegia. Paraplegia 1978; 16:51–58.

128. Giangregorio L, Blimkie CJ: Skeletal adaptations to alterations in weight-bearing activity: a comparison of models of disuse osteoporosis. Sports Med 2002; 32:459–476.

129. Bauman WA, Spungen AM: Metabolic changes in persons after spinal cord injury. Phys Med Rehabil Clin N Am 2000; 11:109–140.

130. Frey-Rindova P, de Bruin ED, Stussi E et al: Bone mineral density in upper and lower extremities during 12 months after spinal cord injury measured by peripheral quantitative computed tomography. Spinal Cord 2000; 38:26–32.

131. de Bruin ED, Frey-Rindova P, Herzog RE et al: Changes of tibia bone properties after spinal cord injury: effects of early intervention. Arch Phys Med Rehabil 1999; 80:214–220.

132. Rodgers MM, Glaser RM, Figoni SF et al: Musculoskeletal responses of spinal cord injured individuals to functional neuromuscular stimulation-induced knee extension exercise training. J Rehabil Res Dev 1991; 28:19–26.

133. Belanger M, Stein RB, Wheeler GD et al: Electrical stimulation: can it increase muscle strength and reverse osteopenia in spinal cord injured individuals? Arch Phys Med Rehabil 2000; 81:1090–1098.

134. Eser P, de Bruin ED, Telley I et al: Effect of electrical stimulation-induced cycling on bone mineral density in spinal cord-injured patients. Eur J Clin Invest 2003; 33:412–419.

135. Ben M, Harvey L, Denis S et al: Does 12 weeks of regular standing prevent loss of ankle mobility and bone mineral density in people with recent spinal cord injuries? Aust J Physiother 2005; 51:251–256.

136. Sheel AW, Reid WD, Townson AF et al: Respiratory management following spinal cord injury. In Eng JJ, Teasell RW, Miller WC et al (eds): Spinal Cord Injury Rehabilitation Evidence. Vancouver, 2006:8.1–8.30.

137. McCarthy EF, Sundaram M: Heterotopic ossification: a review. Skeletal Radiol 2005; 34:609–619.

138. van Kuijk AA, Geurts AC, van Kuppevelt HJ: Neurogenic heterotopic ossification in spinal cord injury. Spinal Cord 2002; 40:313–326.

139. Vanden Bossche L, Vanderstraeten G: Heterotopic ossification: a review. J Rehabil Med 2005; 37:129–136.

140. Banovac K, Banovac F: Heterotopic ossification. In Kirshblum S, Campagnolo DI, DeLisa JA (eds): Spinal Cord Medicine. Philadelphia, Lippincott Williams & Wilkins; 2002:108–122.

141. Snoecx M, De Muynck M, Van Laere M: Association between muscle trauma and heterotopic ossification in spinal cord injured patients: reflections on their causal relationship and the diagnostic value of ultrasonography. Paraplegia 1995; 33:464–468.

142. Sobus KM, Alexander MA, Harcke HT: Undetected musculoskeletal trauma in children with traumatic brain injury or spinal cord injury. Arch Phys Med Rehabil 1993; 74:902–904.

143. Michelsson JE, Rauschning W: Pathogenesis of experimental heterotopic bone formation following temporary forcible exercising of immobilized limbs. Clin Orthop Relat Res 1983; 176:265–272.

144. Michelsson JE, Ganroth G, Andersson LC: Myositis ossificans following forcible manipulation of the leg. A rabbit model for the study of heterotopic bone formation. J Bone Joint Surg (Am) 1980; 62:811–815.

145. Daud O, Sett P, Burr RG et al: The relationship of heterotopic ossification to passive movements in paraplegic patients. Disabil Rehabil 1993; 15:114–118.

146. Crawford CM, Varghese G, Mani MM et al: Heterotopic ossification: are range of motion exercises contraindicated? J Burn Care Rehabil 1986; 7:323–327.

147. Linan E, O'Dell MW, Pierce JM: Continuous passive motion in the management of heterotopic ossification in a brain injured patient. Am J Phys Med Rehabil 2001; 80:614–617.

148. Garber SL, Rintala DH, Hart KA et al: Pressure ulcer risk in spinal cord injury: predictors of ulcer status over 3 years. Arch Phys Med Rehabil 2000; 81:465–471.

149. Fuhrer MJ, Garber SL, Rintala DH et al: Pressure ulcers in community-resident persons with spinal cord injury: prevalence and risk factors. Arch Phys Med Rehabil 1993; 74:1172–1177.

150. Johnson RL, Gerhart KA, McCray J et al: Secondary conditions following spinal cord injury in a population-based sample. Spinal Cord 1998; 36:45–50.

151. Consortium for Spinal Cord Medicine Clinical Practice Guidelines: Pressure ulcer prevention and treatment following spinal cord injury: a clinical practice guideline for health-care professionals. J Spinal Cord Med 2001; 24:S40–101.

152. Bergstrom N, Allman RM, Alvarez OM et al: Treatment of Pressure Ulcers. Clinical Guideline Number 15. Rockville, MD, US Department of Health and Human Services. Public Health Service, Agency for Health Care Policy and Research. AHCPR Publication No. 95–0652; 1994.

153. Stinson MD, Porter-Armstrong A, Eakin P: Seat-interface pressure: a pilot study of the relationship to gender, body mass index, and seating position. Arch Phys Med Rehabil 2003; 84:405–409.

154. Folkedahl BA, Frantz R: Prevention of Pressure Ulcers. Iowa City, IA, University of Iowa Gerontological Nursing Interventions Research Center, Research Dissemination Core, 2002.

155. de Groot PC, van Kuppevelt DH, Pons C et al: Time course of arterial vascular adaptations to inactivity and paralyses in humans. Med Sci Sports Exerc 2003; 35:1977–1985.

156. Cullum N, McInnes E, Bell-Syer SEM et al: Support surfaces for pressure ulcer prevention. The Cochrane Database of Systematic Reviews. 2004: Issue 3. Art. No.: CD001735. DOI: 10.1002/14651858.CD001735.pub2.

157. Regan M, Teasell RW, Keast D et al: Pressure ulcers following spinal cord injury. In Eng JJ, Teasell RW, Miller WC et al (eds): Spinal Cord Injury Rehabilitation Evidence. Vancouver, 2006:20.1–20.26.

158. Coggrave MJ, Rose LS: A specialist seating assessment clinic: changing pressure relief practice. Spinal Cord 2003; 41:692–695.

159. Axelson P, Yamada Chesny D, Minkel J et al: The Manual Wheelchair Training Guide. Minden, NV, PAX Press, 1998.

160. Koczure L, Strine C, Peischl D: Case presentations: practical applications in wheelchair technology. Phys Med Rehabil: State of the Art Reviews 2000; 14:323–338.

161. Axelson P, Minkel J, Perr A et al: The Powered Wheelchair Training Guide. Minden, NV, PAX Press, 2002.
162. Bergen AF: The prescriptive wheelchair: an orthotic device. In O'Sullivan SB, Schmitz TJ (eds): Physical Rehabilitation: Assessment and Treatment. Philadelphia, FA Davis Company, 2000:1061–1092.
163. Ball M: The future is now. Sport'n Spokes 2000.
164. Taylor SJ: Powered mobility evaluation and technology. Top Spinal Cord Inj Rehabil 1995; 1:23–36.
165. Kreutz D: Manual wheelchairs: prescribing for function. Top Spinal Cord Inj Rehabil 1995; 1:1–16.
166. Bolin I, Bodin P, Kreuter M: Sitting position — posture and performance in C5–C6 tetraplegia. Spinal Cord 2000; 38:425–434.
167. Engström B: Ergonomics, Seating and Positioning. Sweden, ETAC, 1993.
168. Conine TA, Hershler C, Daechsel D et al: Pressure ulcer prophylaxis in elderly patients using polyurethane foam or Jay wheelchair cushions. Int J Rehabil Res 1994; 17:123–137.
169. Brienza DM, Karg PE, Geyer MJ et al: The relationship between pressure ulcer incidence and buttock–seat cushion interface pressure in at-risk elderly wheelchair users. Arch Phys Med Rehabil 2001; 82:529–533.
170. Ragan R, Kernozek TW, Bidar M et al: Seat-interface pressures on various thicknesses of foam wheelchair cushions: a finite modeling approach. Arch Phys Med Rehabil 2002; 83:872–875.
171. Ham R, Aldersea P, Porter D: Wheelchair Users and Postural Seating: A Clinical Approach. New York, Churchill Livingstone, 1998.
172. Geyer MJ, Brienza DM, Karg P et al: A randomized control trial to evaluate pressure-reducing seat cushions for elderly wheelchair users. Adv Skin Wound Care 2001; 14:120–132.
173. Miller GE, Seale JL: The mechanics of terminal lymph flow. J Biomech Eng 1985; 107:376–380.
174. Martz E, Livneh H, Priebe MM et al: Predictors of psychosocial adaptation among people with spinal cord injury or disorder. Arch Phys Med Rehabil 2005; 86:1182–1192.
175. Bombardier CH, Richards JS, Krause JS et al: Symptoms of major depression in people with spinal cord injury: implications for screening. Arch Phys Med Rehabil 2004; 85:1749–1756.
176. Kennedy P, Lude P, Taylor N: Quality of life, social participation, appraisals and coping post spinal cord injury: a review of four community samples. Spinal Cord 2006; 44:95–105.
177. Fuhrer MJ, Rintala DH, Hart KA et al: Depressive symptomatology in persons with spinal cord injury who reside in the community. Arch Phys Med Rehabil 1993; 74:255–260.
178. Elliott TR, Frank RG: Depression following spinal cord injury. Arch Phys Med Rehabil 1996; 77:816–823.
179. Kennedy P, Duff J, Evans M et al: Coping effectiveness training reduces depression and anxiety following traumatic spinal cord injuries. Br J Clin Psychol 2003; 42:41–52.
180. Dryden DM, Saunders LD, Rowe BH et al: Depression following traumatic spinal cord injury. Neuroepidemiology 2005; 25:55–61.
181. Faber RA: Depression and spinal cord injury. Neuroepidemiology 2005; 25:53–54.
182. Elfstrom ML, Ryden A, Kreuter M et al: Relations between coping strategies and health-related quality of life in patients with spinal cord lesion. J Rehabil Med 2005; 37:9–16.
183. Frank RG, Kashani JH, Wonderlich SA et al: Depression and adrenal function in spinal cord injury. Am J Psychiatry 1985; 142:252–253.
184. Clay DL, Hagglund KJ, Frank RG et al: Enhancing the accuracy of depression diagnosis in patients with spinal cord injury using Bayesian analysis. Rehabil Psychol 1995; 40:171–180.
185. Fereroff J, Lipsey J, Starkstein S et al: Phenomenological comparisons of major depression following stroke, myocardial infarction or spinal cord lesions. J Affect Disord 1991; 22:83–89.
186. Tate DG, Forchheimer M, Maynard F et al: Comparing two measures of depression in spinal cord injury. Rehabil Psychol 1994; 38:53–61.
187. Tate D, Forchheimer M, Maynard F et al: Predicting depression and psychological distress in persons with spinal cord injury based on indicators of handicap. Am J Phys Med Rehabil 1994; 73:175–183.
188. Hartkopp A, Bronnum-Hansen H, Seidenschnur AM et al: Suicide in a spinal cord injured population: its relation to functional status. Arch Phys Med Rehabil 1998; 79:1356–1361.
189. Rish BL, Dilustro JF, Salazar AM et al: Spinal cord injury: a 25-year morbidity and mortality study. Mil Med 1997; 162:141–148.
190. De Vivo MJ, Black KJ, Richards JS et al: Suicide following spinal cord injury. Paraplegia 1991; 29:620–627.
191. Gerhart KA: Quality of life: the danger of differing perceptions. Top Spinal Cord Inj Rehabil 1997; 2:78–84.
192. Ernst FA: Contrasting perceptions of distress by research personnel and their spinal cord injured subjects. Am J Phys Med 1987; 66:12–15.
193. Consortium for Spinal Cord Medicine: Depression Following Spinal Cord Injury: A Clinical Practice Guideline for Primary Care Physicians. Washington, DC, Paralyzed Veterans of America, 1998.

194. Orenczuk S, Slivinski J, Teasell RW: Depression following spinal cord injury. In Eng JJ, Teasell RW, Miller WC et al (eds): Spinal Cord Injury Rehabilitation Evidence. Vancouver, 2006: 10.1–10.19.

195. Weitzenkamp DA, Gerhart KA, Charlifue SW et al: Spouses of spinal cord injury survivors: the added impact of caregiving. Arch Phys Med Rehabil 1997; 78:822–827.

196. Post MW, Bloemen J, de Witte LP: Burden of support for partners of persons with spinal cord injuries. Spinal Cord 2005; 43:311–319.

197. Holicky R, Charlifue SW: Ageing with spinal cord injury: the impact of spousal support. Disabil Rehabil 1999; 21:250–257.

198. Kreuter M, Sullivan M, Dahllof AG et al: Partner relationships, functioning, mood and global quality of life in person with spinal cord injury and traumatic brain injury. Spinal Cord 1998; 36:252–261.

199. Elovic E, Kirshblum S: Epidemiology of spinal cord injury and traumatic brain injury: the scope of the problem. Top Spinal Cord Inj Rehabil 1999; 5:1–20.

200. Michael DB, Guyot DR, Darmody WR: Coincidence of head and cervical spine injury. J Neurotrauma 1989; 6:177–189.

201. Davidoff GN, Roth EJ, Richards JS: Cognitive deficits in spinal cord injury: epidemiology and outcome. Arch Phys Med Rehabil 1992; 73:275–284.

202. Macciocchi SN, Bowman B, Coker J et al: Effect of co-morbid traumatic brain injury on functional outcomes of persons with spinal cord injuries. Am J Phys Med Rehabil 2004; 83:22–26.

203. McGlinchey-Berroth R, Morrow L, Ahlquist M et al: Late-life spinal cord injury and aging with a long term injury: characteristics of two emerging populations. J Spinal Cord Med 1995; 18:183–193.

204. Whiteneck GG, Charlifue SW, Gerhart KA et al (eds): Aging with Spinal Cord Injury. New York, Demos, 1993.

205. Menter RR: Issues of aging with spinal cord injury. In Whiteneck GG, Charlifue SW, Gerhart KA et al (eds): Aging with Spinal Cord Injury. New York, Demos, 1993:9–21.

206. Krause J, Broderick L: A 25-year longitudinal study of the natural course of aging after spinal cord injury. Spinal Cord 2005; 43:349–356.

207. Fehr L, Langbein WE, Edwards LC et al: Diagnostic wheelchair exercise testing. Top Spinal Cord Inj Rehabil 1997; 3:34–48.

208. Gerhart KA, Bergstrom E, Charlifue SW et al: Long-term spinal cord injury: functional changes over time. Arch Phys Med Rehabil 1993; 74:1030–1034.

209. Menter RR, Whiteneck GG, Charlifue SW et al: Impairment, disability, handicap and medical expenses of persons aging with spinal cord injury. Paraplegia 1991; 29:613–619.

Contents

Step one: assessing
impairments, activity
limitations and participation
restrictions 36

Step two: setting goals 40

Step three: identifying key
impairments 46

Step four: identifying and
administering treatments . . .47

Step five: measuring
outcomes 47

Physiotherapy as part of the
multi-disciplinary team 48

A framework for physiotherapy management

The overall purpose of physiotherapy for patients with spinal cord injury is to improve health-related quality of life. This is achieved by improving patients' ability to participate in activities of daily life. The barriers to participation which are amenable to physiotherapy interventions are impairments that are directly or indirectly related to motor and sensory loss. Impairments prevent individuals from performing activities such as walking, pushing a wheelchair and rolling in bed. During the acute phase, immediately after injury when patients are restricted to bed, the key impairments physiotherapists can prevent or treat are pain, poor respiratory function, loss of joint mobility and weakness (see Chapters 8–11). Once patients commence rehabilitation physiotherapists can also address impairments related to poor skill and fitness (see Chapters 7 and 12).

It is possible to define the role and purpose of physiotherapy for patients with spinal cord injury within the framework of the International Classification of Functioning, Disability and Health (ICF). The ICF was introduced by the World Health Organization in 2001[1] and is a revised version of the International Classification of Impairment, Disability and Handicap.[2] The ICF defines components of health from the perspective of the body, the individual and society (see Figure 2.1). One of its primary purposes is to provide unified and standard language for those working in the area of disability.[1,3]

The ICF can be used to articulate the goals and purpose of physiotherapy for patients with spinal cord injury. For example, the health condition is spinal cord injury. An associated impairment is poor strength. Poor strength directly impacts on the ability to perform activities such as walking and moving. This in turn has implications for participation, such as working, engaging in family life and participating in community activities. Impairments, activity limitations and participation restrictions are all affected by environmental and personal factors, such as support from family and employers, access to appropriate equipment, financial situation and coping mechanisms. In the ICF framework, such environmental and personal influences are termed contextual factors.

Figure 2.1 The ICF framework. Reproduced with permission from World Health Organization: International Classification of Functioning, Disability and Health: ICF short version. Geneva, World Health Organization, 2001.

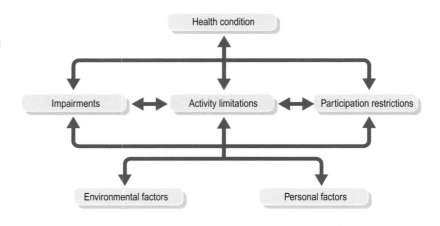

The ICF framework can also be used to describe the process involved in formulating a physiotherapy programme. The process involves five steps:

Step one: assessing impairments, activity limitations and participation restrictions
Step two: setting goals with respect to activity limitations and participation restrictions
Step three: identifying key impairments
Step four: identifying and administering treatments
Step five: measuring outcomes

Each of these steps is described in this chapter and provides the framework for formulating physiotherapy programmes. The focus is primarily on patients undergoing rehabilitation. In the period immediately after injury when patients are restricted to bed it is not feasible to assess activity limitations and participation restrictions, and it may not be appropriate to set goals in these domains.

Step one: assessing impairments, activity limitations and participation restrictions

Assessment is the first step in devising an appropriate physiotherapy programme. The assessment forms the basis of the goal-setting process. It identifies participation restrictions, activity limitations, and impairments.

Initially, various sources need to be used to extract details such as age, cause of injury, time since injury, neurological status, orthopaedic status, other injuries and complications, socio-economic background, medical and surgical management since injury, prior medical history, family support, employment status and living arrangements. These provide key insights into patients' problems, and help direct the subsequent physical assessment.

Assessing activity limitations and participation restrictions

There are several well-accepted assessment tools used to measure activity limitations and participation restrictions,[4,5] including the Functional Independence Measure (FIM®),[6-8] Spinal Cord Independence Measure,[9-11] and Quadriplegic Index of

Function[12-14] (see Table 2.1). They all measure independence across a range of domains, reflecting different aspects of activity limitations and participation restrictions. For example, they assess ability to dress, maintain continence, mobilize, transfer and feed. Some have been specifically designed for patients with spinal cord injury, and others are intended for use across all disabilities.

More physiotherapy-specific assessments of activity limitations and participation restrictions quantify different aspects of mobility and motor function. For example, some assess the ability to walk (e.g. the WISCI, 10 m Walk Test, the Motor Assessment Scale, 6-minute Walk Test, Timed Up and Go), ability to use the hands (e.g. the Grasp and Release test, Sollerman test, Carroll test, Jebsen test) and ability to mobilize in a wheelchair[15,16] (see Table 2.1). There is as yet no consensus on the most appropriate tests, and currently physiotherapists tend to use a battery of different assessments, including non-standardized, subjective assessments of the way patients move.

TABLE 2.1   Assessment tools for measuring activity limitations and participation restrictions

	Brief description
General	
Functional Independence Measure (FIM®)[65,66]	The FIM assesses activity limitations. It contains 18 items across six domains: self-care, sphincter control, transfers, locomotion, communication and social cognition. Each item is scored on a seven-point ordinal scale ranging from total assistance (one) to complete independence (seven).
Spinal Cord Independence Measures (SCIM)[9,10]	The SCIM was developed specifically for patients with spinal cord injury and contains 16 items covering self-care (four items), respiration and sphincter management (four items), and mobility (eight items). The original SCIM was modified in 2001[67] and more recently a questionnaire version has been devised.
Barthel Index[68-72]	The Barthel Index contains 15 self-care, bladder and bowel, and mobility items. Transfers and mobility items (both wheelchair and ambulation) encompass 30%, and toileting and bathing a further 10% of the total score.
Craig Handicap and Reporting Technique (CHART)[73-78]	The CHART was specifically designed for patients with spinal cord injury to measure community integration. It consists of 27 items which cover five domains: physical independence (three questions), mobility (nine questions), occupation (seven questions), social integration (six questions) and economic self-sufficiency (two questions). Each item is assessed on a behavioural criteria (i.e. hours out of bed). It is administered via interview or questionnaire.
Clinical Outcomes Variable Scale (COVS)[79,80]	The COVS consists of 13 items scored on a seven-point scale and measures mobility in activities such as rolling, lying to sitting, sitting balance, transfers, ambulation, wheelchair mobility and arm function. Lower scores reflect poorer levels of mobility. Although originally developed for a general rehabilitation population, COVS discriminates across lesion level, injury completeness and walking status in patients with spinal cord injury.
PULSES[69,81]	The PULSES assesses activity limitation and participation restriction of those with chronic illness and covers six domains: physical condition (P), upper limb function (U), lower limb function (L), sensation (S), excretory function (E) and support factors (S). The scoring for each item ranges from one (independent) to four (fully dependent).

(continued)

TABLE 2.1 (continued)	
	Brief description
Quadriplegic Index of Function (QIF)[14]	The QIF was specifically designed for patients with tetraplegia. It contains 10 items, three of which encompass mobility (transfers 8%, wheelchair mobility 14% and bed activities 10%). Each item is scored on a five-point scale. There is a shorter form of the original QIF.
The Katz Index of ADL[82]	The Katz Index of ADL assesses independence in six activities including bathing, dressing, toileting, transferring, continence and feeding. Each activity is scored on a two-point scale, and summated into an overall score (represented by letters from A to G). There are no mobility items.
SF-36® Health Survey[83,84]	The SF-36 measures health-related quality of life in eight domains (physical functioning, role limitations due to physical problems, bodily pain, general health, vitality, social functioning, role limitations due to emotional problems, mental health). These can be summarized into two measures (physical and mental). The SF-36 has been used in patients with spinal cord injury.[85–88]
Sickness Impact Profile (SIP-136)[89]	The SIP-136 is a generic measure of the impact of disability on physical status and emotional well-being. It is administered via a 136-item questionnaire which requires 'yes' or 'no' responses. It has 12 domains including mobility and ambulation items. A shorter version (68 items) is also available.[90] It has three main domains including a physical domain which assesses ambulation, mobility and body care.
Canadian Occupational Performance Measure (COPM)[91–94]	The COPM was designed to assess patients' perspectives about changes in activity limitations and participation restrictions. The COPM is administered in a semi-structured interview where patients are required to identify specific activity limitations and participation restrictions. Patients use a 10-point scale to rate each identified problem with respect to importance, performance and satisfaction. The COPM is primarily used to monitor change.
The Physical Activity Recall Assessment for People with Spinal Cord Injury (PARA-SCI)[95,96]	The PARA-SCI is a self-report measure of physical activity. It was designed for patients with spinal cord injury and is administered via a semi-structured interview. The time spent on all physical activities related to leisure and daily living is recorded. Each activity is graded for intensity.
Valutazione Funzionale Mielolesi (VFM)[97,98]	The VFM questionnaire was developed specifically for patients with spinal cord injury to assess activity limitations. It covers bed mobility, eating, transfers, wheelchair use, grooming and bathing, dressing and social and vocational skills.
The Tufts Assessment of Motor Performance (TAMP)[99–101]	The TAMP was developed to measure gross and fine motor performance of the upper and lower limbs. It consists of 105 tasks grouped into 31 domains including fine hand function and independence with dressing, mobility, transfers and wheelchair skills. Each item is rated on a seven-point scale.
Needs Assessment Checklist (NAC)[28]	The NAC was designed specifically for patients with spinal cord injury to measure the success of rehabilitation. It consists of 199 items grouped into nine domains including activities of daily living, skin management, bladder management, bowel management, mobility, wheelchair and equipment, community preparation, discharge coordination and psychological issues. It does not differentiate between the ability to direct others to help and the ability to independently perform activities.
	(continued)

TABLE 2.1 (continued)	
	Brief description
Gait-related	
Walking Index for Spinal Cord Injury (WISCI)[102–104]	The WISCI was developed specifically for patients with spinal cord injury. It measures ability to walk 10 m and need for physical assistance, orthoses and walking aids on an incremental scale ranging from zero (unable to stand or walk) to 20 (ambulates without orthoses, aids or physical assistance).
The Spinal Cord Injury Functional Ambulation Inventory (SCI-FAI)[105]	The SCI-FAI is an observational gait assessment which uses an ordinal scale to rate nine different aspects of walking. It includes a 2-minute walk test.
The Walking Mobility Scale[106–108]	The Walking Mobility Scale is a five-point scale that classifies ability to walk into the following categories: physiological ambulators, limited household ambulators, independent household ambulators, limited community ambulators and independent community ambulators.
Timed Up and Go[109,110]	The Timed Up and Go test measures the time taken to stand up from a chair, walk 3 m, turn around and walk back to sit down on the chair. No physical assistance is given.
10 m Walk Test[65,111,112]	The 10 m Walk Test measures speed of walking (m.sec^{-1}). Patients are instructed to walk 14 m at their preferred speed but time is only recorded for the middle 10 m.
6-minute Walk Test[65,113]	The 6-minute Walk Test is a measure of endurance. Patients are instructed to walk as far as possible in 6 minutes, taking rests whenever required. The distance covered and the number of rests required are recorded.
Functional Standing Test (FST)[114]	The FST measures patients' ability to reach while standing. It consists of 20 items requiring manipulation and lifting of different objects. Orthoses can be worn and the tasks are done as quickly as possible. Some of the tasks are from the Jebsen Test of Hand Function.[115]
Modified Benzel Classification[116]	The Modified Benzel Classification is a seven-point scale that classifies patients according to both neurological and ambulatory status. Neurological classification is based on ASIA and ambulatory classification is crudely based on key gait parameters including ability to walk 25–250 feet (~ 7–75 m).
Upper limb function	
Capabilities of Upper Extremity Instrument (CUE)[117]	The CUE is a measure of upper limb function. It was specifically designed for patients with tetraplegia and is administered via a self-report questionnaire. Patients rate their ability to perform 32 different tasks on a seven-point scale.
The Tetraplegic Hand Activity Questionnaire (THAQ)[118]	The THAQ was designed to measure patients' perceptions about their hand and upper limb function. Patients are required to rate 153 motor tasks according to their ability to perform the task (four-point scale), need for an aid (four-point scale) and importance of the task (three point scale).
The Common Object Test (COT)[119]	The COT was designed to evaluate the usefulness of neuroprostheses. Patients are required to perform 14 motor tasks. Each task is divided into its sub-tasks and scored on a six-point scale according to the amount of assistance required.
Grasp and Release Test (GRT)[120]	The GRT is a test of hand function. It was initially designed to evaluate the usefulness of neuroprostheses in patients with C5 and C6 tetraplegia.

(continued)

TABLE 2.1 (continued)	
	Brief description
	The test requires patients to use either a palmar or lateral grasp to manipulate six different objects. Patients are assessed on the speed at which they can complete the tasks as well as their success rate.
Wheelchair mobility Quebec User Evaluation of Satisfaction with Assistive Technology (QUEST)[121,122]	The QUEST is a 12-item questionnaire which assesses patients' satisfaction with assistive technology, including wheelchairs. Each item is rated on a six-point scale ranging from 'not at all satisfied' to 'very satisfied'. Eight items relate to the device and four items to service provision.
Modified Functional Reach Test (mFRT)[123]	The mFRT assesses patients' ability to reach forward while seated. The maximal distance reached following three trials is recorded.
Timed Motor Test (TMT)[124]	The TMT was designed for children with spinal cord injury. It consists of six items and children are assessed on the time taken to complete each task. The tasks include putting on clothing, transferring and manoeuvring a manual wheelchair.
Five Additional Mobility and Locomotor Items (5-AML)[125,126]	The 5-AML was specifically designed for patients who are wheelchair-dependent. It contains five items assessing patients' ability to transfer, move about a bed and mobilize in a manual wheelchair. It is used in conjunction with the FIM.
Wheelchair Circuit Test (WCT)[127]	The WCT contains nine items and assesses different aspects of wheelchair mobility and the ability to transfer and walk. Three items require propelling a wheelchair on a treadmill.
Wheelchair Skills Test (WST)[15,128,129]	The WST is a 57-item test to assess ability to mobilize in a manual wheelchair. It includes simple tasks such as applying brakes, and complex tasks such transferring and ascending kerbs. Each item is scored on a three-point scale reflecting competency and safety. A questionnaire version is also available.[130]

Assessing impairments

The physical assessment also includes an assessment of impairments. These are similar to standard assessments used by physiotherapists in other populations. They include assessments of strength, sensation, respiratory function, cardiovascular fitness and pain. Details of how to assess impairments in patients with spinal cord injury can be found in subsequent chapters (see Chapters 8–12).

Step two: setting goals

Benefits of goals

Goal setting is an important aspect of a comprehensive physiotherapy and rehabilitation programme.[17–28] The process needs to be patient-centred. Initially, a few key goals of rehabilitation are articulated by the patient and negotiated with the multi-disciplinary team.[17,19,22,23,25,29–33] These goals should be expressed in terms of participation restrictions.[20,25] For example, a key goal of rehabilitation might be to return to work or school. Physiotherapy-specific goals then need to be identified and linked to each participation restriction goal. The physiotherapy-specific goals should be functional and purposeful activities as defined within the activity limitation and participation restriction domains of ICF and, specifically, within the ICF sub-domains of mobility, self-care and domestic life. These sub-domains include tasks such as pushing a manual wheelchair, rolling in bed, moving from lying to sitting, eating, drinking, looking after one's health, and pursuing recreation and leisure interests (see Ref. 34 for examples of ways to articulate functional goals appropriate for patients with spinal cord injury). Physiotherapy-specific goals are formulated in conjunction with the patient and other team members who share responsibility for their attainment. Both short- and long-term goals need to be set.[24,25] These may include goals to be achieved within a week or goals to be achieved over 6 months. In addition, specific goals (or targets) should be set as part of each treatment session[25] (see Chapter 7).

Goals are important for several reasons.[24] They ensure that the expectations of patients and staff are similar and realistic, and provide clear indications of what everyone is expected to achieve.[26] If compiled in an appropriate way, they actively engage patients in their own rehabilitation plan, empowering them and ensuring that their wishes and expectations are met.[26] Without goals, rehabilitation programmes can lack direction, and patients can feel like the passive recipients of mystical interventions.[19,22,23,30,35] Goals also help focus the rehabilitation team on the individual needs of patients, and provide team members with common objectives.[24] Perhaps most importantly, goals provide a source of motivation and enhance adherence.

Goals are also used to monitor the success of therapy and to identify problems. Goals achieved indicate success and goals not achieved indicate failure. Failure may be due to any number of reasons which need exploring. For example, a patient may fail to achieve a goal because of medical complications or because equipment fails to arrive, factors which may be difficult to avoid. Failure to achieve goals may reflect poor therapy attendance. Alternatively, failure may indicate unrealistic goals which need revising. A risk of excessive reliance on goals to measure success is that it encourages the selection of non-challenging goals which have a high likelihood of success.[27]

Guidelines to setting goals

Goals should be SMART. That is, they should be: Specific, Measurable, Attainable, Realistic and Timebound.[36] Physiotherapy-related goals need to be based on predictions of future independence, taking into account contextual factors such as patients' and families' perspectives, priorities and personal ambitions.[19,35,37] Other factors which influence outcome include access to products, technology and support, and personal attributes such as age, personality and anthropometrical characteristics.[37–43] Clearly, however, the strongest predictor of future independence is neurological status.[32,44,45] Neurological status determines the strength of muscles which in turn largely determines patients' ability to move.

A simplistic summary of levels of innervation for key upper and lower limb muscles is provided in Table 2.2 (for more details see Tables A1 and A2 in the Appendix). The summary is simplistic because muscles have been grouped together even though different muscles and parts of the same muscle often receive innervation from different spinal nerve roots. For example, the pectoralis muscles consist of pectoralis minor and the sternocostal and clavicular parts of pectoralis major. These muscles receive innervation from C5 to T1.[46]

TABLE 2.2   The levels at which muscles receive sufficient innervation to enable reasonable movement[46]

C4		Diaphragm
C5	Shoulder	Flexors
		Abductors
	Elbow	Flexors*
C6	Shoulder	Extensors
		Adductors
	Wrist	Extensors*
C7	Elbow	Extensors*
	Wrist	Flexors
	Finger	Extensors
	Thumb	Abductors and adductors
C8	Finger	Flexors*
	Thumb	Flexors and extensors
T1	Finger	Abductors*
		Adductors
T1–T12		Intercostals, abdominals and trunk
L2	Hip	Flexors*
		Adductors
L3	Knee	Extensors*
L4	Hip	Abductors
	Ankle	Dorsiflexors*
L5	Hip	Extensors
	Toe	Extensors*
S1	Knee	Flexors
	Ankle	Plantarflexors*
S2	Toe	Flexors

The ASIA muscles are asterisked (see Appendix for more details).

For some patients, particularly those with motor complete lesions without zones of partial preservation, it is relatively simple to look at the extent of paralysis and identify the *optimal* levels of independence which patients can hope to attain.[32,47–49] For instance, patients with complete T12 paraplegia and paralysis of the lower limbs have the potential to independently dress and transfer. In contrast, patients with complete C4 tetraplegia do not. However, this type of information can only be used as a starting point. Not only will outcomes be affected by contextual and other factors, but also by individual variations in neurological status. Often patients with the same ASIA classification have subtle but important differences in strength. For instance, a patient with C6 tetraplegia and grade 4/5 strength in the wrist extensor muscles will generally attain a higher level of function than a patient with the same level of tetraplegia but grade 3/5 strength in the wrist extensor muscles.[50] This is not only due to the implications of wrist extensor strength for function, but also due to the fact that wrist extensor strength is usually indicative of strength in other muscles which are primarily innervated at the C6 level, such as the latissimus dorsi and pectoralis muscles. Weakness in either of these shoulder girdle muscles has deleterious implications for function.[51]

Setting goals for patients with complete lesions

This section provides a brief overview of typical outcomes attained by patients with ASIA complete lesions and no zones of partial preservation.[32,52] A summary is provided in Table 2.3.

C1–C3 tetraplegia

Patients with C2 and above tetraplegia have total paralysis of the diaphragm and other respiratory muscles and consequently are ventilator-dependent. Patients with C3 tetraplegia retain a small amount of diaphragm function but not usually enough to breathe spontaneously (see Chapter 11).[53] All have paralysis of upper and lower limbs and trunk muscles but are able to move their heads. They are fully dependent

TABLE 2.3 Typical level of independence attained by patients with ASIA complete spinal cord injury

	C1–C3 tetraplegia	C4 tetraplegia	C5 tetraplegia	C6 tetraplegia	C7–C8 tetraplegia	Thoracic paraplegia	Lumbar and sacral paraplegia
Unassisted ventilation	no	yes	yes	yes	yes	yes	yes
Push manual wheelchair	no	no	limited	limited	yes	yes	yes
Hand to mouth activities	no	no	yes	yes	yes	yes	yes
Self-feeding	no	no	limited	yes	yes	yes	yes
Hand function	no	no	no	limited (tenodesis)	limited (tenodesis)	yes	yes
Driving[64]	no	no	no	yes	yes	yes	yes
Rolling	no	no	limited	yes	yes	yes	yes
Horizontal transfer	no	no	limited	yes	yes	yes	yes
Lying to sitting	no	no	limited	yes	yes	yes	yes
Floor to wheelchair	no	no	no	limited	limited	yes	yes
Standing in parallel bars with orthoses	no	no	no	no	limited	yes	yes
Walking with orthoses and aids	no	no	no	no	no	limited	yes

on others for all motor tasks and personal care activities. They mobilize in chin-control power wheelchairs and can use head-, mouth- or voice-activated technology (see Figure 2.2).

C4 tetraplegia

Patients with C4 tetraplegia have partial paralysis of the diaphragm and total paralysis of all four limbs and trunk muscles. They retain a small amount of voluntary control around the shoulders and have good strength in the rhomboid muscles but still mobilize in a chin-control power wheelchair. They can breathe independently but in all other respects their activity limitations are similar to those of patients with C1–C3 tetraplegia.

C5 tetraplegia

Patients with C5 tetraplegia have partial paralysis of the upper limbs but full paralysis of the trunk and lower limb muscles. They have good strength of the deltoid and

Figure 2.2 Patients with C1–C3 tetraplegia mobilize in chin-control wheelchairs and use head-, mouth- or voice-activated technology.

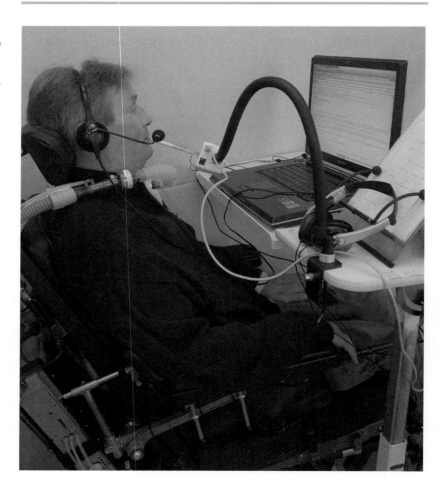

biceps muscles, but poor strength of other shoulder muscles. They have no function in the triceps muscles or any muscles about the wrist or hand. Despite this, they can use a hand-control power wheelchair with the hand passively rested on or secured to the joystick (see Chapter 13). They are unable to perform gross motor tasks such as transferring, rolling or moving from lying to sitting and require assistance for most personal care activities. They can, however, take their hands to their mouth, head and face. They can use the upper limbs to perform simple tasks provided no fine hand control is required and the appliance or utensil is attached to the hand with a splint. Upper limb function is usually possible with splints to stabilize the paralysed wrist. For example, a keyboard can be used with a typing stick attached to the hand and a steering wheel of a car can be turned with adaptations to the wheel (see Chapter 5).[54]

C6 tetraplegia

There is a large functional difference between patients with C5 and C6 tetraplegia. This is due to the preservation of the pectoralis, serratus anterior, latissimus dorsi and wrist extensor muscles. The latissimus dorsi muscle, in combination with the pectoralis and serratus anterior muscles, enables weight bearing through the upper limbs. This provides the potential to lift body weight and transfer (see Chapter 3). The latissimus dorsi muscle also provides some trunk stability.[55] Although not normally considered a trunk muscle, the latissimus dorsi becomes important in the absence of other trunk muscles. Preservation of the pectoralis muscles makes it possible to roll over in bed and provides stability around the shoulder when weight bearing. Serratus anterior is also important for scapula stability.

Patients with C6 tetraplegia have the potential to live independently, provided they are adequately equipped and set up. Some can transfer, roll, move from lying to sitting, dress, bathe and attend to personal hygiene, although all these motor tasks are time-consuming and difficult to master. Patients with C6 tetraplegia mobilize in a manual wheelchair, but most also use a power wheelchair. Voluntary control of the wrist extensor muscles provides crude grasp (tenodesis grip; see Chapter 5). This makes it possible to hold objects between the index finger and thumb, or in the palm of the hand, despite paralysis of the finger and thumb flexor muscles.

C7 tetraplegia

Patients with C7 tetraplegia typically attain higher levels of independence than those with C6 tetraplegia because of the function provided by the triceps, wrist flexor and finger extensor muscles. The triceps muscles are particularly important because they increase the ability to bear weight through a flexed elbow. The triceps muscles also enable patients to carry and hold objects above their heads. Patients with C7 tetraplegia still have paralysis of the finger and thumb flexor muscles so, despite the ability to extend the fingers, they rely on a tenodesis grip for hand function.

C8 tetraplegia

Patients with lesions at C8 have finger and thumb flexor activity, and therefore can actively grasp and release objects. Consequently, hand function is superior to that of patients who rely on a tenodesis grip. Greater strength in the triceps and shoulder muscles enables these patients to more easily attain independence than those with lesions at C6 and C7.

T1 paraplegia

Patients with lesions at T1 have near-normal hand function, although they retain some weakness in the intrinsic and lumbrical muscles affecting fine hand control. They still have extensive paralysis of the trunk muscles and therefore, like those with higher lesions, have difficulty sitting unsupported (see Chapter 3).

Thoracic paraplegia

Patients with thoracic paraplegia have full upper limb movement, varying degrees of paralysis of the trunk and total paralysis of the legs. They are predominantly wheelchair-dependent, although some can walk short distances with extensive bracing and walking aids (see Chapter 6). Patients with high thoracic paraplegia have more extensive paralysis of the trunk muscles than those with lower thoracic paraplegia, primarily affecting their ability to sit unsupported and master complex transfers.

Lumbar and sacral paraplegia

Patients with lumbar and sacral paraplegia have varying extents of paralysis of the lower limbs and do not commonly have complete lesions. Most can walk with or without aids and orthoses although some remain wheelchair-dependent (see Chapter 6).

Setting goals for patients with incomplete lesions

Outcomes for patients with zones of partial preservation, or ASIA C or D incomplete lesions, are less predictable. In these patients, patterns of neurological loss are diverse,[45,56,57] the extent of possible neurological recovery is unclear,[32,45,56,58–60] and consequently accurate and detailed predictions of motor function are difficult.[61–63] Knowledge about levels of independence attainable by patients with complete spinal cord injury is used as a starting reference then modified depending on individual circumstances and neurological status. Some degree of intuition, developed with experience, is needed to generate goals that are realistic and appropriate.

Step three: identifying key impairments

Once goals of treatment are defined in terms of activity limitations and participation restrictions, it is then necessary to determine which impairments prevent the attainment of each goal. That is, key impairments need to be linked to specific activity restrictions and participation limitations. Identification and treatment of impairments without linking them to activity limitations and participation restrictions risks wasting time, money and resources on impairments which are of little consequence. For example, limited hamstring extensibility is an important impairment for some but not all patients. Unless limited hamstring extensibility is linked to activity and participation goals, physiotherapists might be tempted to direct therapeutic attention at increasing the extensibility of the hamstring muscles in some patients unnecessarily (see Chapter 9).

The process of linking impairments to activity restrictions and participation limitations is the same, regardless of whether one is trying to determine the impairments which prevent a patient with incomplete paraplegia from walking, a patient with C6 tetraplegia from rolling, or a patient with T4 paraplegia from transferring. Each motor task is analysed with respect to sub-tasks. For instance, analysis of transferring between a bed and wheelchair for a patient with C6 tetraplegia is done in relation to the sub-tasks of positioning the legs on the bed, moving forward in the wheelchair and transferring between surfaces (see Table 3.8, p. 71). The underlying reasons for the inability to perform any of these sub-tasks need to be identified and expressed in terms of impairments which are responsive to physiotherapy interventions.

The analysis of motor tasks needs to be done within a realistic framework. For instance, the identification of key impairments preventing a patient with incomplete paralysis from walking needs to be done within the context of how that particular patient can best hope to walk (see Chapter 6). Clearly, someone with paralysis of the quadriceps muscles will not walk in the same way as someone with full strength in the quadriceps muscles. Consequently, gait needs to be analysed with respect to the best gait pattern that can be hoped for, not with respect to the normal kinematics and kinetics of gait for an able-bodied individual. This same principle applies across all mobility tasks and, consequently, physiotherapists require a good understanding of how patients with different patterns of paralysis move (see Chapters 3–6).

Only impairments which are amenable to physiotherapy interventions are of real interest. For example, there is little point linking the inability of a patient with paraplegia to get from the floor back into the wheelchair with permanent paralysis of the legs because this will not guide treatment. A far more helpful analysis would be to link the inability to vertically transfer with insufficient upper limb strength because this is an impairment which can be addressed with an appropriately targeted strength-training programme (see Chapter 8).

Step four: identifying and administering treatments

Six key impairments are responsive to physiotherapy intervention and commonly impose activity restrictions and participation limitations. These are largely contained within the Neuromusculoskeletal and Movement-Related Functions domains of ICF. They include:

- poor skill (see Chapter 7)
- poor strength (see Chapter 8)
- poor joint mobility (see Chapter 9)
- pain (see Chapter 10)
- poor respiratory function (see Chapter 11)
- poor cardiovascular fitness (see Chapter 12)

Some interventions administered by physiotherapists are directed at preventing, rather than treating, impairments, activity limitation and participation restrictions. In addition, physiotherapists are often responsible for prescribing mobility equipment such as wheelchairs and cushions. These issues will be discussed throughout subsequent chapters.

Step five: measuring outcomes

Measurement of outcomes is an integral part of any physiotherapy programme. It determines whether the type and extent of physiotherapy intervention should continue, stop or change (see Chapter 14). Outcomes are best expressed in terms of initial goals and, in particular, with respect to activity limitations and participation restrictions. The assessment tools used in the initial examination can be used for this purpose (see p. 36). Alternatively, outcomes can be measured with respect to patient-articulated goals using tools such as the Canadian Outcome Performance Measure (see Table 2.1). Reassessment at the impairment level often provides more sensitive measures of change. Such reassessments are also useful for confirming whether the initial analysis was correct. For example, if an inability to transfer was deemed to be the consequence of poor strength in the shoulder adductor muscles, then improvements in shoulder adductor strength should be accompanied by improvements in the ability to transfer. Measurements which demonstrate an increase in shoulder adductor strength alone are of little relevance if there is no accompanying measurement to demonstrate a change in ability to perform some purposeful motor task.

While there is a temptation to use increasingly sophisticated tools to assess outcomes, there is little to be gained from using expensive technology to detect minuscule changes in impairment or function if the changes are of little clinical relevance. Likewise, there is little to be gained from assessments if they do not influence the clinical decision-making process. For instance, while three-dimensional gait analysis can provide detailed information about angular velocity of the ankle during terminal swing, this information is only useful to clinicians if physiotherapy interventions are sophisticated enough to be able to specifically address terminal velocity of the ankle during swing.

Physiotherapy as part of the multi-disciplinary team

Physiotherapists are members of a multi-disciplinary team, and the overall success of any rehabilitation programme depends on the contribution of all team members. Development of physical independence will be of little avail if patients do not have appropriate accommodation or financial support on discharge home. In the same way, the success of a physiotherapy programme will be undermined if patients return home incontinent or psychologically distressed. The success of rehabilitation is dependent on team members working closely together to ensure continuity and consistency in their individual therapeutic approaches.[24] For example, occupational therapists, nursing staff and physiotherapists are all involved with the day-to-day physical aspects of patients' care. New motor tasks learnt in physiotherapy need to be appropriately practised and reinforced outside formal physiotherapy sessions (see Chapter 7). However, motor tasks need to be taught and reinforced in the same way by all health professions. The application of different treatment approaches to inconsistent goals by different team members can be confusing, frustrating and counter-productive for patients. Inconsistencies of this kind are avoided by close teamwork and clear role delineations.

References

1. World Health Organization: International Classification of Functioning, Disability and Health: ICF short version. Geneva, World Health Organization, 2001.
2. World Health Organization: International Classification of Impairments, Disabilities, and Handicaps: a Manual of Classification Relating to the Consequences of Disease. Geneva, World Health Organization, 1980.
3. Heerkens Y, Van der Brug Y, Ten Napel H et al: Past and future use of the ICF (former ICIDH) by nursing and allied health professionals. Disabil Rehabil 2003; 25:620–627.
4. Marino RJ, Stineman MG: Functional assessment in spinal cord injury. Top Spinal Cord Inj Rehabil 1996; 1:32–45.

5. Dittmar SS, Gresham GE: Functional Assessment and Outcome Measures for the Rehabilitation Health Professional. Gaithersburg, MD, Aspen Publications, 1997.

6. Middleton JW, Truman G, Geraghty TJ: Neurological level effect on the discharge functional status of spinal cord injured persons after rehabilitation. Arch Phys Med Rehabil 1998; 79:1428–1432.

7. Stineman MG, Marino RJ, Deutsch A et al: A functional strategy for classifying patients after traumatic spinal cord injury. Spinal Cord 1999; 37:717–725.

8. Ota T, Akaboshi K, Nagata M et al: Functional assessment of patients with spinal cord injury: measured by the motor score and the Functional Independence Measure. Spinal Cord 1996; 34:531–535.

9. Catz A, Itzkovich M, Agranov E et al: SCIM — spinal cord independence measure: a new disability scale for patients with spinal cord lesions. Spinal Cord 1997; 35:850–856.

10. Catz A, Itzkovich M, Agranov E et al: The spinal cord independence measure (SCIM): sensitivity to functional changes in subgroups of spinal cord lesion patients. Spinal Cord 2001; 39:97–100.

11. Yavuz N, Tezyurek M, Akyuz M: A comparison of two functional tests in quadriplegia: the quadriplegia index of function and the functional independence measure. Spinal Cord 1998; 36:832–837.

12. Marino RJ, Rider-Foster D, Maissel G et al: Superiority of motor level over single neurological level in categorizing tetraplegia. Paraplegia 1995; 33:510–513.

13. Marino RJ, Goin JE: Development of a short-form Quadriplegia Index of Function Scale. Spinal Cord 1999; 37:289–296.

14. Gresham GE, Labi MC, Dittmar SS et al: The Quadriplegia Index of Function (QIF): Sensitivity and reliability demonstrated in a study of thirty quadriplegic patients. Paraplegia 1986; 24:38–44.

15. Kirby RL, Swuste J, Dupuis DJ et al: The wheelchair skills test: a pilot study of a new outcome measure. Arch Phys Med Rehabil 2002; 83:10–18.

16. Kilkens OJ, Post MW, Dallmeijer AJ et al: Wheelchair skills tests: a systematic review. Clin Rehabil 2003; 17:418–430.

17. Baker SM, Marshak HH, Rice GT et al: Patient participation in physical therapy goal setting. Phys Ther 2001; 81:1118–1126.

18. Brincat CA: Managed care and rehabilitation: adapting a true team approach. Top Stroke Rehabil 1999; 6:62–65.

19. Donnelly C, Eng JJ, Hall J et al: Client-centred assessment and the identification of meaningful treatment goals for individuals with a spinal cord injury. Spinal Cord 2004; 42:302–307.

20. Elsworth JD, Marks JA, McGrath JR et al: An audit of goal planning in rehabilitation. Top Stroke Rehabil 1999; 6:51–61.

21. McGrath JR, Adams L: Patient-centered goal planning: a systemic psychological therapy? Top Stroke Rehabil 1999; 6:43–50.

22. Randall KE, McEwen IR: Writing patient-centered functional goals. Phys Ther 2000; 80:1197–1203.

23. Wressle E, Eeg-Olofsson AM, Marcusson J et al: Improved client participation in the rehabilitation process using a client-centred goal formulation structure. J Rehabil Med 2002; 34:5–11.

24. Wade DT: Goal planning in stroke rehabilitation: why? Top Stroke Rehabil 1999; 6:1–7.

25. Wade DT: Goal planning in stroke rehabilitation: what? Top Stroke Rehabil 1999; 6:8–15.

26. Wade DT: Goal planning in stroke rehabilitation: how? Top Stroke Rehabil 1999; 6:16–36.

27. Wade DT: Goal planning in stroke rehabilitation: evidence. Top Stroke Rehabil 1999; 6:37–42.

28. Berry C, Kennedy P: A psychometric analysis of the Needs Assessment Checklist (NAC). Spinal Cord 2002; 41:490–501.

29. Law M, Baptiste S, Mills J: Client-centred practice: what does it mean and does it make a difference? Can J Occup Ther 1995; 62:250–257.

30. Playford ED, Dawson L, Limbert V et al: Goal-setting in rehabilitation: report of a workshop to explore professionals' perceptions of goal-setting. Clin Rehabil 2000; 14:491–496.

31. Saadah MA: Clinical commentary. 'On autonomy and participation in rehabilitation.' Disabil Rehabil 2002; 24:977–982.

32. Consortium for Spinal Cord Medicine: Outcomes Following Traumatic Spinal Cord Injury: Clinical Practice Guidelines for Health Care Professionals. Washington, DC, Paralyzed Veterans of America, 1999.

33. Duff J, Evans MJ, Kennedy P: Goal planning: a retrospective audit of rehabilitation process and outcome. Clin Rehabil 2004; 18:275–286.

34. Laskin JJ, James SA, Cantwell BM: A fitness and wellness program for people with spinal cord injury. Top Spinal Cord Inj Rehabil 1997; 3:16–33.

35. Kennedy P, Evans MJ, Berry C et al: Comparative analysis of goal achievement during rehabilitation for older and younger adults with spinal cord injury. Spinal Cord 2003; 41:44–52.

36. Independent Living Research Utilization: Application of the concept of health and wellness to people with disabilities: from academia to real life. http://www.ilru.org/html/training/webcasts/handouts/2001/10-31-CC/carla1.html. Houston, 2005.

37. Norris-Baker C, Stephens MA, Rintala DH et al: Patient behavior as a predictor of outcomes in spinal cord injury. Arch Phys Med Rehabil 1981; 62:602–608.

38. Grover J, Gellman H, Waters RL: The effect of a flexion contracture of the elbow on the ability to transfer in patients who have quadriplegia at the sixth cervical level. J Bone Joint Surg (Am) 1996; 78:1397–1400.

39. Yarkony GM, Bass LM, Keenan V et al: Contractures complicating spinal cord injury: incidence and comparison between spinal cord centre and general hospital acute care. Paraplegia 1985; 23:265–271.

40. Cifu DX, Steel RT, Kreutzer JS et al: A multicenter investigation of age-related differences in lengths of stay, hospitalization charges, and outcomes for a matched tetraplegia sample. Arch Phys Med Rehabil 1999; 80:733–740.

41. Penrod LE, Hegde SK, Ditunno JF: Age effect on prognosis for functional recovery in acute, traumatic central cord syndrome. Arch Phys Med Rehabil 1990; 71:963–968.

42. Bergstrom EM, Frankel HL, Galer IA et al: Physical ability in relation to anthropometric measurements in persons with complete spinal cord lesion below the sixth cervical segment. Int Rehabil Med 1985; 7:51–55.

43. De Vivo MJ, Kartus PL, Rutt RD et al: The influence of age at time of spinal cord injury on rehabilitation outcome. Arch Neurol 1990; 47:687–691.

44. Fujiwara T, Hara Y, Akaboshi K et al: Relationship between shoulder muscle strength and functional independence measure (FIM) score among C6 tetraplegics. Spinal Cord 1999; 37:58–61.

45. Marino RJ, Ditunno JF, Donovan WH et al: Neurological recovery after traumatic spinal cord injury: data from the Model Spinal Cord Injury Systems. Arch Phys Med Rehabil 1999; 80:1391–1396.

46. Williams PL, Bannister LH, Berry MM et al: Gray's Anatomy, 38th edn. New York, Churchill Livingstone, 1995.

47. Somers MF: Spinal Cord Injury: Functional Rehabilitation, 2nd edn. Upper Saddle River, NJ, Prentice Hall, 2001.

48. Buchanan LE, Nawoczenski DA: Spinal Cord Injury: Concepts and Management Approaches. Baltimore, Williams & Wilkins, 1987.

49. Nixon V: Spinal Cord Injury. A Guide to Functional Outcomes in Physical Therapy Management. London, Heinemann Medical, 1985.

50. Marciello MA, Herbison GJ, Ditunno JF et al: Wrist strength measured by myometry as an indicator of functional independence. J Neurotrauma 1995; 12:99–106.

51. Powers CM, Newsam CJ, Gronley JK et al: Isometric shoulder torque in subjects with spinal cord injury. Arch Phys Med Rehabil 1994; 75:761–765.

52. UAB Model SCI Center: Functional goals following spinal cord injury. In Network SCII (ed): http://www.spinalcord.uab.edu/show.asp?durki = 28922. Birmingham, UAB Model SCI System, 2006.

53. Wicks AB, Menter RR: Long-term outlook in quadriplegic patients with initial ventilator dependency. Chest 1986; 90:406–410.

54. Gittler MS: Acute rehabilitation in cervical spinal cord injuries. Top Spinal Cord Inj Rehabil 2004; 9:60–73.

55. Bogduk N, Johnson G, Spalding D: The morphology and biomechanics of latissimus dorsi. Clin Biomech 1998; 13:377–385.

56. Mange KC, Marino RJ, Gregory PC et al: Course of motor recovery in the zone of partial preservation in spinal cord injury. Arch Phys Med Rehabil 1992; 73:437–441.

57. Mange KC, Dituno JF, Herbison GJ et al: Recovery of strength at the zone of injury in motor complete and motor incomplete cervical spinal cord injured patients. Arch Phys Med Rehabil 1990; 71:562–565.

58. Waters RL, Adkins RH, Yakura JS et al: Motor and sensory recovery following incomplete paraplegia. Arch Phys Med Rehabil 1994; 75:67–72.

59. Waters RL, Adkins RH, Yakura JS et al: Motor and sensory recovery following incomplete tetraplegia. Arch Phys Med Rehabil 1994; 75:306–311.

60. Waters RL, Adkings RH, Yakura JS et al: Motor and sensory recovery following complete tetraplegia. Arch Phys Med Rehabil 1993; 74:242–247.

61. Burns SP, Golding DG, Rolle WA et al: Recovery of ambulation in motor incomplete tetraplegia. Arch Phys Med Rehabil 1997; 78:1169–1172.

62. Ditunno JF, Cohen ME, Hauck WW et al: Recovery of upper-extremity strength in complete and incomplete tetraplegia: a multicenter study. Arch Phys Med Rehabil 2000; 81:389–393.

63. Ditunno JF, Stover SL, Freed MM et al: Motor recovery of the upper extremities in traumatic quadriplegia: a multicenter study. Arch Phys Med Rehabil 1992; 73:431–436.

64. Kiyono Y, Hashizume C, Matsui N et al: Car-driving abilities of people with tetraplegia. Arch Phys Med Rehabil 2001; 82:1389–1392.

65. Finch E, Brooks D, Stratford PW et al: Physical Rehabilitation Outcome Measures: A Guide to Enhanced Clinical Decision Making, 2nd edn. Hamilton, ON, BC Decker, 2002.

66. Keith RA, Granger CV, Hamilton BB et al: The functional independence measure: a new tool for rehabilitation. In Eisenberg MG, Grzesiak RC (eds): Advances in Clinical Rehabilitation. New York, Springer, 1987:6–18.

67. Catz A, Itzkovich M, Steinberg F et al: The Catz-Itzkovich SCIM: a revised version of the Spinal Cord Independence Measure. Disabil Rehabil 2001; 23:263–268.
68. Collin C, Wade DT, Davies S et al: The Barthel ADL Index: a reliability study. Int Disabil Stud 1988; 10:61–63.
69. Granger CV, Albrecht GL, Hamilton BB: Outcome of comprehensive medical rehabilitation: measurement by PULSES Profile and the Barthel Index. Arch Phys Med Rehabil 1979; 60:145–154.
70. Yarkony GM, Roth EJ, Heinemann AW et al: Spinal cord injury rehabilitation outcome: the impact of age. J Clin Epidemiol 1988; 41:173–177.
71. Yarkony GM, Roth EJ, Heinemann AW et al: Benefits of rehabilitation for traumatic spinal cord injury: Multivariate analysis in 711 patients. Arch Neurol 1987; 44:93–96.
72. Yarkony GM, Roth EJ, Heinemann AW et al: Rehabilitation outcomes in C6 tetraplegia. Paraplegia 1988; 26:177–185.
73. Whiteneck GG, Charlifue SW, Gerhart JA et al: Quantifying handicap: a new measure of long-term rehabilitation outcomes. Arch Phys Med Rehabil 1992; 73:519–526.
74. Menter RR, Whiteneck GG, Charlifue SW et al: Impairment, disability, handicap and medical expenses of persons aging with spinal cord injury. Paraplegia 1991; 29:613–619.
75. Gerhart KA, Bergstrom E, Charlifue SW et al: Long-term spinal cord injury: functional changes over time. Arch Phys Med Rehabil 1993; 74:1030–1034.
76. Fuhrer MJ, Rintala DH, Hart KA et al: Depressive symptomatology in persons with spinal cord injury who reside in the community. Arch Phys Med Rehabil 1993; 74:255–260.
77. Tate D, Forchheimer M, Maynard F et al: Predicting depression and psychological distress in persons with spinal cord injury based on indicators of handicap. Am J Phys Med Rehabil 1994; 73:175–183.
78. Prince JM, Manley MS, Whiteneck GG: Self-managed versus agency-provided personal assistance care for individuals with high level tetraplegia. Arch Phys Med Rehabil 1995; 76:919–923.
79. Campbell J, Kendall M: Investigating the suitability of the clinical outcome variables scale (COVS) as a mobility outcome measure in spinal cord injury rehabilitation. Physiother Can 2003; 55:135–144.
80. Seaby L, Torrance G: Reliability of a physiotherapy functional assessment used in a rehabilitation setting. Physiother Can 1989; 41:264–270.
81. Mattison PG, Aitken RC, Prescott RJ: Rehabilitation status — the relationship between the Edinburgh Rehabilitation Status Scale (ERSS), Barthel Index, and PULSES profile. Int Disabil Stud 1991; 13:9–11.
82. Katz S, Stroud MW: Functional assessment in geriatrics. A review of progress and directions. J Am Geriatr Soc 1989; 37:267–271.
83. Andresen EM, Meyers AR: Health-related quality of life outcomes measures. Arch Phys Med Rehabil 2000; 81:S30–S45.
84. Ware JE: SF-36 health survey update. Spine 2000; 25:3130–3139.
85. Andresen EM, Fouts BS, Romeis JC et al: Performance of health-related quality-of-life instruments in a spinal cord injured population. Arch Phys Med Rehabil 1999; 80:877–884.
86. Forchheimer M, McAweeney M, Tate DG: Use of the SF-36 among persons with spinal cord injury. Am J Phys Med Rehabil 2004; 83:390–395.
87. Haran MJ, Lee BB, King MT et al: Health status rated with the Medical Outcomes Study 36-Item Short-Form Health Survey after spinal cord injury. Arch Phys Med Rehabil 2005; 86:2290–2295.
88. Leduc BE, Lepage Y: Health-related quality of life after spinal cord injury. Disabil Rehabil 2002; 24:196–202.
89. Post MW, Gerritsen J, Diederikst JP et al: Measuring health status of people who are wheelchair-dependent: validity of the Sickness Impact Profile 68 and the Nottingham Health Profile. Disabil Rehabil 2001; 23:245–53.
90. de Bruin AF, Diederiks JP, de Witte LP et al: Assessing the responsiveness of a functional status measure: the Sickness Impact Profile versus the SIP68. J Clin Epidemiol 1997; 50:529–540.
91. Dedding C, Cardol M, Eyssen IC et al: Validity of the Canadian Occupational Performance Measure: a client-centred outcome measurement. Clin Rehabil 2004; 18:660–667.
92. Law M, Baptiste S, McColl M et al: The Canadian Occupational Performance Measure: An outcome measure for occupational therapy. Can J Occup Ther 1990; 57:82–87.
93. Law M, Cadman D, Rosenbaum P et al: Neurodevelopmental therapy and upper-extremity inhibitive casting for children with cerebral palsy. Dev Med Child Neurol 1991; 33:379–387.
94. Law M, Baptiste S, Carswell AC et al (eds): Canadian Occupational Performance Measure, 3rd edn. Toronto, ON, CAOT Publications ACE, 1998.
95. Martin Ginis KA, Latimer AE, Hicks AL et al: Development and evaluation of an activity measure for people with spinal cord injury. Med Sci Sports Exerc 2005; 37:1099–1111.
96. Latimer AE, Martin Ginis KA, Craven BC et al: The physical activity recall assessment for people with spinal cord injury: validity. Med Sci Sports Exerc 2006; 38:208–216.

97. Taricco M, Apolone G, Colombo C et al: Functional status in patients with spinal cord injury: a new standardized measurement scale. Arch Phys Med Rehabil 2000; 81:1173–1180.

98. Taricco M, Colombo C, Adone R et al: The social and vocational outcome of spinal cord injury patients. Paraplegia 1992; 30:214–219.

99. Gans BM, Haley SM, Hallenborg SC et al: Description and interobserver reliability of the Tufts Assessment of Motor Performance. Am J Phys Med Rehabil 1988; 67:202–210.

100. Haley SM, Ludlow LH, Gans BM et al: Tufts assessment of motor performance: an empirical approach to identifying motor performance categories. Arch Phys Med Rehabil 1991; 72:359–66.

101. Haley SM, Ludlow LH: Applicability of the hierarchical scales of the Tufts Assessment of Motor Performance for school-aged children and adults with disabilities. Phys Ther 1992; 72:191–206.

102. Ditunno PL, Dittunno JF. Walking index for spinal cord injury (WISCI II): scale revision. Spinal Cord 2001; 39:654–656.

103. Ditunno JF, Ditunno PL, Graziani V et al: Walking Index for Spinal Cord Injury (WISCI): an international multicenter validity and reliability study. Spinal Cord 2000; 38:234–243.

104. Morganti B, Scivoletto G, Ditunno P et al: Walking index for spinal cord injury (WISCI): criterion validation. Spinal Cord 2005; 43:27–33.

105. Field-Fote EC, Fluet GG, Schafer SD et al: The Spinal Cord Injury Functional Ambulation Inventory (SCI-FAI). J Rehabil Med 2001; 33:177–181.

106. Hussey RW, Stauffer ES: Spinal cord injury: requirements for ambulation. Arch Phys Med Rehabil 1973; 54:544–547.

107. Hoffer MM, Feiwell E, Walker JM et al: Functional ambulation in patients with myelomeningocele. J Bone Joint Surg (Am) 1973; 55:137–148.

108. Nene AV, Hermens HJ, Zilvold G: Paraplegic locomotion: a review. Paraplegia 1996; 34:507–524.

109. Podsiadlo D, Richardson S: The timed 'Up & Go': a test of basic functional mobility for frail elderly persons. J Am Geriatr Soc 1991; 39:142–148.

110. Siggeirsdottir K, Jonsson BY, Jonsson HJ et al: The timed 'Up and Go' is dependent on chair type. Clin Rehabil 2002; 16:609–616.

111. van Herk I, Arendzen JH, Rispens P: Ten-metre walk, with or without a turn? Clin Rehabil 1998; 21:30–35.

112. van Loo MA, Moseley AM, Bosman JM et al: Inter-rater reliability and concurrent validity of walking speed measurement after traumatic brain injury. Clin Rehabil 2003; 17:775–779.

113. Butland RJ, Pang J, Gross ER et al: Two-, six-, and 12-minute walking tests in respiratory disease. BMJ 1982; 284:1607–1608.

114. Triolo RJ, Bevelheimer T, Eisenhower G et al: Inter-rater reliability of a clinical test of standing function. J Spinal Cord Med 1995; 18:14–22.

115. Jebsen RH, Taylor N, Trieschmann RB et al: An objective and standardized test of hand function. Arch Phys Med Rehabil 1969; 50:311–399.

116. Giesler F, Coleman WP, Grieco G et al: Measurements and recovery patterns in a multicenter study of acute spinal cord injury. Spine 2001; 26:S68–S86.

117. Marino RJ, Shea JA, Stineman MG: The capabilities of upper extremity instrument: reliability and validity of a measure of functional limitation in tetraplegia. Arch Phys Med Rehabil 1998; 79:1512–1521.

118. Land NE, Odding E, Duivenvoorden HJ et al: Tetraplegia Hand Activity Questionnaire (THAQ): the development, assessment of arm–hand function-related activities in tetraplegic patients with a spinal cord injury. Spinal Cord 2004; 42:294–301.

119. Stroh KC, Van Doren C: An ADL test to assess hand function with tetraplegic patients. J Hand Ther 1994; 7:47–48.

120. Wuolle KS, Van Doren CL, Thrope GB et al: Development of a quantitative hand grasp and release test for patients with tetraplegia using a hand neuroprosthesis. J Hand Surg (Am) 1994; 19:209–218.

121. Demers L, Weiss-Lambrou R, Ska B: Development of the Quebec User Evaluation of Satisfaction with Assistive Technology (QUEST). Assist Technol 1996; 8:3–13.

122. Demers L, Weiss-Lambrou R, Ska B: Item analysis of the Quebec User Evaluation of Satisfaction with Assistive Technology (QUEST). Assist Technol 2000; 12:96–105.

123. Lynch SM, Leahy P, Barker SP: Reliability of measurements obtained with a modified functional reach test in subjects with spinal cord injury. Phys Ther 1998; 78:128–133.

124. Chafetz R, McDonald C, Mulcahey MJ et al: Timed motor test for wheelchair users: initial development and application in children with spinal cord injury. J Spinal Cord Med 2004; 27:S38–43.

125. Middleton JW, Harvey LA, Batty J et al: Five additional mobility and locomotor items to improve responsiveness of the FIM in wheelchair-dependent individuals with spinal cord injury. Spinal Cord 2006; 44:495–504.

126. Harvey LA, Batty J, Fahey A: Reliability of a tool for assessing mobility in wheelchair-dependent paraplegics. Spinal Cord 1998; 36:427–431.

127. Kilkens OJ, Post MW, van der Woude LH et al: The wheelchair circuit: reliability of a test to assess mobility in persons with spinal cord injuries. Arch Phys Med Rehabil 2002; 83:1783–1788.

128. Best KL, Kirby RL, Smith C et al: Comparison between performance with a pushrim-activated power-assisted wheelchair and a manual wheelchair on the Wheelchair Skills Test. Disabil Rehabil 2006; 28:213–220.

129. Faculty of Medicine Dalhousie University (2005): Wheelchair skills program. http://www.wheelchairskillsprogram.ca.

130. Mountain AD, Kirby RL, Smith C: The wheelchair skills test, version 2.4: validity of an algorithm-based questionnaire version. Arch Phys Med Rehabil 2004; 85:416–423.

"

Understanding how people with paralysis perform motor tasks

CHAPTER 3

Transfers and bed mobility of people with lower limb paralysis

57

CHAPTER 4

Wheelchair mobility

79

CHAPTER 5

Hand function of people with tetraplegia

93

CHAPTER 6

Standing and walking with lower limb paralysis

107

"

Contents

Sitting unsupported 57
Rolling 57
Rolling 60
Lying to long sitting 61
Vertical lift 64
Transfers 68
Vertical transfers 74
Other factors which
influence the ability to
perform mobility tasks 74

Transfers and bed mobility of people with lower limb paralysis

This chapter describes how people who are wheelchair dependent transfer and move about in bed. It is not feasible to describe all the ways that people with different levels of spinal cord injuries transfer and move. Instead, the approach taken here is to describe the most common strategies used by people with C6 tetraplegia and thoracic paraplegia. People with C6 tetraplegia and thoracic paraplegia utilize strategies adopted by most people with spinal cord injury. People with C6 tetraplegia are of particular interest because paralysis of the triceps muscles has important implications for movement and because C6 is a common level of spinal cord injury.

The key mobility tasks are sitting unsupported, rolling, moving from lying to sitting and transferring. The most common way of performing each task is described in terms of sub-tasks. Sub-tasks can be thought of as critical steps. The text is supplemented by video clips freely available at www.physiotherapyexercises.com.

Sitting unsupported

Sitting unsupported is important because it is an integral part of transferring and dressing.[1-4] It is also used when reaching and grasping for objects while sitting on the front edge of a commode, toilet or wheelchair.[5] For example, reaching for something in a high cupboard requires moving to the front edge of the wheelchair and reaching upwards and laterally.

The seated position is not inherently stable. It is even less stable when reaching or using the hands to grasp, manipulate and lift objects. Reaching forwards or sideways displaces the centre of mass, causing a tendency to fall. In able-bodied people the tendency to fall is counteracted by trunk and leg muscle activity. Appropriate muscle activity occurs subconsciously in response to proprioceptive feedback about body position. However, patients with spinal cord injury have limited proprioception and are unable to use the legs and trunk to maintain an upright position. Instead, they must adopt alternate strategies.

One strategy is to use upper limb muscles to help stabilize the trunk in an upright position.[1,5,6] The muscles capable of providing trunk stability are the latissimus dorsi,

Figure 3.1 A patient with C6 tetraplegia sitting unsupported with the knees flexed. When reaching to the left the patient makes compensatory postural adjustments with the right arm.

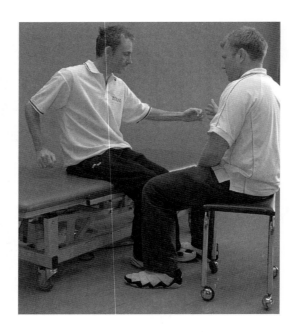

pectoralis and serratus anterior muscles. All these muscles have insertions on the trunk or scapula, and while not normally considered postural muscles, they can take on this role in patients with trunk paralysis. Their importance helps explain why patients with C6 tetraplegia attain a higher level of independence than those with C5 tetraplegia (see Chapter 2). Patients with C6 tetraplegia have reasonable strength in these shoulder muscles but patients with C5 tetraplegia do not. Consequently, patients with C5 tetraplegia have great difficulty sitting unsupported and cannot normally perform associated mobility tasks.

Patients with thoracic paraplegia and C6 tetraplegia also use compensatory postural adjustments to sit unsupported.[1,3,7,8] Small postural adjustments are normally used by able-bodied people during performance of seated tasks. For example, when reaching sideways in sitting, able-bodied people laterally flex the trunk and neck away from the direction in which they are reaching. This minimizes sideway displacement of the centre of mass. Patients with spinal cord injury exaggerate postural adjustments to compensate for the loss of leg and trunk muscles. Thus to reach sideways with one arm they abduct the contralateral arm (see Figure 3.1). Similarly, to reach forwards with one arm they reach backwards behind the body with the other arm while at the same time extending the neck.

Compensatory postural adjustments do not occur spontaneously. Not surprisingly, patients with spinal cord injury and extensive paralysis of the trunk muscles initially have difficulty sitting unsupported. Patients with C6 tetraplegia have added difficulties because not only do they have extensive leg and trunk paralysis, but they also have upper limb weakness affecting their ability to 'catch' themselves when falling. For example, paralysis of the triceps muscles limits the ability to rapidly extend a protective arm and paralysis of the hand muscles prevents grasping stable objects to prevent a fall. With time and practice most learn compensatory postural adjustments enabling unsupported sitting.

Patients with spinal cord injury and extensive trunk paralysis usually find it easier to sit with the knees extended (see Figure 3.2). This is because the paralysed

Figure 3.2 A patient with C6 tetraplegia sitting unsupported with the knees extended. In this position passive tension in the paralysed hamstring muscles helps maintain the trunk in an upright position. The patient is leaning forwards to position the centre of mass of the trunk (circle) anterior to the hip joints. This prevents a backwards fall.

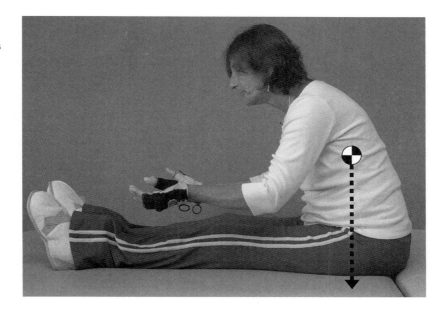

Figure 3.3 The paralysed hamstring muscles cannot prevent a forward fall if they are highly extensible.

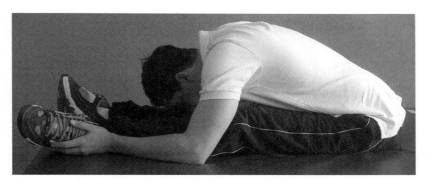

hamstring muscles generate passive tension when the knees are extended. In turn, passive tension in the hamstring muscles generates hip extensor torques which prevent the trunk falling forwards.[9] Patients will not fall backwards provided they are leaning far enough forward to position the centre of mass of the trunk anterior to the hip joints. This strategy for sitting is dependent on appropriate extensibility in the hamstring muscles. If the hamstring muscles are *inextensible* the hips cannot flex sufficiently to position the trunk's centre of mass anterior to the hip joints. Consequently, the patient falls backwards. On the other hand if the hamstring muscles are *highly extensible* they do not constrain a forward fall (see Figure 3.3). Needless to say, the hamstring muscles can do nothing to prevent a sideways fall.

The paralysed hamstring muscles do not generate passive tension when the knees are flexed. Consequently, they cannot help maintain an upright sitting position when sitting over the side of a bed or on the front edge of a wheelchair (see Figure 3.1). It is therefore more difficult to sit over the side of a bed or on the front edge of a wheelchair than it is to sit in long sitting. In addition, some surfaces are more difficult to sit upon than others.[3,10] For example, cushions which are very compliant (i.e. those filled with gel, air or fluid) are more difficult to sit on unsupported than relatively firm surfaces (see Chapter 13).[3]

Rolling

Rolling is used to dress and change position at night. It is also a prerequisite for getting from lying to sitting.

Able-bodied people roll by placing the leading arm across the body and using trunk and leg muscles to initiate rotation of the body. Patients with thoracic paraplegia and C6 tetraplegia cannot use trunk and leg muscles, so instead rely solely on the head and upper limbs to roll. They roll by rapidly swinging the arms across the body (see Table 3.1). This generates angular momentum which is transferred to the paralysed lower segments of the body, facilitating rotation. The position of the legs and head influence the ease of rolling. Most patients have less difficulty rolling if the ankles are crossed and the head is lifted off the bed. Rolling is also easier if the trunk is slightly stiff with loss of passive rotation.

Patients with C6 tetraplegia have added difficulties rolling because paralysis of the triceps muscles limits their ability to maintain elbow extension. Without appropriate strategies, the elbows flex as the arms move across the body and patients may hit themselves in the face. This is avoided by externally rotating the shoulders, minimizing shoulder flexion, and performing the whole task with sufficient speed to ensure the elbows have little opportunity to flex. Contrary to what some may intuitively think it is not possible to roll with the elbows fully flexed. The shortened upper

TABLE 3.1 A patient with C6 tetraplegia rolling onto the side (some practice strategies are described)

	Sub-task	Practice strategies
 Figure 3.4a	1. Pre-swing: The head and both arms are rotated away from the direction of the roll.	*Practice of this sub-task can be made easier if:* • a small weight is placed in the hands • elbow extension splints are used
 Figure 3.4b	2. Swing: The head and both arms are thrown across the body.	• a pillow is placed behind the trunk • the ankles are crossed • the leading hip is supported in 45° flexion • elbow extension splints are used

limbs cannot generate sufficient angular momentum to roll the body, and hand position limits arm swing.

Patients unable to roll in bed can use bed rails or loops attached to the side of the bed to pull themselves from side to side. Alternatively, they must rely on assistance from others.

Lying to long sitting

The ability to move from lying to long sitting is an essential part of dressing and transferring. However, the widespread use of electric beds which move patients into sitting has lessened the importance of attaining independence with this task.

Two strategies are used to move from lying to sitting. One involves rolling on to the side and then sitting up from a side-lying position (see Tables 3.2 and 3.3). This

	Sub-task	Practice strategies
TABLE 3.2 A patient with paraplegia moving from lying to sitting (some practice strategies are described)		
Figure 3.5a	1. Rolling onto the side: see Table 3.1.	*Practice of this sub-task can be made easier if:* • see Table 3.1
Figure 3.5b	2. Lifting the upper trunk off the bed: The left arm is horizontally abducted and weight is borne through both hands.	• a pillow is placed under the chest • the sub-task is practised in reverse
Figure 3.5c	3. Moving into the upright position: The elbows are extended.	• a pillow is placed under the chest • the sub-task is practised in reverse

TABLE 3.3 A patient with C6 tetraplegia moving from lying to sitting (some practice strategies are described)

	Sub-task	Practice strategies
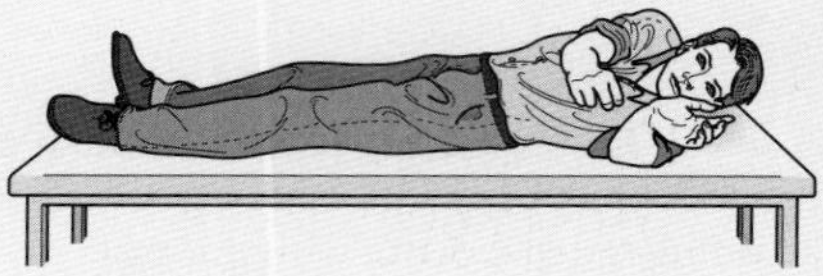 **Figure 3.6a**	1. Rolling onto the side: see Table 3.1.	*Practice of this sub-task can be made easier if:* • see Table 3.1
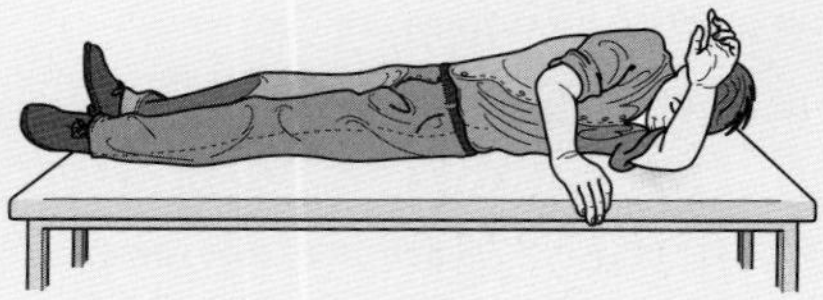 **Figure 3.6b**	2. Lifting the upper trunk off the bed: The left arm is horizontally abducted and weight is borne through the left elbow.	• a pillow is placed under the chest • the sub-task is practised in reverse
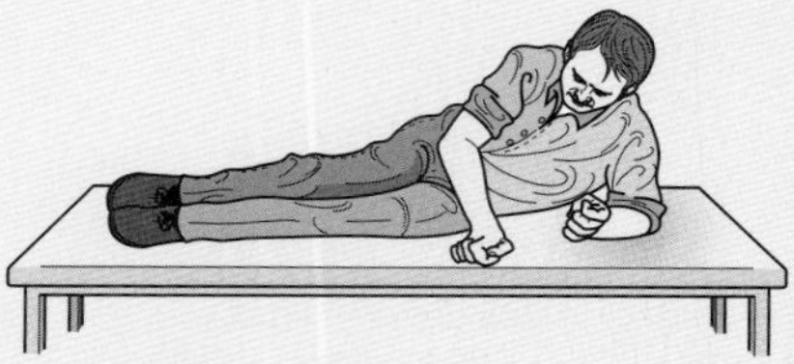 **Figure 3.6c**	3. Supporting the upper trunk: The right hand is placed on the bed to help prevent a forward collapse of the trunk. Alternatively, both elbows are placed on the bed. *(The top arm can bear some weight even though the elbow is flexed and the triceps muscles are paralysed.)*	• a pillow is placed under the chest
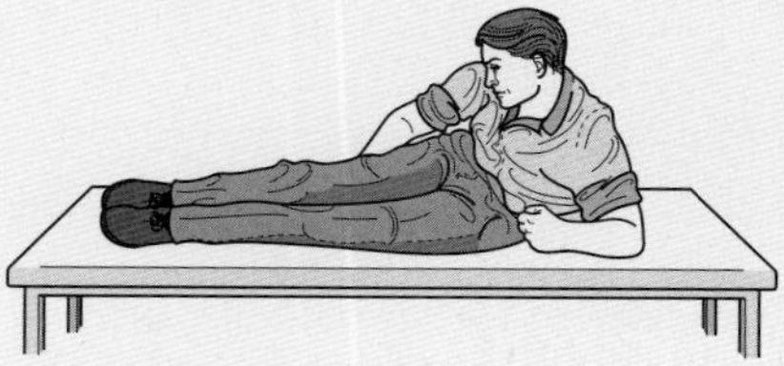 **Figure 3.6d**	4. Positioning the top hand under the leg: The right wrist is extended and hooked behind the right knee.	• a pillow or block is placed under the left elbow (see p. 140, Figure 7.1b)

(continued)

TABLE 3.3 (continued)

	Sub-task	Practice strategies
		Practice of this sub-task can be made easier if:
Figure 3.6e	5. Shuffling the bottom elbow around the body: The right arm is adducted with the wrist anchored behind the knee. This momentarily removes weight from the left elbow. At this instant the left elbow is shuffled a small distance towards the feet. This procedure is repeated several times to 'walk' the left elbow up towards the knees. (see p. 139, Figure 7.1 for a variation of this sub-task)	• a pillow or block is placed under the left elbow (see p. 140, Figure 7.1b) • the sub-task is practised in reverse
Figure 3.6f	6. Moving into the upright position: The right arm is adducted with the wrist anchored behind the knee. The left arm is abducted. The action at both arms pulls/pushes the trunk into the midline.	• a pillow or block is placed under the left elbow (see p. 140, Figure 7.1b) • the sub-task is practised in reverse

approach is cumbersome but relatively easy. Paralysis of the triceps muscles adds complexity because it limits the ability to push down through the hands to lift the body. Patients with C6 tetraplegia overcome this problem by maintaining the side-lying position and 'walking' one or both elbows around the body towards the knees (see Table 3.3, Figure 3.6e). From this position, the top arm is hooked under the top leg to pull up into sitting.

Another strategy for moving from lying to sitting involves using the upper arms to push directly into sitting from the supine position (see Figure 3.7). Patients with paraplegia place the hands behind the body. They then push down through the hands and use elbow extension to lift the trunk. Paralysis of the abdominal muscles makes it difficult to initially position the hands behind the body. Patients with C6 tetraplegia can also move directly from the supine position into sitting; however, a different technique is used which requires awkward positioning of the shoulders. Consequently, few patients master the technique and it often causes shoulder pain. It is therefore probably best avoided.

Figure 3.7 A patient with thoracic paraplegia moving directly into sitting from the supine position.

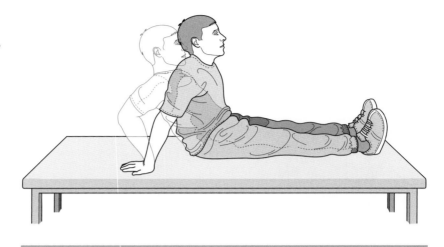

Vertical lift

The ability to vertically lift is an important task for patients to master early.[11] Vertical lifts are used to relieve pressure, transfer, dress, and move about the bed. Patients need to be able to lift while sitting in bed with the knees extended and while sitting in their wheelchairs with their knees flexed (see Tables 3.4–3.6). Lifting with the knees extended is often easier because patients can use the paralysed hamstring muscles to help maintain an upright position.

To vertically lift, the hands are placed next to the hips, usually on the seating surface but occasionally on adjacent surfaces. The patient then pushes down through the hands to lift the trunk on the stabilized arms. There are three components to the lift: elbow extension, shoulder depression and shoulder flexion.[12] Once the elbows are extended, further lift is achieved by depressing the scapulas on the trunk and by inclining the trunk forwards on the fixed shoulders (see Figure 3.10c).[13] The vertical lift is controlled by the latissimus dorsi, anterior deltoid, pectoralis major and lower trapezius muscles.[13–15] The glenohumeral joint is stabilized in adduction throughout the lift by the shoulder adductors and rotator cuff muscles.[12,14–16]

Patients with C6 tetraplegia and paralysis of the triceps muscles have the added difficulty of preventing elbow collapse while lifting. They overcome this problem by externally rotating the shoulders, supinating the forearms and placing the elbows in a hyper-extended position. This upper limb position places the trunk's centre of mass posterior to the elbow joint. In turn, this creates a tendency for the elbows to extend under the weight of the body even though the triceps muscles are paralysed. Elbow collapse is also prevented by contraction of the anterior deltoid muscles. These muscles generate torques which rotate the shoulders into flexion. Shoulder flexion can extend the elbows if the forearms are stabilized. Stability in the forearms is achieved by wrist flexor torques generated as patients lean forwards. The wrist flexor torques originate from the stretch of the paralysed wrist flexor muscles and other soft tissues spanning the front of the wrists.[15,17–21] In this way, elbow extension is a product of the torques generated by the trunk's centre of mass, the active contraction of the shoulder flexor muscles and the passive stretch of the structures

TABLE 3.4 **A patient with paraplegia lifting in a wheelchair (some practice strategies are described)**

	Sub-task	Practice strategies
		Practice of this sub-task can be made easier if:
Figure 3.8a	1. Positioning the hands: The hands are placed on the apex of the back wheels.	
Figure 3.8b	2. Lifting the body: The elbows are extended and the shoulders adducted and depressed.	• the vertical position of the back wheels is adjusted to optimize elbow position • the thickness of the cushion is adjusted to optimize elbow position

spanning the front of the wrist. This is sometimes called 'passive' elbow extension because elbow extension is not due to the direct action of the triceps muscles (see Figure 3.11).

It is often stated that patients with paralysis of the triceps muscles can only bear weight through the upper limbs if the elbows are hyper-extended. However, this is not correct. While it is true that patients with paralysis of the triceps muscles tend to lift with their elbows hyper-extended, and that they are unable to bear large amounts of body weight through a flexed elbow, they can bear some weight through a flexed elbow.[17] That is, they can push through the hands even if the elbows are slightly flexed. Elbow collapse is prevented as described above. A similar strategy is used in

TABLE 3.5 A patient with C6 tetraplegia lifting in a wheelchair (some practice strategies are described)

	Sub-tasks	Practice strategies
Figure 3.9a	1. Positioning the hands: One hand is placed on the apex of the wheel and the other on the seat.	*Practice of this sub-task can be made easier if:* • the width of the seat is increased so the hand can be easily positioned next to the hips (between the wheel and the seat)
Figure 3.9b	2. Lifting the body: The shoulders are adducted and depressed. The elbows are 'passively' extended (see p. 68 and Figure 3.11).	• the vertical position of the back wheels is adjusted to optimize elbow position • the thickness of the cushion is adjusted to optimize elbow position • the cushion is firm (this prevents the hands sinking into the cushion when lifting)

other tasks which involve bearing small amounts of weight through flexed elbows (for example, see Figure 3.6c).

Some believe that vertical lifting is easier for patients with long arms and short trunks. However, the importance of the relative length of the arms and trunk may be overstated.[22,23] Patients with short arms and long bodies compensate by leaning well forward when lifting with the knees extended.[13,24]

TABLE 3.6 A patient with C6 tetraplegia lifting on a plinth (some practice strategies are described)

	Sub-task	Practice strategies
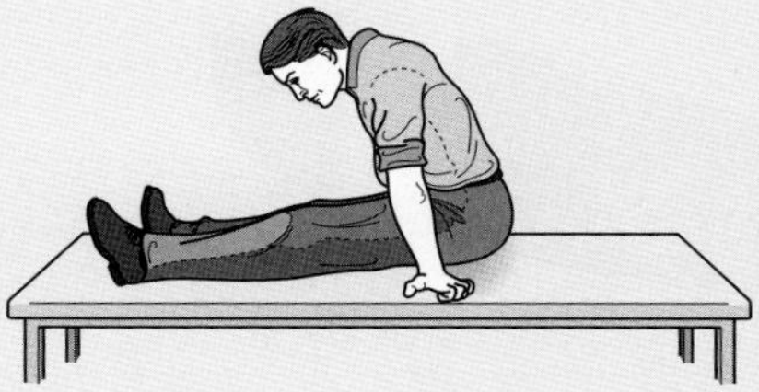 Figure 3.10a	1. Positioning the hands: The hands are placed next to and in front of the hips.	*Practice of this sub-task can be made easier if:* • elbow extension splints are used to help prevent elbow collapse • very high blocks are placed under the arms and the patient lifts through fully flexed elbows (see p. 142, Figure 7.2c) • small blocks are placed under the hands or under the buttocks (depending on the ratio of arms and trunk lengths; see p. 147, Figure 7.6)
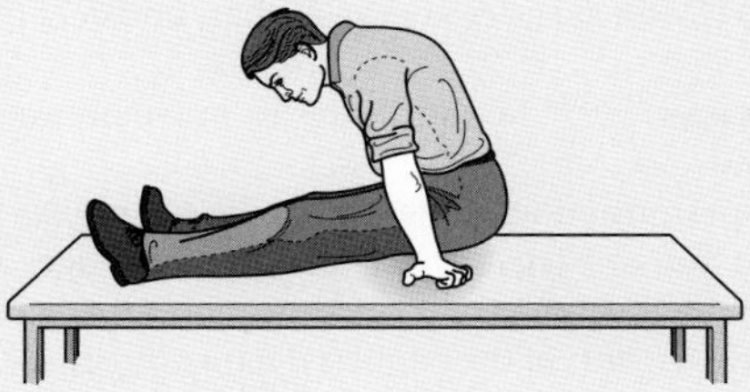 Figure 3.10b	2. Lifting the body: The shoulders are depressed. The elbows are 'passively' extended (see p. 68 and Figure 3.11).	As above
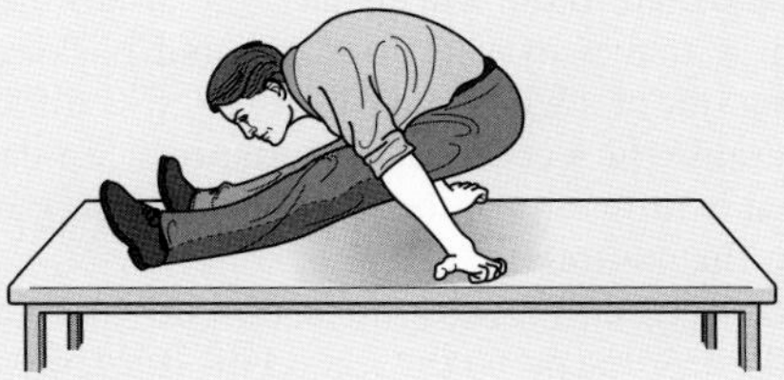 Figure 3.10c	3. Rotating the trunk: The trunk is rotated forwards about the wrists and shoulders.	• The feet are stabilized to prevent a forward slide

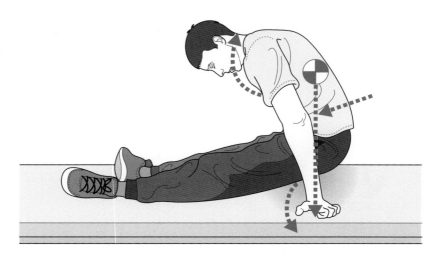

Figure 3.11 A patient with C6 tetraplegia prevents elbow collapse by externally rotating the shoulders and placing the elbows in a hyper-extended position. This upper limb position places the trunk's centre of mass (circle) posterior to the elbow joints. Shoulder and wrist flexor torques also help stabilize the elbow.

Transfers

The term 'transfer' refers to movement between surfaces while maintaining a seated upright position. It includes moving to and from wheelchair, car, toilet, bath, commode and bed. Generally transfers onto lower surfaces are easier than transfers onto higher surfaces.

A range of strategies are used to transfer.[11,22,25] Key strategies to move between a wheelchair and bed are described below.

Transfers to and from a bed can be performed with the legs up (see Table 3.8) or down (see Table 3.7) or with one leg up and one leg down. There are advantages and disadvantages of each approach. The main advantage of transferring with the legs up is that the extended knees increase passive tension in the paralysed hamstring muscles, helping to maintain the trunk in an upright position (see pp. 58–59). Transferring with the legs up when moving in and out of bed also avoids the need to lift or lower the legs when precariously perched on the edge of the bed. Instead, the legs are lifted or lowered when patients are sitting supported in the wheelchair. The disadvantage of transferring with the legs up is that it makes moving forwards and backwards difficult. For example, when transferring out of a wheelchair into bed, it is difficult to move forwards during the transfer because the feet dig into the mattress. Similarly, when transferring into the wheelchair it is difficult to move the buttocks back into the wheelchair because the feet drag on the mattress.

Transferring *with the legs down* can be done either with the feet on the footplates of the wheelchair or positioned on the floor. Some prefer the feet on the floor because it better enables weight to be borne through the legs (see Figure 3.12d). It does, however, create an increased tendency to slide off the front edge of the wheelchair (see Figure 3.12c). If the feet remain on the footplates care needs to be taken to ensure the wheelchair does not tip forwards when patients sit on the front edge of the seat. The likelihood of a forward tip can be minimized by rotating the front castors forwards (see Chapter 13, Figure 13.10). The castors will naturally rotate forwards if prior to transferring the wheelchair is reversed into position.[26]

There are two strategies commonly used to lift laterally between surfaces.[11,22] The first strategy involves inclining the trunk forwards and rotating the trunk about the

TABLE 3.7 A patient with paraplegia transferring from wheelchair to bed with the legs down and using the rotatory strategy (some practice strategies are described)

	Sub-task	Practice strategies
		Practice of this sub-task can be made easier if:
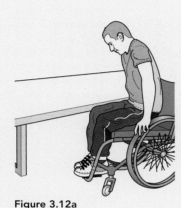 **Figure 3.12a**	1. Moving to the front edge of the wheelchair: The elbows are extended and the shoulders adducted and depressed to vertically lift the body (see Table 3.4). The shoulders are then extended to push the trunk and legs forwards on the seat.	• a firm cushion is used (this prevents the buttocks from sinking into the cushion) • the back of the wheelchair is raised so gravity assists the forward movement • the cushion cover and the patient's lower limb clothing are slippery • the feet are placed on the ground (this increases the tendency to slide forwards) • the vertical position of the back wheels is adjusted to optimize elbow position • the thickness of the cushion is adjusted to optimize elbow position
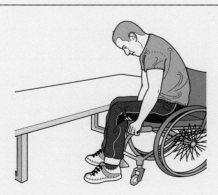 **Figure 3.12b**	2. Positioning the feet on the floor: The left arm lifts the right leg onto the ground. The right arm is used to hold the trunk upright. The mirror of this procedure is used to position the left leg on the floor.	

(continued)

TABLE 3.7 (continued)

	Sub-task	Practice strategies
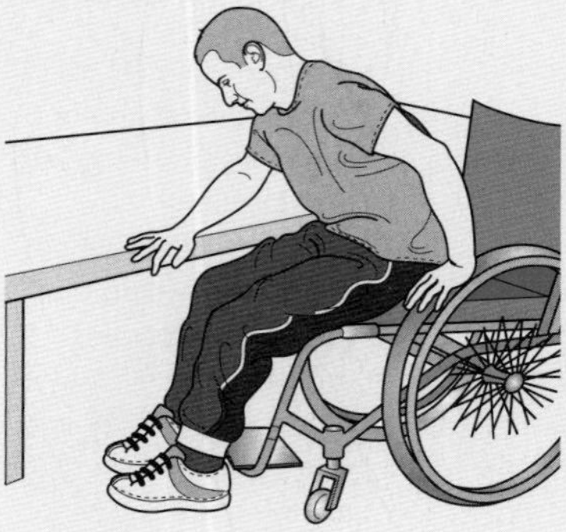 **Figure 3.12c**	3. Positioning the hands: The right hand is placed on the bed and the left hand on the front corner of the wheelchair.	*Practice of this sub-task can be made easier if:* • the wheelchair is positioned as close as possible to the bed • the bed is slightly lower than the wheelchair • additional beds are placed in front and to the side of the patient (this decreases the fear of falling)
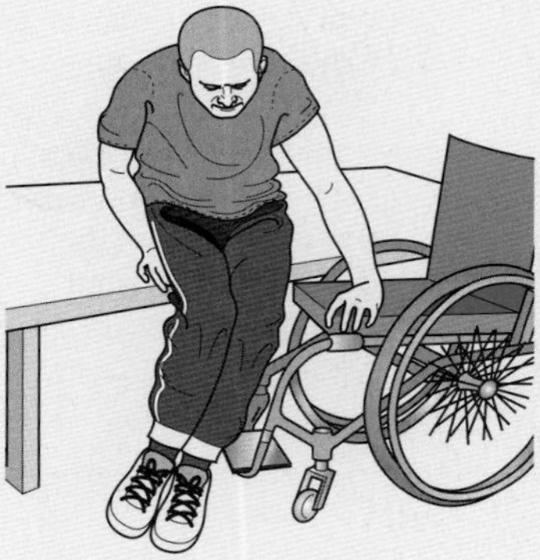 **Figure 3.12d**	4. Lifting *and* shifting the body onto the bed: The elbows are extended and the shoulders adducted and depressed to vertically lift the body (see Table 3.4). The right shoulder is adducted and the left shoulder is abducted to laterally shift the body.	• the wheelchair is positioned as close as possible to the bed • the bed is slightly lower than the wheelchair • the cushion is firm (this prevents the hands sinking into the cushion when lifting) • a slideboard is used
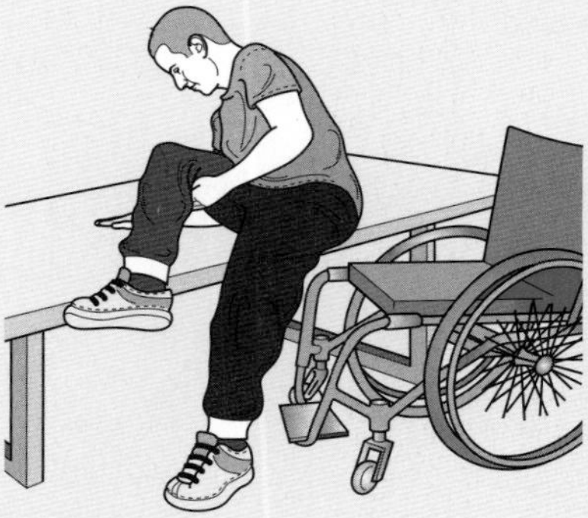 **Figure 3.12e**	5. Lifting the legs onto the bed: Weight is borne through the right elbow while the left arm is used to lift each leg onto the bed.	• the feet are placed on a raised stool to decrease the height the legs need to be lifted • a strap is used to help lift the legs

shoulders. This is called the *rotatory* strategy. With the rotatory strategy, the head goes down and the buttocks go up (see Table 3.7). One advantage of this strategy is that weight can be borne through the paralysed legs (see Figure 3.12d). In the second strategy, the patient maintains a more upright position while moving laterally (see Figure 3.13d). This is called the *translatory* strategy.[11,22] The translatory strategy is more commonly adopted by patients with poor shoulder strength and limited ability to rotate the trunk about the shoulders.

Both the rotatory and translatory strategies require generation of large torques by the pectoralis, latissimus dorsi, serratus anterior muscles and the anterior deltoid

---

TABLE 3.8 **A patient with C6 tetraplegia moving laterally from wheelchair to bed with the legs up using the translatory strategy (some practice strategies are described)**

	Sub-task	Practice strategies
		Practice of this sub-task can be made easier if:
 Figure 3.13a	1. Moving to the front edge of the wheelchair: The head and trunk are extended over the back of the wheelchair. The hands are pushed in behind the back. The hips are levered forwards by external rotation of the shoulders and extension of the wrists. The sides and top of the backrest are used as a fulcrum.	• a firm cushion is used (this prevents the buttocks from sinking into the cushion) • the back of the wheelchair is raised so gravity assists the forward movement • the cushion cover and the patient's lower limb clothing are slippery • the feet are placed on the ground (this increases the tendency to slide forwards) • the backrest of the wheelchair is lowered
 Figure 3.13b	2. Lifting the first leg onto the bed: The left arm is hooked around the back of the wheelchair to prevent a forward fall. The right arm is used to lift the leg onto the bed. The leg is held with a wrist extension hook.	• the feet are placed on a raised stool to decrease the height the legs need to be lifted • a strap is used to help lift the legs

(continued)

TABLE 3.8 (continued)

	Sub-task	Practice strategies
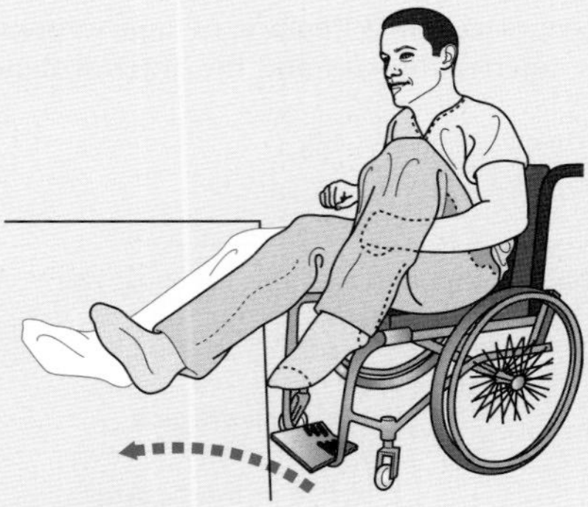 **Figure 3.13c**	3. Lifting the second leg onto the bed: As above.	*Practice of this sub-task can be made easier if:* As above
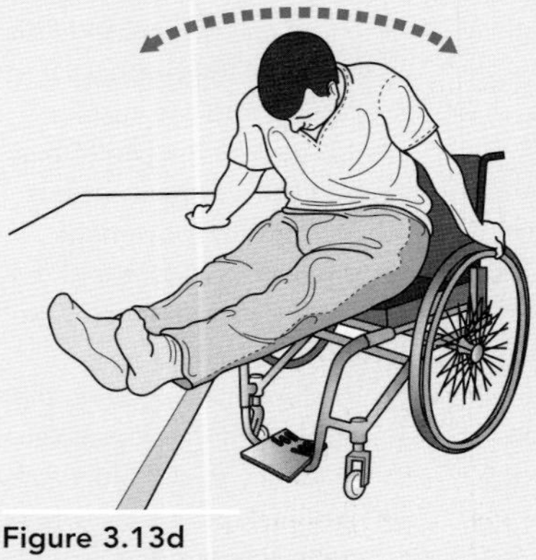 **Figure 3.13d**	4. Positioning the hands: The left hand is placed on the bed and the right hand on the apex of the far wheel. Passive stretch of the hamstring muscles prevents a forward fall.	• the wheelchair is positioned as close as possible to the bed • the bed is slightly lower than the wheelchair • additional beds are placed to the front and to the side of the patient (this decreases the fear of falling)
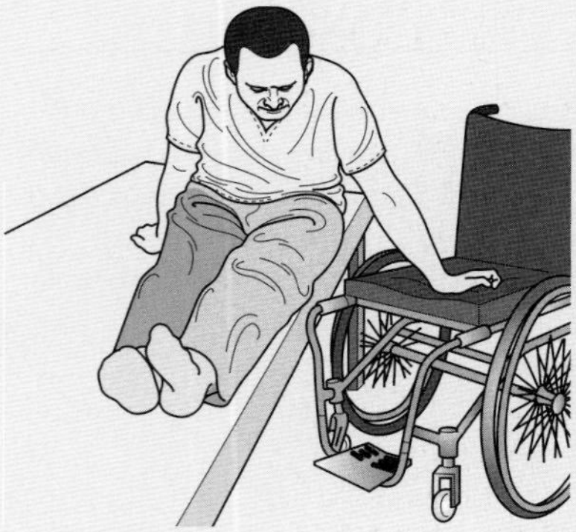 **Figure 3.13e**	5. Lifting *and* shifting the body onto the bed: The shoulders are externally rotated and depressed and the elbows are 'passively' extended to vertically lift the body (see p. 68 and Figure 3.11). The left shoulder is adducted and the right shoulder is abducted to shift the body laterally.	• the wheelchair is positioned as close as possible to the bed • the bed is slightly lower than the wheelchair • additional beds are placed to the front and to the side of the patient (this decreases the fear of falling) • the cushion is firm (this prevents the hands sinking into the cushion when lifting) • a slideboard is used • a slide sheet or slideboard is placed under the feet • the shoes are removed and a slide sheet or slideboard is placed under the feet

muscles.[14] Surprisingly, during lateral transfers the biceps muscles of patients with paraplegia are more active than the triceps muscles, despite the clear need for elbow extension. This underscores the importance of the biceps muscle, along with the anterior deltoid and pectoralis muscles, for generating shoulder flexor torques to extend the elbow and rotate the trunk.[13,15,20,21]

A critical aspect of transfers is ensuring that the buttocks do not touch the back wheels of the wheelchair when moving laterally. Repeated knocking and scraping of the buttocks on the wheel can cause skin damage and, ultimately, pressure ulcers. To avoid skin damage it is important patients transfer on and off the front edge of the wheelchair (see Figure 3.12c). Skin can also be damaged if patients repeatedly land heavily at the end of transfers or drop their feet onto hard surfaces (e.g. metal footplates). Patients should practise controlling both these aspects of transfers.

Slideboards can be used to bridge the gap between transfer surfaces (see Figure 3.14). They are used by patients with limited ability to lift upwards and sideways and can be used either for training purposes or for long-term use. It is best if the slideboard is positioned on an angle between the two transfer surfaces. This encourages patients to rotate around as they move sidewards. It also discourages patients from sliding off the back edge of the slideboard and scraping their buttocks on the wheel. Patients often struggle with positioning slideboards under the buttocks because this requires shifting weight while at the same time manipulating the slideboard. The task of positioning the slideboard is best done when sitting supported in

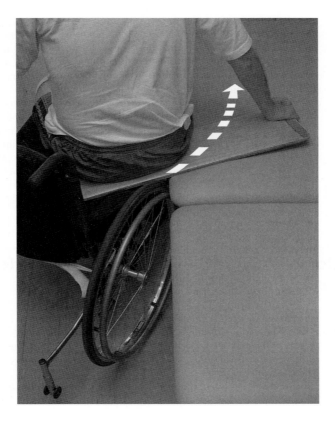

Figure 3.14 Slideboards can be used to bridge the gap between transfer surfaces. The slideboard is positioned on an angle between the two transfer surfaces and the patient rotates around as moving sidewards. This ensures patients do not slide off the back edge of the slideboard and scrape their buttocks on the wheel.

the back of the wheelchair. However, patients then need to ensure that the slide-board does not move forwards out of position as they move forwards in the wheel-chair. This can be avoided by placing one hand on the slideboard when moving forwards.

Paralysis of the triceps muscles makes transferring difficult for patients with C6 tetraplegia. These patients cannot lift their entire body weight through flexed elbows. Consequently, full weight bearing is done through hyper-extended elbows. This limits options for hand placement and makes transferring onto higher surfaces particularly difficult.

The limited hand function of patients with C6 tetraplegia also makes transfers difficult. They cannot easily use their hands to lift and move their legs. Nor can they grasp parts of the wheelchair to hold themselves upright. A passive tenodesis grip is not strong enough to hold and lift a leg. Consequently, rather than grasping the leg with a tenodesis grip, patients with C6 tetraplegia actively extend the wrist to create a 'hook' with the back of the hand. The hook is used to cradle the leg so that it can be lifted (see Figure 3.13b). Similarly, the elbow is commonly hooked onto the back of the wheelchair while leaning forwards (see Figure 3.13b).

Vertical transfers

Vertical transfers involve lifting the body from the ground to a wheelchair (or lower-ing the body from a chair to the ground). Only some patients with paraplegia and the exceptional patient with C6 tetraplegia master this transfer. However, the ability to transfer between floor and wheelchair has important functional implications. It enables patients to get back into their wheelchairs following a fall (this is particu-larly important for patients likely to participate in wheelchair sports). It also enables patientsto get on and off the ground for specific work or leisure activities (for example, at picnics).

The most common way of moving from the floor to the wheelchair is with the wheelchair initially positioned to the side of the patient (see Table 3.9). One hand is positioned up on the front corner of the seat and the other on the ground beside the hips. The lift upwards and sidewards requires the generation of large torques about the shoulder. Less commonly, patients transfer from the floor to the wheelchair with the wheelchair initially positioned behind them. This latter strategy requires very awkward positioning of the shoulders (see Chapter 8, Figure 8.1). Moving from the wheelchair to the floor is done with the same techniques but in reverse.

Other factors which influence the ability to perform mobility tasks

Many factors influence the ease of mastering mobility tasks. The most obvious is body weight: heavier patients have more difficulty lifting themselves than lighter patients. In patients with extensive paralysis less obvious factors take on an important role. For instance, the extensibility of the hamstring muscles is an important determinant of patients' ability to sit unsupported with the knees extended (see p. 59).

Sometimes patients require extremely good extensibility over and above that required by able-bodied individuals. For example, a patient with C6 tetraplegia requires

TABLE 3.9 A patient with paraplegia moving from the floor to wheelchair using the side approach (some practice strategies are described)

	Sub-task	Practice strategies
		Practice of this sub-task can be made easier if:
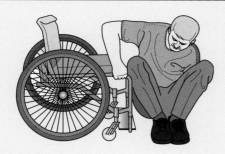 Figure 3.15a	1. Positioning the legs: The body is positioned at right angles to the chair. The hips and knees are fully flexed and the feet are positioned alongside the foot plates.	• a strap is placed around the ankles and/or knees • the wheelchair is secured to prevent it rolling away
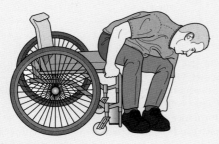 Figure 3.15b	2. Positioning the hands: The right hand is placed on the front corner of the seat. The left hand is placed on the ground next to the hips. *(The right forearm needs to be perpendicular to the ground.)*	• the height of the wheel-chair seat is lowered • the patient sits on a step • a block is placed under the right hand
Figure 3.15c	3. Lifting *and* rotating the body onto the wheelchair: The right arm is adducted to pull the body laterally. The left arm is abducted and depressed to lift and move the body laterally.	• the height of the seat is lowered • the patient sits on a step • a block is placed under the left hand • the cushion is removed • the sub-task is prac-tised in reverse

(continued)

TABLE 3.9 (continued)

	Sub-task	Practice strategies
		Practice of this sub-task can be made easier if:
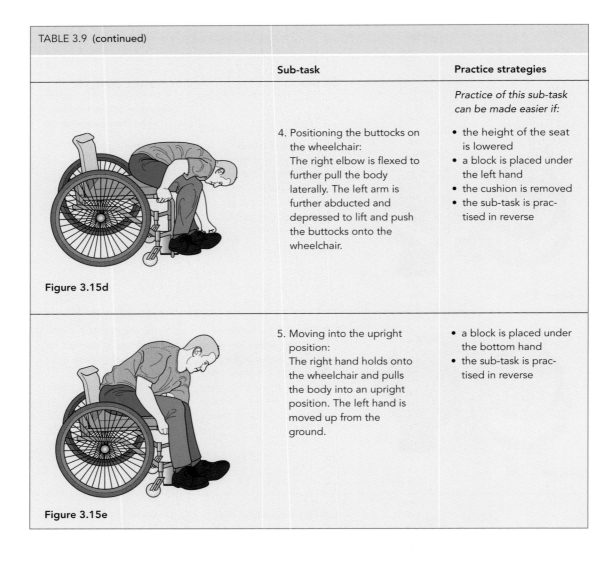Figure 3.15d	4. Positioning the buttocks on the wheelchair: The right elbow is flexed to further pull the body laterally. The left arm is further abducted and depressed to lift and push the buttocks onto the wheelchair.	• the height of the seat is lowered • a block is placed under the left hand • the cushion is removed • the sub-task is practised in reverse
Figure 3.15e	5. Moving into the upright position: The right hand holds onto the wheelchair and pulls the body into an upright position. The left hand is moved up from the ground.	• a block is placed under the bottom hand • the sub-task is practised in reverse

very good extensibility in the back to get into the awkward side-lying position required to move from lying to sitting (see Table 3.3). Even slight back stiffness that would normally have no functional consequence can prevent patients mastering this skill. Paradoxically, back stiffness can assist rolling.[27]

Spasticity can assist or hinder performance of mobility tasks. A clear example in which spasticity assists task performance can be seen in patients with C6 tetraplegia transferring between a wheelchair and bed. Often the most difficult aspect of this transfer is getting the legs up onto the bed (see Figure 3.13b). Some patients overcome this problem by tapping the quadriceps muscles to elicit a leg extension spasm. As the leg extends under the influence of the spasm the patient swivels the leg onto the bed, overcoming the necessity to physically lift the leg with weakened arms. In contrast even small torques generated by spasticity can sometimes hinder task performance, especially in patients with little potential to counteract any adverse effects of unwanted spasticity.

References

1. Potten YJ, Seelen HA, Durukker J et al: Postural muscle responses in the spinal cord injured person during forward reaching. Ergonomics 1999; 42:1200–1215.
2. Chen C, Yeung K, Bih L et al: The relationship between sitting stability and functional performance in patients with paraplegia. Arch Phys Med Rehabil 2003; 84:1276–1281.
3. Aissaoui R, Boucher C, Bourbonnais D et al: Effect of seat cushion on dynamic stability in sitting during a reaching task in wheelchair users with paraplegia. Arch Phys Med Rehabil 2001; 82:274–281.
4. Kamper D, Barin K, Parnianpour M et al: Preliminary investigation of the lateral postural stability of spinal cord-injured individuals subject to dynamic perturbations. Spinal Cord 1999; 37:40–46.
5. Seelen HA, Vuurman EF: Compensatory muscle activity for sitting posture during upper extremity task performance in paraplegic persons. Scand J Rehabil Med 1991; 23:89–96.
6. Seelen HA, Potten YJ, Huson A et al: Impaired balance control in paraplegic subjects. J Electromyogr Kinesiol 1997; 7:149–160.
7. Seelen HA, Janssen-Potten YJ, Adams JE: Motor preparation in postural control in seated spinal cord injured people. Ergonomics 2001; 44:457–472.
8. Do MC, Bouisset S, Moynot C: Are paraplegics handicapped in the execution of a manual task? Ergonomics 1985; 28:1363–1375.
9. Janssen-Potten YJ, Seelen HA, Drukker J et al: The effect of footrests on sitting balance in paraplegic subjects. Arch Phys Med Rehabil 2002; 83:642–648.
10. Ferguson-Pell MW: Seat cushion selection. J Rehabil Res Dev 1990; Clinical Supplement:49–73.
11. Allison GT: The ability to transfer in individuals with spinal cord injury. Crit Rev Phys Rehabil Med 1997; 9:131–150.
12. Reyes ML, Gronley JK, Newsam CJ et al: Electromyographic analysis of shoulder muscles of men with low-level paraplegia during a weight relief raise. Arch Phys Med Rehabil 1995; 76:433–439.
13. Gagnon D, Nadeau S, Gravel D et al: Biomechanical analysis of a posterior transfer maneuver on a level surface in individuals with high and low-level spinal cord injuries. Clin Biomech 2003; 18:319–331.
14. Perry J, Gronley JK, Newsam CJ et al: Electromyographic analysis of the shoulder muscles during depression transfers in subjects with low-level paraplegia. Arch Phys Med Rehabil 1996; 77:350–355.
15. Harvey LA, Crosbie J: Biomechanical analysis of a weight relief manoeuvre in C5 and C6 quadriplegia. Arch Phys Med Rehabil 2000; 81:500–505.
16. Perry J: Normal upper extremity kinesiology. Phys Ther 1978; 58:265–278.
17. Harvey L, Crosbie J: Effect of elbow flexion contractures on the ability of people with C5 and C6 tetraplegia to lift. Physiother Res Int 2001; 62:78–82.
18. Harvey LA, Crosbie J: Weight bearing through flexed upper limbs in quadriplegics with paralyzed triceps brachii muscles. Spinal Cord 1999; 37:780–785.
19. Zerby SA, Herbison GJ, Marino RJ et al: Elbow extension using the anterior deltoids and the upper pectorals. Muscle Nerve 1994; 17:1472–1474.
20. Marciello MA, Herbison GJ, Cohen ME et al: Elbow extension using anterior deltoids and upper pectorals in spinal cord-injured subjects. Arch Phys Med Rehabil 1995; 76:426–432.
21. Gefen JY, Gelmann AS, Herbison GJ et al: Use of shoulder flexors to achieve isometric elbow extension in C6 tetraplegic patients during weight shift. Spinal Cord 1997; 35:308–313.
22. Allison GT, Singer KP, Marshall RN: Transfer movement strategies of individuals with spinal cord injuries. Disabil Rehabil 1996; 18:35–41.
23. Bergstrom EM, Frankel HL, Galer IA et al: Physical ability in relation to anthropometric measurements in persons with complete spinal cord lesion below the sixth cervical segment. Int Rehabil Med 1985; 7:51–55.
24. Allison GT, Singer KP: Assisted reach and transfers in individuals with tetraplegia: towards a solution. Spinal Cord 1997; 35:217–222.
25. Forslund EG, Granström A, Levi R et al: Transfer from table to wheelchair in men and women with spinal cord injury: coordination of body movement and arm forces. Spinal Cord 2007; 45:41–48.
26. Faculty of Medicine Dalhousie University (2005): Wheelchair skills program. http://www.wheelchairskillsprogram.ca.
27. Tanaka S, Yoshimura O, Kobayashi R et al: Three-dimensional measurement of rolling in tetraplegia patients. Spinal Cord 2000; 38:683–686.

CHAPTER

4

Contents

Mobilizing with power
wheelchairs 80

Mobilizing with manual
wheelchairs 80

Providing assistance for
people in manual
wheelchairs 90

Wheelchair mobility

Wheelchair mobility is fundamental to the independence of people who are unable to walk. This chapter describes ways of mobilizing with power and manual wheelchairs. It also provides details of how people in manual wheelchairs negotiate obstacles such as kerbs, ramps, grassy slopes and stairs.

Neurological loss is an important determinant of wheelchair mobility. The level of wheelchair mobility typically attained by people with tetraplegia and paraplegia can be summarized as follows:

People with C1–C4 tetraplegia. People with C1–C4 tetraplegia use a chin-control or mouth-operated power wheelchair. Most also use manual wheelchairs pushed by others when going to places where they are likely to need lifting up and down stairs, or if the wheelchair needs to be stowed in the boot of a car.

People with C5 tetraplegia. People with C5 tetraplegia primarily use a hand-control power wheelchair. They can push a manual wheelchair on flat smooth surfaces but require assistance elsewhere.

People with C6–C8 tetraplegia. Most people with C6–C8 tetraplegia primarily use a manual wheelchair. Few attain advanced levels of wheelchair mobility and most require assistance to negotiate awkward terrains. Some may, at least initially, have difficulty performing apparently simple tasks such as turning the wheelchair. Those with C8 tetraplegia attain a higher level of mobility than those with C6 tetraplegia because of superior hand and upper limb function. Nearly all use a power wheelchair when traversing long distances or uneven and difficult terrains.

People with paraplegia. Most people with paraplegia rely solely on a manual wheelchair. They attain more advanced levels of wheelchair mobility than people with low levels of tetraplegia, and most can negotiate ramps and uneven ground with practice. Some that are young and agile can negotiate stairs, kerbs and grassy slopes, and can perform other difficult manouvres.[1,2]

Mobilizing with power wheelchairs

Patients dependent on power wheelchairs can readily negotiate flat ground and most ramps, but not other obstacles. Driving a power wheelchair requires practice especially for patients with C1–C4 tetraplegia who use chin- or mouth-control mechanisms. Patients with C5 tetraplegia who are capable of using hand-control mechanisms generally have less difficulty learning to control power wheelchairs, although poor shoulder strength can make control difficult.

There are many types of mouth-, chin- and hand-control mechanisms which can be triggered in different ways.[3] Control mechanisms can be electronically programmed to vary power-related features of the wheelchair including sensitivity, acceleration, cut-out and speed (see Chapter 13).[4]

Patients need to practise driving their wheelchairs on the types of terrains they are likely to encounter. This is important not only because it provides context-specific learning of mouth-, chin- or hand-control mechanisms, but also because it provides an opportunity to learn which environmental situations can and cannot be safely negotiated. For instance, wheelchairs can topple during negotiation of highly cambered surfaces or while descending and ascending steep grassy slopes. Initially patients need to practise in a safe environment such as a basketball court or physiotherapy gymnasium. Patients can then progress to more difficult environments.

Initially close supervision may be necessary when negotiating difficult terrains. The physiotherapist may need to stand alongside the wheelchair ready to stabilize it if necessary. Most power wheelchairs have 'kill' switches for training purposes. These are controlled by the physiotherapist and when activated instantly cut power to the wheelchair.

The ability to control an electrical wheelchair also relies on correct positioning in the wheelchair. Patients with high levels of tetraplegia do not have the ability to reposition themselves and consequently are dependent on how others position them. Subtle changes in position, especially a change in the alignment of the arms or heads with respect to the control mechanism, can render a patient incapable of driving the wheelchair. Changes in position may occur if patients slide forwards on their cushions or if they are jolted or knocked while traversing bumpy ground. The trunk can also be pitched forwards when descending steep slopes.[5] Chest or arm straps and moulded backrests can be used to help maintain an appropriate position. The tilt of the wheelchair and the angle of the backrest can also be manipulated to place patients in a less vertical and more stable position (see Chapter 13).

Mobilizing with manual wheelchairs

When patients first sit in manual wheelchairs they need to be taught basic skills such as how to apply and release the brakes, remove the arm rests and footplates, and turn the wheelchair. They can practise manoeuvring and reversing in tight spaces and negotiating around obstacles. There are also some simple tricks patients can be taught which are particularly important for those with tetraplegia and limited upper limb strength.[1] For example, an arm placed on the wall can be used to help turn a corner (see Figure 4.1).

The wheelstand as the basis of advanced mobility

The wheelstand (also called a 'wheelie') is the basis of advanced wheelchair mobility.[3] It involves rotating the wheelchair on its back axle so the front castors lift up off

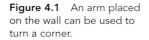

Figure 4.1 An arm placed on the wall can be used to turn a corner.

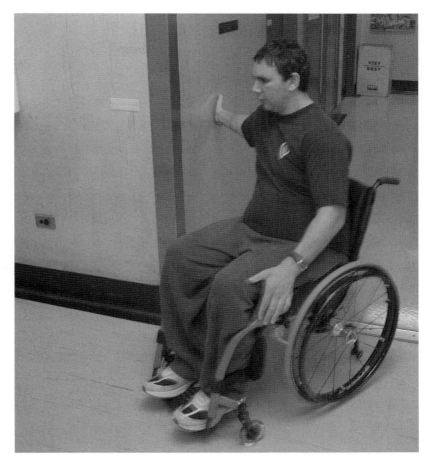

the ground (see Figure 4.2). The ability to perform this manoeuvre enables patients to descend grassy slopes, negotiate kerbs and small obstacles, and turn in tight spaces.

Training advanced wheelchair skills requires appropriate supervision to ensure patient safety. Physiotherapists must anticipate how patients may fall and position themselves appropriately to intervene if necessary. For example, patients are most likely to fall backwards when learning to descend a kerb backwards, and they are most likely to fall forwards when learning to ascend a kerb forwards. In both scenarios, physiotherapists need to stand at the kerb anticipating how the patient is most likely to fall and ready to provide assistance if necessary. Therapists need to guard against potential falls without interfering with the patient's attempts at performing the wheelchair skill. A spotter training strap can be used for this purpose.[6,7] The strap is attached to the under-frame of the wheelchair (see Figure 4.3). The physiotherapist holds one end of the strap, pulling on it if the wheelchair rotates too far backwards. This returns the wheelchair onto its four wheels, averting a backward fall. The physiotherapist still needs to stand close to the wheelchair so the weight of a backward-tipping wheelchair can be shared between the strap and the physiotherapist's thigh. The spotter training strap can also be used when patients practise controlling a

Figure 4.2   The amount of tilt required to perform a wheelstand depends on the location of the wheelchair's rear axle (i.e. the wheelbase, WB). If the axle is located posteriorly, as in (a), the front castors need to lift well off the ground to attain the balanced position. In contrast, if the axle is located more anteriorly, as in (b), the front castors only need to just lift off the ground.

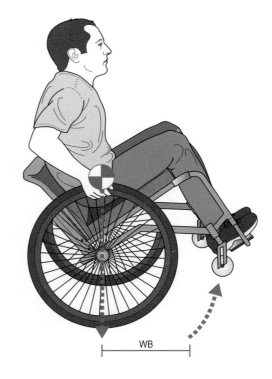

(a)

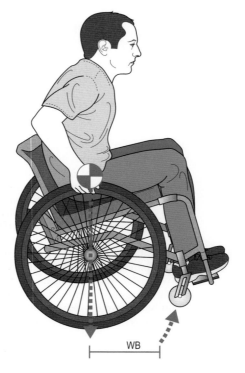

(b)

Figure 4.3 A spotter training strap. This can be used to prevent a backwards fall in patients learning to perform wheelstands.[7]

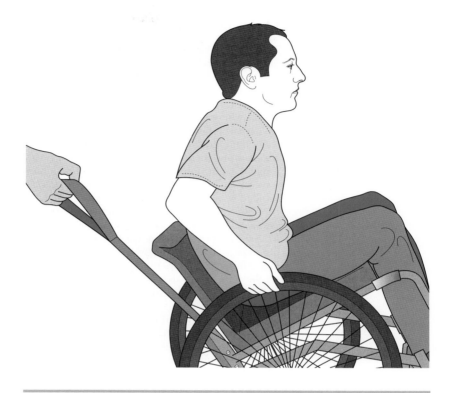

wheelchair down a slope. In this instance the strap is used as a breaking device in case the patient loses control of the wheelchair.

Sometimes 'anti-tip' bars are used to prevent the wheelchair toppling backwards (see Chapter 13, Figure 13.15). Anti-tip bars can prevent injury but they cannot be used while performing advanced wheelchair skills. For this reason 'anti-tip' bars need to be temporarily removed or rotated out of position during training sessions. Once patients develop sufficient wheelchairs skills 'anti-tip' bars can be permanently removed.

Moving into a wheelstand

A wheelchair can be moved into a wheelstand by exploiting the wheelchair's inertia. When the wheelchair accelerates forwards its inertia tends to rotate the wheelchair about the axes of its stationary back wheels, lifting the front castors off the ground.[2,3,6,8]

Initially patients find it easiest to perform wheelstands by rolling the wheelchair backwards and then applying a small, quick forward push on the wheel rims. It takes some practice to tip the wheelchair up to the balance point, yet not tip the wheelchair over backwards. With practice, and provided the wheelchair is sufficiently 'tippy', a forward 'flick' of the wheels is all that is required. Skilled users can apply the 'flick' and tip the wheelchair into a wheelstand as the wheelchair is moving forwards.

The ability to move into a wheelstand while moving forwards is important for more advanced wheelchair skills. For example, this is an essential component of getting up and over kerbs (see Figure 4.9).[1]

Maintaining a wheelstand

To maintain a balanced wheelstand, the centre of mass of the wheelchair and patient needs to sit precisely over the point of contact between the back wheels and ground, and therefore over the back axle.[6,8] If the centre of mass falls either anterior or posterior to this point, the wheelchair will tend to rotate away from the balanced position. If the wheelchair rotates forwards without a response from the patient the front castors will return to the ground and usually no harm will be done. However, if the wheelchair rotates backwards without a response from the patient, the wheelchair will fall backwards with the risk of injury. Patients can keep the centre of mass over the axles, and therefore maintain the balanced position, by rotating the back wheels. Rotation repositions the wheels under the combined centre of mass. For example, a forward fall is avoided by pushing on the back wheels and a backwards fall is avoided by pulling on the back wheels.[1,8] The balanced position is maintained by continuously making such adjustments. Without these adjustments, it is almost impossible to stay in a balanced wheelstand for more than a few seconds.

There are two quite different strategies used to maintain a balanced position. The *first strategy*, typically used by unskilled patients, involves merely responding to deviations from the balance point. As patients starts to fall forwards they push forwards on the rims and as they start to fall backwards they pull backwards on the rims. Novices typically make unnecessarily large responses, overcompensating and causing a fall in the opposite direction.

A *second strategy* is adopted by more skilled patients. It involves continuously but subtly rotating the wheelchair backwards and forwards around the balance point.[6,8] It is speculated that this makes it easier to balance because the point at which the back wheels contact the ground constantly moves, creating a dynamic and large base of support.[6,8] A more convincing explanation might be that patients use forces through the hands to monitor the tendency of the wheelchair to rotate out of the balanced position. This may be a more sensitive way of detecting early signs of moving out of the balanced position than relying on vision or the sense of falling.

What determines the ease of getting into a wheelstand?

The characteristics of the wheelchair determine how easy or hard it is to perform a wheelstand (see Chapter 13). In some wheelchairs, the front castors only just need to lift off the ground to attain a balanced wheelstand position (see Figure 4.2b). That is, only a small arc of rotation is required and it is relatively easy to move into a wheelstand position. In other wheelchairs, large arcs of rotation are required and a wheelstand position is more difficult to attain and is dependent on the front castors lifting well off the ground (see Figure 4.2a).

The arc of rotation is primarily determined by the length of the wheelbase. That is, the distance between the front and back wheels.[9] If the wheelbase is long, the weight of the wheelchair and patient sits well in front of the back wheels and a large arc of rotation is required to attain a balanced wheelstand position. In contrast, if the wheelbase is short, weight is shifted posteriorly and only a small arc of rotation is required. In most adjustable wheelchairs, the wheelbase can be changed by moving the back wheels on the wheelchair frame.[3,10,11] The further forwards the back wheels are positioned, the 'tippier' the wheelchair and the easier it is to get into a balanced wheelstand position (see Chapter 13).

The weight of the patient and wheelchair, as well as the distribution of weight, are also important. Lots of weight sitting well anterior of the back wheels makes it difficult to get into a wheelstand regardless of the wheelbase. For this reason it is difficult to perform wheelstands in heavy hospital wheelchairs with footplates positioned away from the body and it is relatively easy to perform wheelstands in lightweight sports wheelchairs with footplates tucked under the body, even if the wheelbases are identical. Similarly a bag of personal belongings carried on the back of a wheelchair will increase its 'tippiness'. The weight distribution can also be altered by changing the inclination of the seat. For example, tilting the back of the seat downwards shifts weight posteriorly, making it easier to get into a wheelstand position.

While on the one hand 'tippy' wheelchairs are easy to rotate, on the other hand, they are dangerous if patients are unable to control them and are at risk of inadvertently flipping them over backwards. This is most likely to happen when pushing up steep slopes or performing sudden manoeuvres (see Chapter 13). The appropriate amount of wheelchair 'tippiness' depends on patients' wheelchair skills and their ability to lean forwards when pushing up inclines. Recently-injured patients can rarely manage 'tippy' wheelchairs. Instead they require stable wheelchairs with the back wheels positioned posteriorly on the frame. As patients' wheelchair skills improve they can trial increasingly 'tippy' wheelchairs until they find the amount of 'tippiness' that suits their lifestyle and needs.

Descending stairs and kerbs

Descending a kerb backwards

Kerbs can be descended either forwards or backwards, although it is generally easier to descend kerbs backwards. The wheelchair needs to be aligned symmetrically at the edge of the kerb. Patients then push backwards over the kerb while leaning forwards (see Figure 4.4).

Descending stairs backwards

Descending stairs is one of the simplest wheelchair skills to master because it is not dependent on a wheelstand. However, it is frightening and requires good upper limb strength. Stairs need to be descended backwards with a rail. Initially patients align themselves symmetrically at the top of the stairs. One hand holds the rail and the other hand holds the rim of the wheel. Both hands are used to lower the wheelchair down the steps (see Figure 4.5).

Descending a kerb forwards

Descending kerbs forwards requires more skill. Patients need to move into a wheelstand position on the top edge of the kerb. This position is maintained while rolling forwards over the kerb (see Figure 4.6). Novices tend to move out of the wheelstand prior to dropping the back wheels over the kerb. This drops the front of the wheelchair and throws the patient forwards.

Descending stairs forwards

Skilled patients can descend a couple of stairs forwards without a rail. The technique is the same as descending a kerb but it is associated with considerable risk and not generally encouraged (see Figure 4.7).

Figure 4.4 Moving down a
kerb backwards.

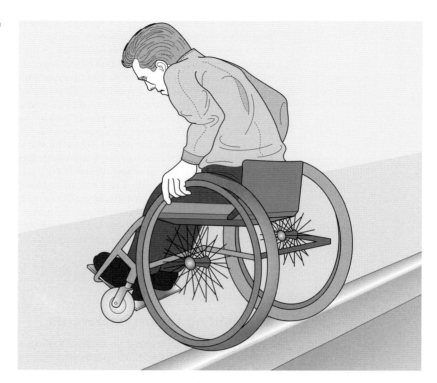

Figure 4.5 Descending a
flight of stairs backwards.

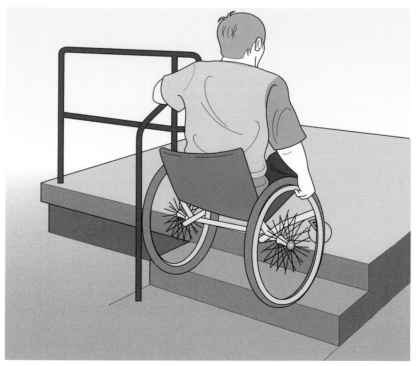

Figure 4.6 Descending a kerb forwards.

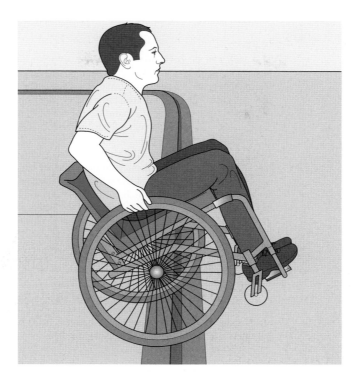

Figure 4.7 Descending a couple of stairs forwards.

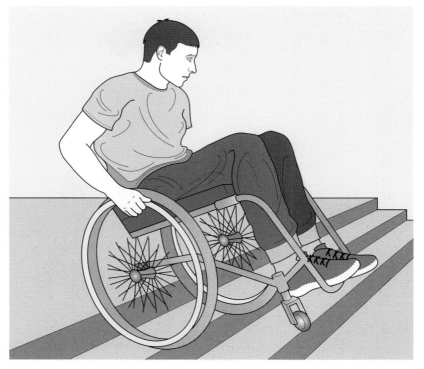

Ascending kerbs

This skill can be performed either with or without the help of a street pole (see Figures 4.8 and 4.9). To ascend a kerb *with a street pole* patients need to initially perform a wheelstand to get the front castors up on the kerb. One hand is placed on the pole and the other hand on the back wheel. The hand on the pole is used to pull the wheelchair upwards and the hand on the wheel is used to push the wheelchair forwards. Done together, the wheelchair moves up and over the kerb.

Getting up a kerb *without a street pole* is one of the more advanced wheelchair skills. It requires approaching the kerb with speed and moving into a wheelstand just prior to the kerb without stopping. Momentum is used to lift the wheelchair over the kerb. The height of the wheelstand needs to be sufficient for the front castors to clear the kerb and the front castors need to land down on the top of the kerb before the back wheels hit.[1] At this point the patient leans forwards and continues to push up and over the kerb. If the patient fails to lift the front castors up high enough to clear the kerb, the wheelchair will come to a sudden stop and the patient will be thrown forwards.

Descending grassy slopes in a wheelstand position

Steep grassy slopes need to be descended in a wheelstand (see Figure 4.10). If patients attempt to roll down grassy slopes on all four wheels the front castors will

Figure 4.8 Ascending a kerb with a street pole.

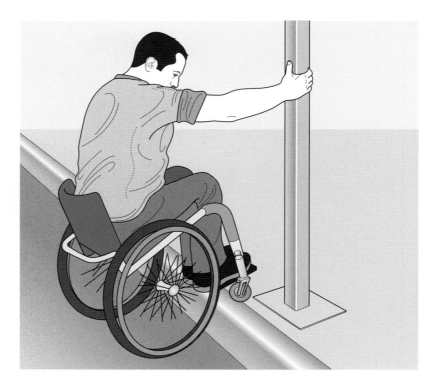

Figure 4.9 Ascending a kerb without a street pole.

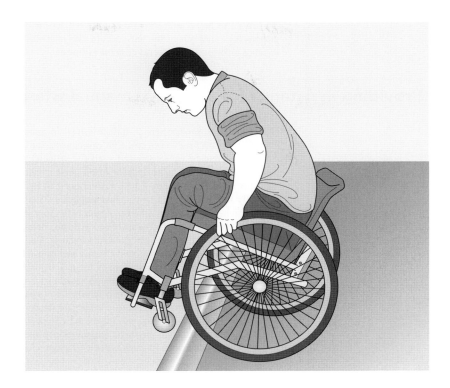

Figure 4.10 Descending a grassy slope.

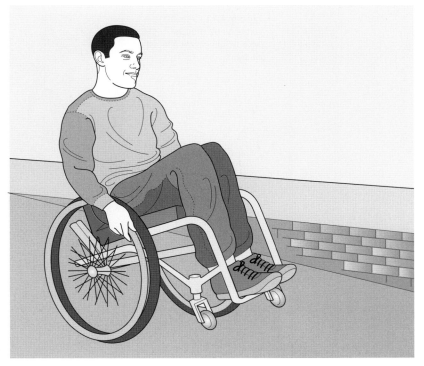

dig into the grass and the wheelchair will come to a sudden stop, toppling the patient forwards out of the wheelchair. The technique used to descend grassy slopes is often also used to descend concrete slopes.

Providing assistance for people in manual wheelchairs

Unbeknown to most, there is skill involved in assisting patients in manual wheelchairs. It is therefore important that carers are appropriately trained and educated.

Most obstacles are negotiated with the wheelchair held in the wheelstand position. For this reason 'anti-tip bars' often need to be temporarily removed or rotated out of position (see Figure 13.5). Carers need to be particularly careful not to inadvertently tip patients out of their wheelchairs. This is most likely to happen when guiding wheelchairs down steep slopes. The footplates can hit the ground at the transition between the slope and level ground, bringing the wheelchair to an unexpected halt and throwing the patient forwards. Patients most vulnerable are those unable to use their hands to hold themselves in the wheelchair.

To descend stairs, the wheelchair is turned around so the patient descends backwards (see Figure 4.11).[2] Two or three assistants are required; one (or two) at the back and one at the front. The wheelchair is lowered down each step in a slow and controlled way. A similar technique is used to descend kerbs.

To ascend a flight of stairs, the wheelchair is pulled backwards up the steps (see Figure 4.12). Again, two or three assistants are required. Initially, the wheelchair needs to be rotated onto its back wheels. The wheelchair is then pulled up each step,

Figure 4.11 Assisting a patient in a manual wheelchair *down* a flight of stairs.

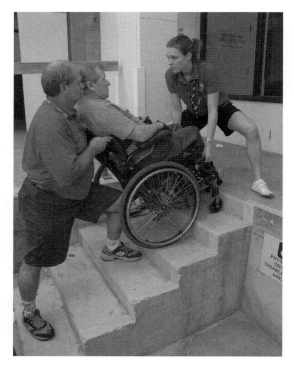

Figure 4.12 Assisting a patient in a manual wheelchair *up* a flight of stairs.

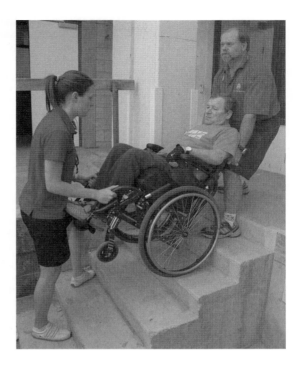

Figure 4.13 Assisting a patient in a manual wheelchair up a kerb.

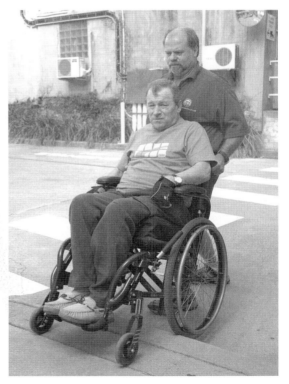

one at a time, while maintaining the wheelstand position. If possible, patients should assist by pulling on the wheels.

To ascend kerbs, the wheelchair is pushed forwards up and over the kerb. Initially, the wheelchair is tipped on its back wheels, so that the front castors can clear the kerb. Then the assistant pushes and lifts the back wheels up and over the kerb (see Figure 4.13). It is important that the assistant does not try to jolt the back wheels up the kerb. If jolting fails to get the wheelchair up the kerb, the wheelchair will come to a sudden halt, thrusting the patient forwards.

References

1. Croteau C: Wheelchair Mobility. A Handbook. Worcester, MA, Park Press Publishing, 1998.
2. Axelson P, Yamada Chesny D, Minkel J et al: The Manual Wheelchair Training Guide. Minden, NV, PAX Press, 1998.
3. Ham R, Aldersea P, Porter D: Wheelchair Users and Postural Seating: A Clinical Approach. New York, Churchill Livingstone, 1998.
4. Batavia M, Batavia AI, Friedman R: Changing chairs: anticipating problems in prescribing wheelchairs. Disabil Rehabil 2001; 23:539–548.
5. Axelson P, Minkel J, Perr A et al: The Powered Wheelchair Training Guide. Minden, NV, PAX Press, 2002.
6. Kirby RL, Smith C, Seaman R et al: The manual wheelchair wheelie: A review of our current understanding of an important motor skill. Dis Rehabil: Ass Tech 2006; 1:119–127.
7. Kirby RL, Lugar JA: Spotter strap for the prevention of wheelchair tipping. Arch Phys Med Rehabil 1999; 80:1354–1356.
8. Bonaparte JP, Kirby RL, MacLeod DA: Proactive balance strategy while maintaining a stationary wheelie. Arch Phys Med Rehabil 2001; 82:475–479.
9. Kreutz D: Manual wheelchairs: prescribing for function. Top Spinal Cord Inj Rehabil 1995; 1:1–16.
10. Tomlinson J: Managing maneuverability and rear stability of adjustable manual wheelchairs: an update. Phys Ther 2000; 80:904–911.
11. Engström B: Ergonomics, Seating and Positioning. Sweden, ETAC, 1993.

Contents

Hand function and
principles of therapy 93
Tenodesis grip 98
Reconstructive
surgery and electrical
stimulation 104

Hand function of people with tetraplegia

Loss of hand function is often more important to people with tetraplegia than loss of lower limb function and the inability to walk.[1,2] This reflects the importance of hand function for independence. The purpose of this chapter is to describe how people with different patterns of paralysis use their hands and to outline some of the splints and adaptive equipment commonly prescribed. The use of surgery and electrical stimulation to improve hand function will also be discussed.

The same generic framework advocated for devising physiotherapy programmes in Chapter 2 can be used for hand management. Initially, goals of treatment are negotiated with the patient. Goals need to also be set in conjunction with occupational therapists and other team members who share responsibility for their attainment. Goals are expressed with respect to activity limitations such as taking a spoon to the mouth and using a keyboard. Goals can also be expressed with respect to participation restrictions such as dining out with friends or returning to work. Once realistic goals are defined, impairments preventing the attainment of each goal are identified but only with respect to impairments which physiotherapy can address. These typically include poor strength, joint mobility and skill.

The hand function of patients with tetraplegia is primarily limited by neurological status (see Appendix). Below is a summary of the hand function typically attained by a patient with different ASIA motor complete lesions.

Hand function and principles of therapy

C4 and above tetraplegia

Patients with C4 and higher levels of tetraplegia have no upper limb function.

Therapy for these patients is directed at preventing contractures. It is important to prevent contractures because they can be unsightly and create problems with hygiene and personal care. Contractures of the hand are probably best avoided with prolonged stretch and regular passive movements (see Chapter 9). Prolonged stretch can be

Figure 5.1 A splint which flexes the MCP and extends the IP joints of the fingers can be used to prevent MCP hyper-extension contractures and IP flexion contractures. Alternatively, it can be used to promote a tenodesis grip in patients with C6 tetraplegia. The thumb can be held against the index finger with tape or a thumb piece incorporated into the splint.

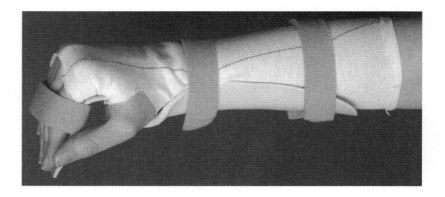

administered with splints. In patients *without* contractures, the appropriate type of splint is determined by the type of contractures patients are most likely to develop. For example, patients with total paralysis of the hands commonly develop metacarpophalangeal (MCP) joint hyper-extension and interphalangeal (IP) joint flexion contractures. Therefore the appropriate splint is one which immobilizes these joints in a stretched position, namely MCP joint flexion and IP joint extension (see Figure 5.1). A less aggressive 'functional' splint which places the hand in a neutral position does not stretch these joints and is probably less effective for preventing these types of contractures. In patients *with* existing contractures, the appropriate type of splint is determined on a case-by-case basis but the splint needs to provide a substantial stretch to affected joints.

C5 tetraplegia

Patients with C5 tetraplegia have anti-gravity strength in their biceps muscles. Often, but not always, they have sufficient strength in their deltoids and other shoulder muscles to lift a hand to the face. However, these patients have paralysis of all wrist and hand muscles and consequently are unable to grasp objects. Instead, objects can be manipulated by clamping them between the wrists (see Figure 5.2), balancing them on an upturned hand (see Figure 5.3) or using orthoses which attach objects to the hand (see Figure 5.4). Splints are commonly used to support the wrist (see Figure 5.5).

Poor shoulder strength and passive joint mobility commonly limit the hand function of patients with C5 tetraplegia. In addition, hand function is limited by lack of skill, particularly in patients soon after spinal cord injury. That is, patients do not know how to use their paralysed hands in purposeful ways. Therapy is therefore directed at each of these three impairments using the principles outlined in Chapters 7–9.

An important additional aspect of hand management for these patients is the provision of appropriate aids, splints and orthoses (some examples of commonly prescribed hands splints are provided in Figures 5.3–5.5). This is generally the responsibility of occupational therapists. Hand function of some patients can also be improved with surgery or electrical stimulation (see p. 104).

C6 and C7 tetraplegia

Patients with C6 and C7 tetraplegia have reasonable shoulder strength and can readily bring the hand to the mouth. They have paralysis of all finger and thumb flexor

Figure 5.2 A patient with C5 tetraplegia clamps an object between the wrists.

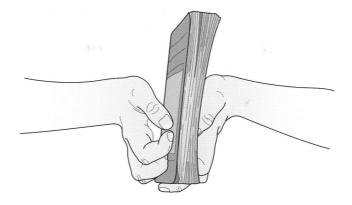

Figure 5.3 A patient with C5 tetraplegia balances objects on an upturned hand.

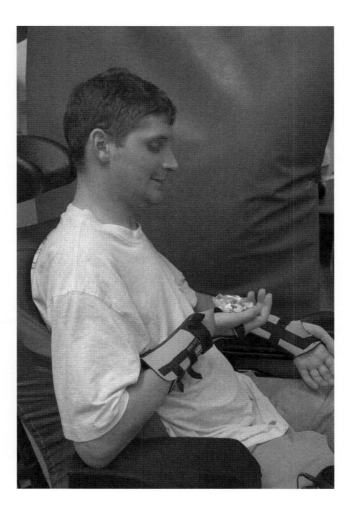

Figure 5.4 (a) A splint which enables patients with C5 tetraplegia to feed. (b) It has a fork attached to it and it stabilizes the wrist. (Images reproduced with permission from www.spinalis.se/tips; Spinalis, Karolinska Hospital, Sweden, 2006.)

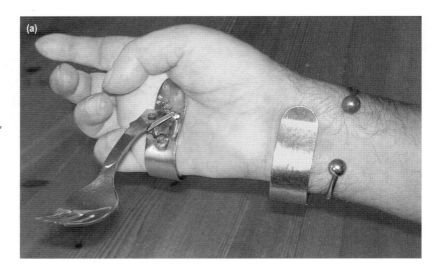

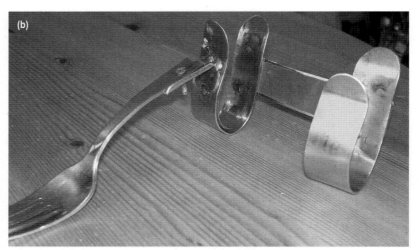

Figure 5.5 A splint to support the wrist of patients with C5 tetraplegia.

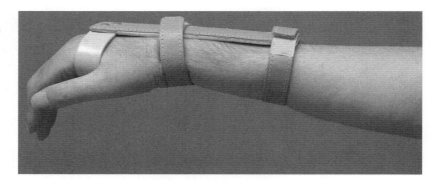

Figure 5.6 Patients with C6 tetraplegia commonly use small splints to write.

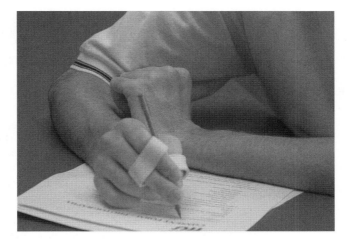

Figure 5.7 Patients with C6 tetraplegia commonly use palmar bands to attach utensils such as typing sticks to the hand. (Image reproduced with permission from www.spinalis.se/tips; Spinalis, Karolinska Hospital, Sweden, 2006.)

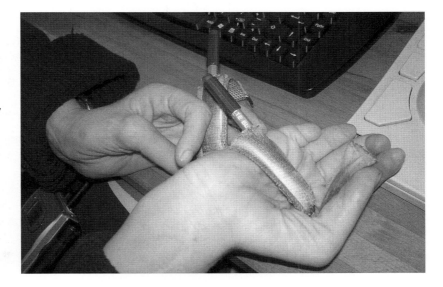

muscles but they retain good strength in their wrist extensor muscles. Those with C7 tetraplegia also have some strength in their wrist flexor and finger extensor muscles. Most patients with C6 and C7 tetraplegia rely on a tenodesis grip for crude hand function (see below). Hand splints, aids, electrical stimulation and surgery are other important aspects of overall hand management (see Figures 5.6 and 5.7).[3]

C8 tetraplegia

Patients with C8 tetraplegia have some strength, but not full strength, in their finger and thumb flexor muscles. They therefore do not use a tenodesis grip. They do, however, have paralysis of their intrinsic hand muscles. Consequently, they have limited fine hand control. Therapy is primarily directed at strengthening finger and thumb flexor muscles, preventing contractures and practising hand activities. Hand orthoses, aids, electrical stimulation and surgery are also aspects of hand management for these patients.

Tenodesis grip

A tenodesis grip is a method of grasping used by patients with C6 and C7 tetraplegia who have paralysis of finger and thumb flexor muscles but active wrist extension. The tenodesis grip relies on passive tension generated in the paralysed extrinsic finger and thumb flexor muscles (flexor digitorum superficialis, flexor digitorum profundus and flexor pollicis longus) with wrist extension.[3–8] The open hand is placed around an object with the wrist flexed. The wrist is then actively extended, increasing the passive tension in the paralysed finger and thumb flexor muscles and pulling the fingers and thumb into flexion. In this way, objects can be grasped between the paralysed thumb and index finger or in the palm of the hand (see Figures 5.8 and 5.9). A tenodesis grip provides crude but nonetheless useful hand function.[7] Some patients can enhance the effectiveness of their tenodesis grip by eliciting spasm in the extrinsic thumb and finger flexor muscles with wrist extension.

The tenodesis grip can be used to grasp objects between the thumb and index finger using either a lateral key or pincer grip. In the *lateral key grip* the pad of the thumb contacts the side of the index finger (see Figure 5.8b) and in the *pincer grip* the tip of the thumb contacts the tip of the index finger (see Figure 5.9b). The type of grip

Figure 5.8 A tenodesis grip (lateral key grasp). (a) The fingers and thumb passively open when the wrist falls into flexion. (b) Active wrist extension generates passive tension in the extrinsic finger and thumb flexor fingers, flexing the fingers and thumb.

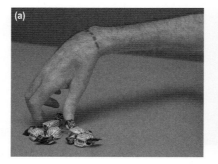
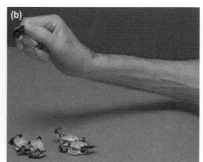

Figure 5.9 A palmar (a) and pincer (b) tenodesis grip. The fingers passively flex as the wrist extends, enabling objects to be held in the palm of the hand.

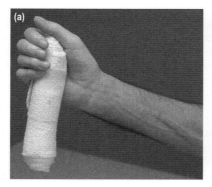
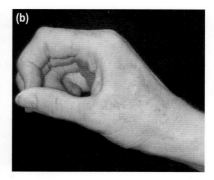

attained is primarily determined by the extensibility of the thumb adductor muscles. A pincer grip is attained if the thumb adductors are extensible and a lateral key grip is attained if the thumb adductors are inextensible. The point of contact between the thumb and index finger also depends to a lesser degree on the relative lengths of the thumb and index finger, and the extensibility of the extrinsic finger flexor muscles.[3,4]

A lateral key grip is generally considered easier to achieve because it requires less precision to ensure the thumb hits the side of the index finger. Provided the thumb hits anywhere along the medial aspect of the finger, some type of grip will be attained. In contrast, a pincer grip is reliant on the thumb meeting the index finger at precisely the tip of the finger. If there is slight overstretching of the thumb adductor muscles, the thumb will miss its target. When a pincer grip can be attained it provides better fine control than a lateral key grip; however, it is less powerful than a lateral key grip. Sometimes it is advantageous to promote a pincer grip in one hand and a lateral key grip in the other.

While the tenodesis grip is primarily used by patients with C6 and C7 tetraplegia, some patients with C5 tetraplegia can also use a crude type of tenodesis grip. Patients with C5 tetraplegia have paralysis of the wrist extensor muscles so they cannot actively extend the wrist to close the hand. They may, however, be able to use forearm supination to manipulate the position of the wrist. With the forearm in pronation, gravity pulls the wrist into flexion. With supination, gravity pulls the wrist into extension. Thus manipulation of the forearm can be used to change wrist position which in turn opens and closes the hand. This type of grip is sometimes called a *passive* tenodesis grip because wrist position is passively manipulated by forearm rotation. However, the terminology is not ideal because it implies that the tenodesis grip of patients with C6 and C7 tetraplegia is *active* and hence due to something more than the passive mechanical properties of the hand.

The passive tenodesis grip of people with C5 tetraplegia is of limited functional use and most patients gain superior upper limb function from splints which stabilize the wrist (see Figure 5.5). A passive tenodesis grip cannot be used in conjunction with these splints because the splints prevent passive wrist extension. However, strategies appropriate for promoting a tenodesis grip in patients with C6 and C7 tetraplegia are also appropriate for promoting a passive tenodesis grip in people with C5 tetraplegia.

Splinting and taping to promote a tenodesis grip

The effectiveness of a tenodesis grip is often compromised because of excessive extensibility in the extrinsic thumb and finger flexor muscles. When these muscles are too extensible, wrist extension produces only weak thumb and finger flexion. The best way to increase the 'strength' of the tenodesis grip is to induce shortening (i.e. decrease extensibility) of the extrinsic thumb and finger flexors.

Splinting and taping are widely used to encourage loss of extensibility in the extrinsic finger and thumb flexor muscles and promote a tenodesis grip. However, it remains unclear whether either intervention can decrease the passive extensibility of the extrinsic finger and thumb flexor muscles and improve hand function.[8,9] This controversy is discussed in more detail below.

Splinting and taping programmes to promote a tenodesis grip may need to be withheld if patients are likely to have hand surgery. Often the effectiveness of hand surgery relies on good extensibility in the finger and thumb flexor muscles. However, the difficulty with this approach is that often the decision about hand surgery is not made until 1 or 2 years after injury. Consequently, it is not always clear which patients will and will not ultimately be suitable candidates. In addition, some patients suitable for hand surgery do not elect to have it (see p. 104 for further discussion).[2] The dilemma for therapists is whether they should compromise hand function by with-holding strategies designed to promote a tenodesis grip on the basis that patients *may* have hand surgery in the future.

A theoretical basis for splints designed to promote a tenodesis grip

Animal studies have convincingly shown that immobilization of muscles at short lengths induces shortening (see Chapter 9). On this basis, it has been argued that the best way to promote a tenodesis grip is with a splinting or taping regime which immobilizes the extrinsic finger and thumb flexor muscles in their shortened positions. To achieve this, one of two splinting regimens is probably best adopted. The *more conservative approach* is to splint the hand in a relatively neutral position with the MCP joints fully flexed, the IP and wrist joints extended and the thumb flexed against the side of the index finger (see Figure 5.1). This type of splint immobilizes the extrinsic finger and thumb flexor muscles in a relatively shortened position but discourages extension contractures of the MCP joints and flexion contractures of the IP joints.

A *second more aggressive approach* is to flex the MCP and proximal IP joints of the fingers with the thumb positioned against the side of the index finger. This is typically done by applying tape across the back of the fingers and thumb (see Figure 5.10). The wrist is held in an extended position with a splint. The flexed position of the fingers places the extrinsic finger flexor muscles in a shortened position. However, it also substantially increases the risk of undesirable flexion contractures of the proximal IP joints. If this second approach is used, the hand needs to be carefully monitored and patients should spend at least some time of each day with the proximal IP joints in full extension. In addition, passive movements to the proximal IP joints should be regularly administered. Whenever the IP joints are extended, the wrist and MCP joints need to be flexed to avoid stretch of the extrinsic finger flexor muscles (see Figure 5.11).

The thumb requires special consideration. While it is important to maintain full passive mobility of the finger IP joints, this is not the case for the thumb. It is beneficial to hand function if the thumb IP joint becomes stiff in extension. This ensures that the pad of the thumb pushes against the side of the index finger rather than curls under the finger (see Figure 5.12). Therapists can facilitate the development of

Figure 5.10 Wrist splints with tape applied across the back of the fingers and thumb are used to promote a tenodesis grip.

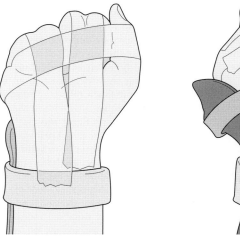
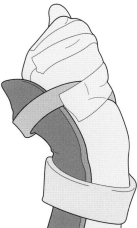

Figure 5.11 Passive movements of the fingers need to be performed with the wrist held in flexion to avoid excessive stretch on the extrinsic finger flexor muscles.

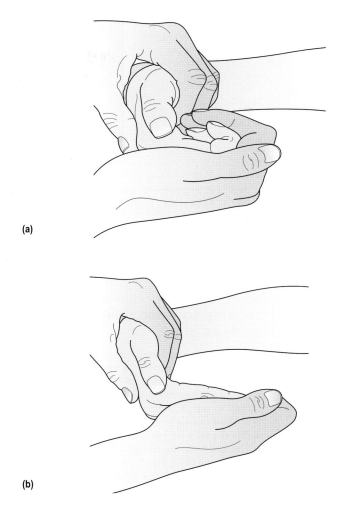

(a)

(b)

Figure 5.12 Flexion of the thumb IP joint causes it to curl under rather than contact the side of the index finger.

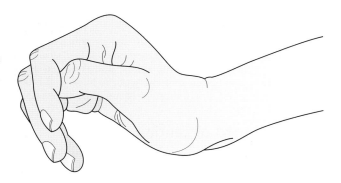

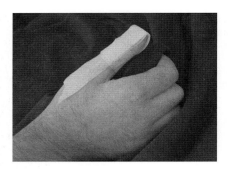

Figure 5.13 A simple way of encouraging stiffness of the thumb IP joint is to immobilize the thumb in extension with tape.

stiffness (i.e. contracture) in the thumb IP joint by splinting the joint in extension for prolonged periods of time (see Figure 5.13). This can be easily done with tape. Of course, care needs to be taken to ensure taping does not restrict circulation or cause a pressure ulcer. A more permanent and effective solution is surgical stabilization of the thumb IP joint (see discussion on surgical options below).

How long to wear splints designed to promote a tenodesis grip?

Splints need to be worn for long enough to have the desired therapeutic effects without unnecessarily impeding independence. Some therapists believe that the rapid facilitation of an effective tenodesis grip warrants short-term restriction of function imposed by an aggressive splinting regime. A more compromising approach is to apply splints only at night so the hands can be used during the day.

The length of time required to achieve an effective tenodesis grip is variable. It probably depends on many factors such as pattern of denervation and presence of spasticity and oedema. Changes in muscle extensibility may occur at differing rates within the same hand. For example, a patient may have sufficient loss of extensibility in the extrinsic finger flexor muscles but not thumb flexor muscles. Even within the extrinsic finger flexor muscles, the medial component of these muscles may have sufficient loss of extensibility before the lateral component, resulting in good passive flexion of the index and middle fingers but not the ring and little fingers.[3] These factors should be considered and splinting individualized to the needs of each patient. For example, if the extrinsic finger flexor muscles have optimal extensibility but the extrinsic thumb flexor muscles do not, then a splint which continues to immobilize the thumb but not the fingers is appropriate.[9] Such a splint may incorporate a thumb loop connected to a wrist band, immobilizing the carpometacarpal and MCP joints of the thumb in flexion (see Figure 5.14). Similarly if the medial components of the extrinsic finger flexor muscles have optimal extensibility but the lateral components do not, a splint that just incorporates the ring and little fingers may be indicated.

Interim results from animal studies suggest that regular use of electrical stimulation may hasten shortening of the finger and thumb flexor muscles. However, the clinical efficacy of this type of intervention has not yet been established.

A word of caution

It is important to avoid excessive loss of extensibility in the finger or thumb flexor muscles because this will be detrimental to hand function. As soon as an effective

Figure 5.14 A thumb loop to hold the extrinsic thumb flexor muscle in a shortened position.

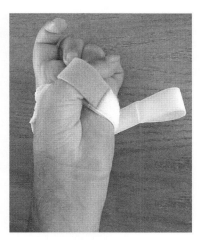

tenodesis grip is attained, therapeutic intervention may need to be directed at maintaining rather than reducing muscle extensibility. This may or may not require regular use of splints.

Some patients are at risk of excessive loss of extensibility of the finger or thumb flexor muscles. They include those patients with incomplete spinal cord injury resulting in paralysis of the finger extensor but not finger flexor muscles and patients with marked spasticity in the finger flexor muscles. It is inappropriate to splint the hands of these patients to encourage loss of extensibility. Instead, these patients may need different types of splints designed to maintain or even increase extensibility of the finger and thumb flexor muscles (e.g. some may benefit from a splint which immobilizes the MCP and IP joints in extension). This highlights the importance of anticipating and predicting losses of extensibility, individualizing therapy to patients' needs, monitoring change and understanding the implications of loss of extensibility for function. These issues are discussed in more detail in Chapter 9.

A tenodesis grip should not be promoted in patients with incomplete injuries unless it is clear that they are not going to regain active movement of the finger and thumb flexor muscles (see Chapter 1 for time frame). It is important that normal extensibility and full range of motion is maintained in all muscles and joints.

Flexor-hinge splints

Flexor-hinge splints mechanically supplement the tenodesis grip of patients with C6 and C7 tetraplegia.[10] These splints enclose the wrist and hand and mechanically guide the tips of the index and second fingers into contact with the tip of the thumb when the wrist is actively extended (see Figure 5.15).[3] The fingers and thumbs are mechanically pulled into extension when the wrist flexes. Such splints are said to 'train' a tenodesis grip, although this terminology may be inappropriate because it implies that the action of the fingers and thumb with wrist extension depends primarily on something other than the passive mechanical properties of the hand. This would seem unlikely. It is possible that flexor-hinge splints protect the extrinsic thumb flexor and extrinsic finger flexor muscles from stretch, thereby helping to reduce extensibility. Regardless of the underlying mechanisms of action, some patients with C6 and C7 tetraplegia find flexor-hinge splints provide superior hand function and routinely use

Figure 5.15 A flexor-hinge splint. The splint opens the hand when the wrist is flexed (a) and closes the hand when the wrist is extended (b).

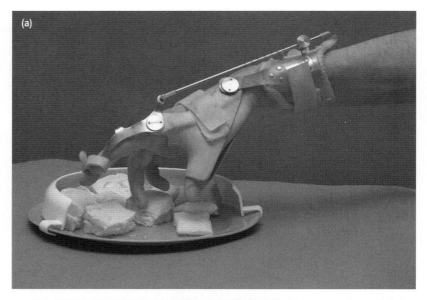

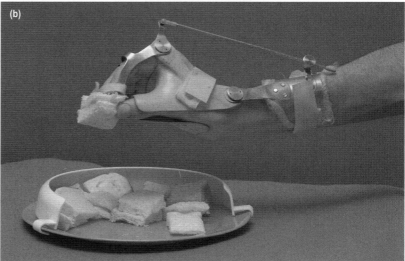

them. Most, however, find the splints bulky, expensive and cosmetically unappealing. For these reasons they are less commonly used today than 20 years ago.

Reconstructive surgery and electrical stimulation

Many surgical procedures are used to improve the hand and upper limb function of people with tetraplegia.[11] Moberg,[12] a Swedish hand surgeon, is generally considered the pioneer in this field. He devised widely used procedures to improve the lateral key grip of patients with C6 tetraplegia. These procedures typically involve arthrodesis of the thumb IP joint and surgical tenodesis of the extrinsic thumb flexor and extrinsic finger flexor muscles. Over the last 10 years an increasing number of sophisticated surgical procedures to improve hand function have been introduced.[13] Tendon transfers from non-paralysed muscles to paralysed muscles are particularly common. These procedures enable a non-paralysed muscle to pull on the tendon of a paralysed muscle. The two most common tendon transfers are from the non-paralysed deltoid muscle to the paralysed triceps muscle or from the non-paralysed brachioradialis muscle to the paralysed extensor carpi radialis muscle, providing active elbow and wrist extension respectively. Tendon transfers can also be used to provide or strengthen the lateral key grip of patients with C6 and C7 tetraplegia. The tendon of the non-paralysed extensor carpi radialis longus muscle is transferred to the paralysed flexor digitorum profundus muscle, and the tendon of non-paralysed brachioradialis is transferred to paralysed flexor pollicis longus muscle.

Electrical stimulation can be used to stimulate paralysed muscles of the hand and upper limb. It is primarily used in people with C5 or C6 tetraplegia to provide finger and thumb movement for grasp and release.[11,14-16] Stimulation can be applied with surface or implanted electrodes and is usually controlled by patients' voluntary wrist or shoulder movements. Some electrical stimulation systems are incorporated into gloves or splints which stimulate key muscles.[14,17-19] More sophisticated devices are surgically implanted, providing more refined hand function.[17,20,21] Reconstructive surgery is commonly used to augment the effects of electrical stimulation. Physiotherapy involves training patients to use these devices and working with other team members to optimize stimulation parameters.

Despite the apparent success of reconstructive surgery and electrical stimulation for hand function, only a small percentage of patients opt for these interventions.[22] There may be numerous reasons for this, but ease of use and social acceptance would appear to be key factors.[16] It may also be that patients are reluctant to opt for invasive interventions which are associated with hospitalization and long periods of recovery.

References

1. Hanson RW, Franklin MR: Sexual loss in relation to other functional losses for spinal cord injured males. Arch Phys Med Rehabil 1976; 57:291–293.
2. Snoek GJ, IJzerman MJ, Hermens HJ et al: Survey of the needs of patients with spinal cord injury: impact and priority for improvement in hand function in tetraplegics. Spinal Cord 2004; 42:526–532.
3. Johanson ME, Murray WM: The unoperated hand: the role of passive forces in hand function after tetraplegia. Hand Clin 2002; 18:391–398.
4. Harvey L: Principles of conservative management for a non-orthotic tenodesis grip in tetraplegics. J Hand Ther 1996; 9:238–242.
5. Curtin M: An analysis of tetraplegic hand grips. Br J Occup Ther 1999; 62:444–450.
6. Doll U, Maurer-Burkhard B, Spahn B et al: Functional hand development in tetraplegia. Spinal Cord 1998; 36:818–821.
7. Harvey L, Batty J, Jones R et al: Hand function in C6 and C7 quadriplegics 1–16 years following injury. Spinal Cord 2001; 39:37–43.
8. DiPasquale-Lehnerz P: Orthotic intervention for development of hand function with C-6 quadriplegia. Am J Occup Ther 1994; 48:138–144.
9. Harvey L, Simpson D, Pironello D et al: Does three months of nightly splinting reduce the extensibility of the flexor pollicis longus muscle in people with tetraplegia? Physiother Res Int, in press.
10. Nickel VL, Perry J, Garrett AL: Development of useful function in severely paralyzed hands. J Bone Joint Surg (Am) 1963; 45:933–952.
11. Bryden AM, Sinnott KA, Mulcahey MJ: Innovative strategies for improving upper extremity function in tetraplegia and considerations in measuring functional outcomes. Top Spinal Cord Inj Rehabil 2005; 10:75–93.

12. Moberg E: Surgical treatment for absent single-hand grip and elbow extension in quadriplegia. Principles and preliminary experience. J Bone Joint Surg (Am) 1975; 57:196–206.

13. Meiners T, Abel R, Lindel K et al: Improvements in activities of daily living following functional hand surgery for treatment of lesions to the cervical spinal cord: Self-assessment by patients. Spinal Cord 2002; 40:574–580.

14. Prochazka A, Gauthier M, Wieler M et al: The bionic glove; an electrical stimulator garment that provides controlled grasp and hand opening in quadriplegia. Arch Phys Med Rehabil 1997; 78:608–614.

15. Peckham PH, Keith MW, Freehafer AA: Restoration of functional control by electrical stimulation in the upper extremity of the quadriplegic patient. J Bone Joint Surg (Am) 1988; 70:144–148.

16. Hummel JM, Snoek GJ, van Til JA et al: A multicriteria decision analysis of augmentative treatment of upper limbs in persons with tetraplegia. J Rehabil Res Dev 2005; 42:635–644.

17. Peckham PH, Gorman PH: Functional electrical stimulation in the 21st century. Top Spinal Cord Inj Rehabil 2004; 10:126–150.

18. Alon G, Dar A, Katz-Behiri D et al: Efficacy of a hybrid upper limb neuromuscular electrical stimulation system in lessening selected impairments and dysfunctions consequent to cerebral damage. J Neurol Rehabil 1998; 12:73–80.

19. Snoek GJ, IJzerman MJ, in't Groen FA et al: Use of the NESS handmaster to restore hand function in tetraplegia: clinical experiences in ten patients. Spinal Cord 2000; 38:244–249.

20. Kilgore KL, Peckham PH, Keith MW et al: An implanted upper-extremity neuroprosthesis. Follow-up of five patients. J Bone Joint Surg (Am) 1997; 79:533–541.

21. Taylor P, Esnouf J, Hobby J: The functional impact of the Freehand System on tetraplegic hand function. Clinical results. Spinal Cord 2002; 40:560–566.

22. Snoek GJ, IJzerman MJ, Post MW et al: Choice-based evaluation for the improvement of upper-extremity function compared with other impairments in tetraplegia. Arch Phys Med Rehabil 2005; 86:1623–1630.

Contents

Standing for therapeutic
purposes 108
Walking with thoracic
paraplegia 110
Walking with partial
paralysis of the lower limbs .118
Electrical stimulation 128

Standing and walking with lower limb paralysis

Approximately 50% of people with spinal cord injury walk.[1-6] For some, walking is their primary form of mobility and for others it is used only for therapeutic purposes, or only for specific tasks which require being upright. Neurological status is the strongest predictor of walking. The level of ambulation typically attained can be summarized as follows:

People with tetraplegia. People with tetraplegia and total paralysis of the lower limbs (i.e. ASIA A or B) can stand with frames, tilt tables or standing wheelchairs. The primary purpose for standing is to obtain the therapeutic benefits associated with being upright and weight bearing through the legs (p. 109).

People with thoracic paraplegia. People with thoracic paraplegia and total paralysis of the lower limbs (i.e. ASIA A or B) can ambulate with walking aids on level ground provided they have good upper limb strength and extensive orthotic support. Gait is slow and the energy cost of walking is high.[7-10] These people usually find it difficult to perform associated tasks such as walking up and down slopes, negotiating steps and uneven terrain, putting the orthoses on and off, and turning in tight spaces.[6,8,11-13] The reliance on walking aids is particularly limiting because it largely prevents the use of the hands when upright for tasks such as cooking and carrying bags.[14] In addition, some do not like the appearance and bulkiness of the orthoses. For all these reasons, most people with thoracic paraplegia and total paralysis of the lower limbs stand only for exercise or specific purposes (e.g. while teaching).[7,14-24] Few people with thoracic paraplegia walk as their primary form of mobility.

People with motor incomplete lesions and lumbosacral paraplegia. Most people with motor incomplete lesions (i.e. ASIA C, D or E) and lumbosacral paraplegia can walk for at least limited distances. The usefulness of walking largely depends on the extent of paralysis because this determines the need for orthoses and aids, and the speed and energy cost of walking.[25] As a guiding rule, people with composite ASIA lower extremity motor scores *less than* 20/50 generally use wheelchairs as their primary form of mobility.[19,25] They may, however, walk around the home or exercise with orthoses and aids.[26,27] Walking is only a realistic and functional alternative to a wheelchair if people have at least sufficient strength in one leg to avoid the need for bilateral splinting of the ankles and knees with knee–ankle–foot orthoses.[4,19,28] People with ASIA lower extremity motor scores *more than* 20/50 generally attain the capacity for community ambulation and are capable of walking at reasonable speeds (e.g. $1.0 \, m.sec^{-1}$; this compares to a comfortable walking speed of between 1.0 and $1.7 \, m.sec^{-1}$ for able-bodied individuals). The ability to hitch and control the pelvis increases the likelihood of attaining a functional level of ambulation.[4,6] People with incomplete tetraplegia who are dependent on walking aids generally require more strength in their lower extremities than those with paraplegia in order to adequately compensate for their upper limb weakness.[26]

Any degree of lower limb paralysis clearly makes walking more difficult than normal. The more extensive the paralysis the more difficult walking becomes and the more likely success will be limited by upper limb weakness, lack of proprioception, excessive weight, or presence of spasticity or contracture.[6,29,30]

People may be able to walk effectively in one context but not in another. For example, a person who is capable of walking unencumbered across the floor of a physiotherapy gymnasium will not necessarily be able to carry bags from a supermarket to a car park. Effective walking depends on attaining some level of automaticity so that attention can be simultaneously directed at other activities while upright.[31,32] It also depends on the ability to ascend slopes, stand up from sitting, and negotiate stairs and uneven ground.[13,33] People eventually tend to choose the most practical and functional way of moving about in the community and they will not opt to walk unless it is as efficient, fast and functional as getting about in a wheelchair. Some are surprised to find that, in many environments, a wheelchair is an efficient form of transport. Of course some environments, such as rugged and mountainous places in developing countries, have such poor wheelchair accessibility that walking provides the only option for mobility.

There are and always will be people who defy the odds and attain remarkable levels of upright mobility despite severe paralysis and dependency on extensive orthotic support and aids. Children generally attain a higher level of upright mobility than adults although it is not clear whether this is solely due to the biomechanical advantages of being a child[34,35] or the extensive support provided by children's schools, parents and therapists.[7,23,36]

The remainder of this chapter summarizes how people with different patterns of paralysis stand and walk.

Standing for therapeutic purposes

All patients, even those with total paralysis of the lower limbs, can be provided with equipment which enables them to stand.

The most convenient way of enabling patients with tetraplegia to stand is with a tilt table. Alternatively, electronic standing wheelchairs and frames can be used.[37,38] The patient is strapped to the tilt table, standing chair or frame to prevent knee, hip and trunk flexion (see Figure 6.1). Patients with thoracic paraplegia and good upper limb strength can stand in relatively simple frames which block knee flexion. A strap behind the hip prevents hip flexion (see Figure 6.2). They can also use knee extension splints and pull up into standing between parallel bars (see Figure 6.3). At home, appropriately placed benches or sinks can be used.

Patients can stand without a strap behind the hips provided they push down through the hands to hold the body upright. Alternatively, they can lean backwards

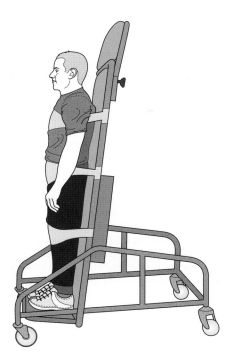

Figure 6.1   Standing with a tilt table.

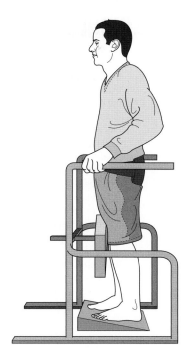

Figure 6.2   Standing in a standing frame. The wedge placed under the feet provides an additional stretch to the ankle plantarflexor muscles.

Figure 6.3   Standing in parallel bars using knee extension splints.

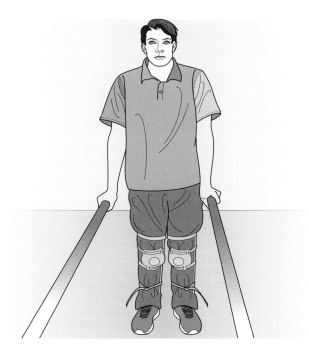

and hyper-extend the lumbar spine. This posture creates a passive hip extension torque that keeps the trunk upright despite paralysis of the hip extensor muscles (see p. 113).

Most patients, regardless of the extent of paralysis, want the opportunity to stand during the initial rehabilitation period. The desire to stand is understandable and, if possible, should be met. At this time, when patients are coming to terms with their paralysis and its implications for mobility, it can be helpful to stand. Standing provides a practical understanding of the complexities of upright mobility and can satisfy patients' needs for 'at least giving it [standing] a go.'

The decision about whether to continue standing after the initial rehabilitation phase is more complex. Some authorities recommended that patients stand for at least 20 minutes, three to five times a week, on an ongoing basis. It is often claimed that regular standing improves psychological status,[39,40] renal function[41] and bone density.[17,42–46] It is also said to help spasticity,[47,48] orthostatic hypotension[49] and joint range of motion.[6,17,50–52] While there is a good theoretical basis to believe that standing has all these beneficial effects, sound evidence is lacking.[37,53] Most work directed at quantifying the benefits of regular standing has been carried out in children[6,54] or is inconclusive.[55,56] The important question as to whether possible benefits justify the inconvenience, effort and cost is yet to be answered.[23] Possibly, to reap therapeutic benefits, patients need to stand more frequently and for longer periods than is generally recommended.

Walking with thoracic paraplegia

Two types of orthoses enable patients with thoracic paraplegia and total paralysis of the lower limbs to walk. They are knee–ankle–foot orthoses and hip–knee–ankle–foot orthoses. Both enable either a reciprocal or jumping gait pattern. Walking aids such as elbow crutches or a frame are essential. Elbow crutches are more versatile than a frame but require a higher level of skill and upright stability.

Bilateral knee–ankle–foot orthoses

Bilateral knee–ankle–foot orthoses provide the cheapest and simplest way to enable patients with thoracic paraplegia to walk. There are various types of knee–ankle–foot orthoses but most incorporate double metal uprights bars and plastic moulded calf and thigh sections (see Figure 6.4).[57] They all stabilize the knee in full extension and ankle in 5–10° dorsiflexion.[6] Different types of knee joints can be used. Most can be unlocked so the knee can be flexed when sitting.[57,58]

Knee–ankle–foot orthoses only compensate for paralysis around the ankle and knee. They provide no stability around the hip or trunk, nor do they provide assistance for hip flexion during swing. They do not stop the pelvis from tilting downwards on the unweighted swing leg. This, combined with fact that the knee is held in extension, makes foot clearance during swing difficult. To overcome problems of foot clearance patients exert downward forces through crutches to 'hitch' (elevate) the pelvis on the swing leg or depress the shoulders.[26,59] Foot clearance during swing is particularly problematic when walking up slopes or stairs.

Figure 6.4 A double metal upright knee–ankle–foot orthosis.

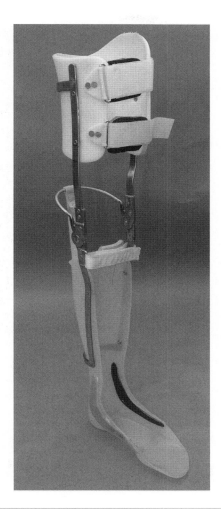

Walking with knee–ankle–foot orthoses

Bilateral knee–ankle–foot orthoses can be used to walk with either a jumping or reciprocal gait pattern. Both strategies rely on forces exerted through walking aids. The legs move in response to these forces. It is important to remember that, unlike parallel bars which are fixed to the ground, patients cannot pull up through walking aids. They can only push down or laterally.

The jumping gait pattern (see Table 6.1) involves placing both crutches in front of the feet and then swinging both legs through simultaneously[15,60] by extending the shoulders. If the feet are moved up *to* the crutches the gait is called a 'swing-*to*' pattern. Alternatively, if the feet are moved past the crutches the gait is called a 'swing-*through*' pattern.[61] Both swing patterns are physically demanding[17,19,26] but provide a quick way of getting around (up to 1.8 m.sec^{-1} in children[62]). In contrast, the reciprocal gait pattern involves moving the feet forwards one at a time. Each leg is swung forwards by elevating the pelvis on the swing side and circumducting the leg (i.e. hip abduction and external rotation combined with pelvic elevation). One crutch

TABLE 6.1   A patient with thoracic paraplegia walking with a swing-through gait pattern using bilateral knee–ankle–foot orthoses[60]

	Sub-tasks
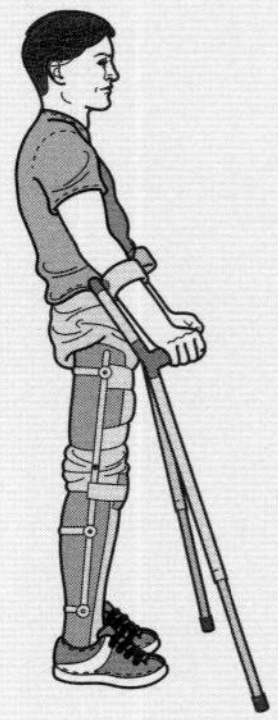 Figure 6.5a	1. Positioning crutches in front of the body: The hips are 'passively' extended to momentarily maintain hip extension while the crutches are moved forward.
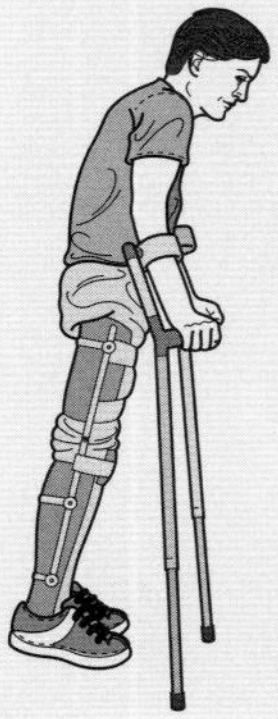 Figure 6.5b	2. Leaning forwards and weight bearing through crutches: The shoulders are depressed and the elbows are extended to lift the feet.
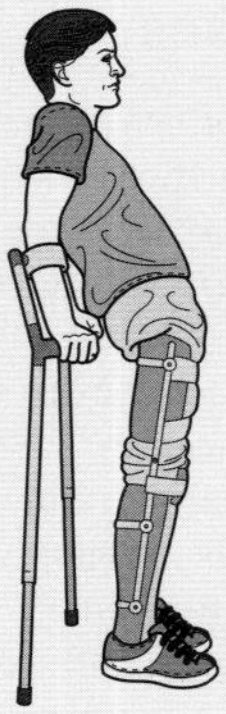 Figure 6.5c	3. The feet are lifted and moved past the crutches: The shoulders are depressed and extended, and the elbows are extended to move the feet up and past the crutches.

Figure 6.6 Hip extension can be maintained when walking with paralysis of the hip extensor muscles and bilateral knee–ankle–foot orthoses by positioning the centre of mass of the trunk and head (circle) behind the hip joint.

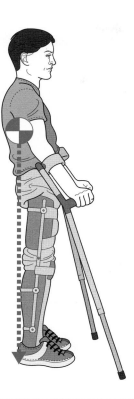

is placed in front of the body while the opposite foot is moved forwards. This is a relatively slow way to ambulate.

While the two gait patterns look very different they share important features. With both gait patterns it is necessary to maintain hip extension during stance. Hip extension can be maintained by pushing down through the hands into crutches. However, this strategy of maintaining hip extension is strenuous and causes discomfort in the hands. In addition, it is important that patients can maintain hip extension without using the hands at least momentarily so they can lift and reposition the crutches to move forwards.

Hip extension can be maintained without using the hands by leaning the trunk backwards and extending the lumbar spine. This positions the centre of mass of the trunk and head behind the hips, creating a torque which passively extends the hips (see Figure 6.6). Excessive hip extension is prevented by the soft tissues spanning the front of the hips. If the centre of mass of the trunk and head moves anterior to the hips with the crutches off the ground, the hips will rapidly flex. The feet can only remain flat on the ground when patients lean backwards if the ankles are dorsiflexed. For this reason the ankles of knee–ankle–foot orthoses are commonly fixed in 5–10° dorsiflexion.[58] Slight modifications to ankle position can make a substantial difference to the ease of standing.[58]

Moving from sit to stand with knee–ankle–foot orthoses

It is difficult to get from sitting to standing with knee–ankle–foot orthoses (see Table 6.2). Most patients place the hands behind the body and lift up into standing with

TABLE 6.2   A patient with thoracic paraplegia moving from sitting to standing using bilateral knee–ankle–foot orthoses

	Sub-tasks
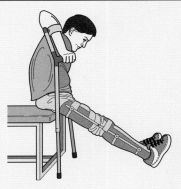 **Figure 6.7a**	1. Positioning the crutches: The crutches are positioned as far posteriorly as possible. The patient leans forwards and bears weight through the upper limbs.
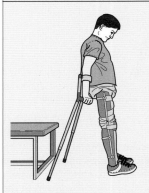 **Figure 6.7b**	2. Lifting into standing: Shoulder depression, shoulder extension and elbow extension are used to lift the body into standing.
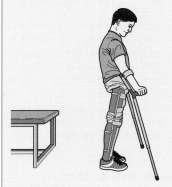 **Figure 6.7c**	3. Positioning the crutches in front of the body: The crutches are repositioned in front of the body.

the knee joints locked in extension. The centre of mass must initially move forwards over the feet. However, the feet cannot be tucked under the chair because the knees are extended. Consequently, the centre of mass needs to move much further forward than it would otherwise if the knees were flexed. The centre of mass cannot be moved sufficiently forward through hip flexion alone. Instead the centre of mass is moved forwards by pushing backwards and downwards through crutches or the arms of a chair. Not surprisingly, patients require good upper limb strength.

There are other strategies which can be used to stand up. For example, some patients find it easier to stand up using the armrests of a chair, rotating in to face the chair as they stand. In this latter technique, patients end up facing the chair in a semi-standing position before grasping walking aids to move into an upright position.[63] It is also possible to stand up with the knee joints unlocked. This requires very good upper limb strength to lift the body into standing. Weight cannot be borne through the feet until the knee joints are locked. A special type of ratchet joint can be built into orthotic knee joints to prevent knee collapse and enable weight to be borne through a flexed knee.[6] These type of joints are not widely used because they are expensive and add weight and complexity to orthoses. Electrical stimulation of the quadriceps and hip extensor muscles can overcome some of these problems and help patients move from sitting to standing.[64]

Hip–knee–ankle–foot orthoses

Hip–knee–ankle–foot orthoses are bilateral knee–ankle–foot orthoses joined together with hip joints.[6] The orthotic hip joints can be placed between the legs or connected laterally to a pelvic or lumbar band or a lumbosacral corset. Orthoses which include extensive trunk bracing are sometimes referred to as *trunk–hip–knee–ankle–foot orthoses*.[36]

By joining two knee–ankle–foot orthoses together, *hip*–knee–ankle–foot orthoses substitute for paralysis of the hip abductor muscles and provide medio-lateral stability during stance. In addition, they prevent the pelvis from tilting down-wards on the unweighted swing leg. This assists foot clearance during swing and reduces the need for the upper limbs to lift the swing leg. However, the torques tend-ing to tilt the pelvis downwards during swing are large, especially in heavy patients. To resist these torques, hip–knee–ankle–foot orthoses need good lateral rigid-ity.[5,34,35,65–67] If the orthosis is insufficiently rigid, swing leg clearance is difficult.

The three most common types of hip–knee–ankle–foot orthoses are the *hip guid-ance orthosis* (HGO; see Figure 6.8), the *reciprocating gait orthosis* (RGO; see Figure 6.9) and the *medial-linkage orthosis* (MLO; see Figure 6.10).[6,11,24,64,65,68–75] Various types of hip and knee joints can be used in all three orthoses.[7,65,73,76–78] A summary of each is given below.

The hip guidance orthosis

The hip guidance orthosis, also called the ParaWalker, was first introduced for children with spina bifida in the 1970s (see Figure 6.8).[79] It consists of two knee–ankle–foot orthoses attached to a rigid body brace with laterally placed hip joints. The hip joints are low friction and restrict flexion and extension, although they can be released to enable sitting. During the swing phase of gait, the leg flexes like a pendulum. That is, hip flexion is achieved solely by the effects of gravity on the unweighted leg. Gravity will only act to flex the hip when the leg is extended with the mass of the leg behind the hip joint.[80]

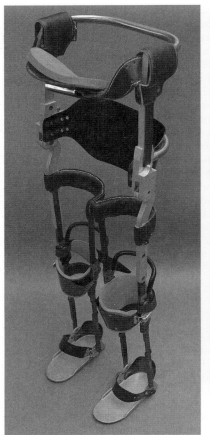

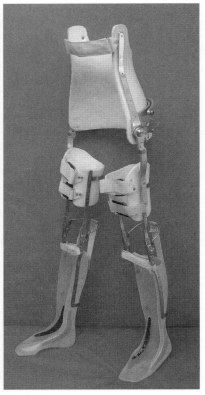

Figure 6.9 A reciprocating gait orthosis.

Figure 6.8 A hip guidance orthosis.

The reciprocating gait orthosis

The reciprocating gait orthosis joins two knee–ankle–foot orthoses to a trunk corset with laterally placed joints (see Figure 6.9). A key feature of the reciprocating gait orthosis is the coupling together of the hip joints, preventing bilateral hip flexion in stance. The hip mechanism was designed so hip extension on one leg could assist hip flexion on the other leg when stepping. However, the effectiveness of this mechanism may be overstated.[81] The hip joints can be unlocked to flex simultaneously.[10,82,83] This is important for sitting.

Early versions of reciprocating gait orthoses coupled the two hip joints together with cables.[84] The cables were attached under high tension so that forces from extension in one leg were transmitted to flexion of the other.[85] In more recent years a pivot bar has replaced the cables.[85] The pivot bar is positioned centrally and at the back of the corset in the lumbar region.[80] Reciprocating gait orthoses incorporating pivot bars are called *isocentric* reciprocating gait orthoses. A variation is the *advanced* reciprocating gait orthosis.[65]

Figure 6.10
A medial-linkage
orthosis.

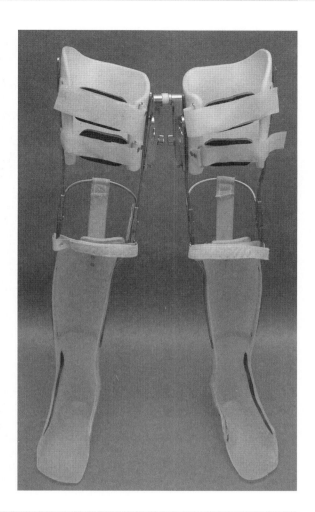

The medial-linkage orthosis

The medial linkage orthosis, also known as the walkabout orthosis, has a hinge-like joint positioned between the legs (see Figure 6.10). The joint limits hip flexion and extension but does not mechanically assist either. Instead, gravity flexes the hip and moves the unweighted leg forward. Hip extension is achieved by leaning the trunk backwards and extending the lumbar spine (see Figure 6.6). Consequently, even slight loss of passive hip extension can be a problem, increasing patients' reliance on their upper limbs to hold the trunk upright. The medial-linkage orthosis is aesthetically more appealing than other types of hip–knee–ankle–foot orthoses but it provides a slower and more energy-consuming gait.[10,11,71,72,86,87]

Walking with hip–knee–ankle–foot orthoses

Typically, patients use a reciprocal gait pattern with either crutches or a frame.[24,65,68,73,74,81,83,88,89] There are various strategies used to walk depending on the

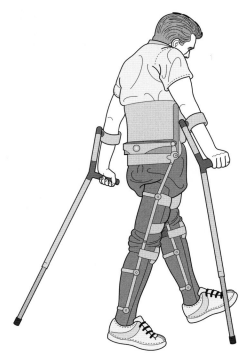

Figure 6.11 A patient with thoracic paraplegia walking with a hip–knee–ankle–foot orthosis. Initially weight needs to be shifted onto the front foot. This is achieved by pushing the body forwards and laterally through a posteriorly-placed walking aid.

type of orthosis and walking aid, and extent of trunk paralysis; however, the underlying principles of all strategies are similar. Initially, weight needs to be shifted from the back leg forwards and laterally onto the front leg. This is achieved by pushing the body forwards and laterally through a posteriorly-placed walking aid (see Figure 6.11). Further unweighting of the back leg is achieved by shoulder depression and pelvic hitch. Once all weight is removed from the back leg, it can be moved forwards either in response to gravity or in response to trunk extension.[81,90]

Moving from the floor or a seated position into standing with hip–knee–ankle–foot orthoses is done in a similar way to standing up with knee–ankle–foot orthoses (see Table 6.2). However, the additional weight and bulk of hip–knee–ankle–foot orthoses makes both these tasks particularly difficult and most patients require assistance.[7,8,70]

Walking with partial paralysis of the lower limbs

The discussion until now has concentrated on standing and walking in patients with total paralysis of the lower limbs. The situation is more complex in patients with partial paralysis of the lower limbs where some muscle groups are paralysed and others are not. For example, some patients with lumbar paraplegia have paralysis around the ankle but retain strength in the quadriceps, and hip flexor and adductor muscles (see Table 2.2, p. 42). The pattern of lower limb paralysis with lumbar paraplegia is highly variable because few patients have complete lesions and muscles are innervated from many spinal nerve roots.

The next section outlines the effects of different patterns of isolated lower limb paralysis on the reciprocal gait pattern and some of the more commonly prescribed orthoses.

Paralysis around the ankle

Paralysis of the dorsiflexor muscles (L4, L5, S1)

The dorsiflexor muscles are primarily responsible for maintaining dorsiflexion during swing and lowering the foot into plantarflexion at heel strike.[61,91,92] Paralysis of the dorsiflexor muscles results in excessive plantarflexion during swing and lack of dorsiflexion at heel strike.[61,68,93] This is commonly called 'foot-drop', although foot-drop also occurs when there is excessive spasticity or contracture in the plantarflexor muscles.

To avoid dragging the toes along the ground during swing, patients increase hip and knee flexion (see Figure 6.12)[93] or hitch the pelvis.[92] Alternatively, they circumduct the entire leg or plantarflex the ankle of the other foot.[92] The precise strategy adopted depends on the strength and mobility at other joints.[92] For example,

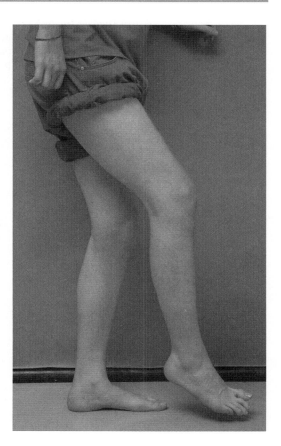

Figure 6.12   Walking with isolated paralysis of the dorsiflexor muscles requires excessive hip and knee flexion to clear the toes.

patients will be unable to plantarflex the contralateral ankle if they have weakness in the plantarflexor muscles of the contralateral leg.

Paralysis of the plantarflexor muscles (L5, S1, S2)

The plantarflexor muscles are primarily active during stance, initially acting eccentrically to control the forward rotation of the tibia over the fixed foot, then acting concentrically to power push-off.[61,94–101] Without control of tibial rotation during mid stance, patients typically move into excessive dorsiflexion. The extent of dorsiflexion is determined by the extensibility of the paralysed plantarflexor muscles (see Figure 6.13).[97,101,102] Excessive dorsiflexion necessitates knee and hip flexion to keep the centre of mass over the base of support (sometimes this is called a 'crouch' gait).[100,101,103,104] In turn, large knee and hip extensor torques are required to prevent collapse.[59,93,105–107] Alternatively, patients avoid the need to use the plantarflexor muscles by remaining plantarflexed throughout stance (see Figure 6.14).[59,61,92,95] Thus the knee hyper-extends and the hip remains flexed.[108] Of course, patients can avoid both scenarios by pushing down through their hands into walking aids and holding themselves upright. Gait then appears more normal, but it is nonetheless physically demanding.[26,95] The lack of push-off limits hip extension at the end of stance and decreases step length.[61,98]

Ankle–foot orthoses (AFO)

There are many ankle–foot orthoses (AFO).[80,109] All restrain ankle motion.[36,58,109,110] Some stabilize the ankle in a fixed position, others allow movement within a certain range and still others assist or resist movement into dorsiflexion or plantarflexion. A patient with isolated paralysis of the dorsiflexor muscles needs only a lightweight

Figure 6.13 The plantarflexor muscles are required at mid stance to prevent excessive forward rotation of the tibia on the fixed foot. Without the ability to restrain the forward rotation of the tibia some patients collapse into excessive dorsiflexion.

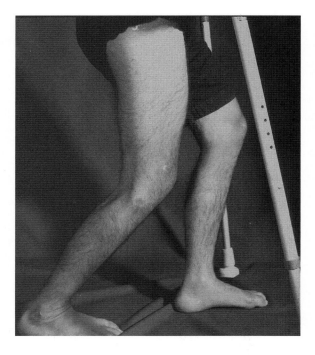

Figure 6.14
Some patients with isolated paralysis of the plantarflexor muscles avoid dorsiflexion during mid stance. The knee hyperextends to keep the trunk's centre of mass (circle) over the ankle joint.

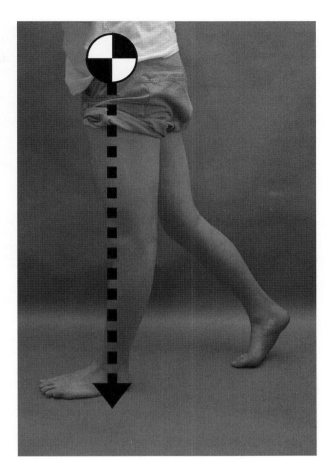

orthosis to resist the small torques tending to plantarflex the ankle during swing. In contrast, a patient with paralysis of the plantarflexor muscles needs a heavy duty orthosis to resist the large torques tending to rotate the tibia over the fixed foot during stance.[95,111]

Posterior leaf spring AFO

The posterior leaf spring AFO is a type of dorsiflexion-assist AFO (see Figure 6.15). It is made from thin, light, thermoplastic material and worn inside a shoe. As the name implies, it assists dorsiflexion. It is primarily used in patients with isolated paralysis of the dorsiflexor muscles. The narrow strip of plastic behind the ankle gives flexibility, allowing the tibia to move over the fixed foot during stance. However, when the foot is off the ground the plastic recoils, preventing foot-drop. Leaf spring AFOs are commercially available in different sizes, or can be individually made by orthotists.[57]

Plastic solid AFO

The plastic solid AFO is also made from thermoplastic material (see Figure 6.16). It provides superior mediolateral stability to the lighter posterior leaf spring AFO.[57] In

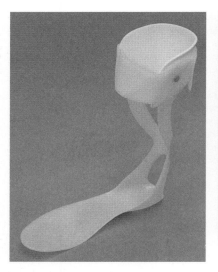

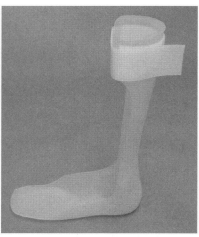

Figure 6.16   A plastic solid AFO appropriate for paralysis of dorsiflexor and plantarflexor muscles.

Figure 6.15   A posterior leaf spring AFO appropriate for paralysis of the dorsiflexor muscles.

addition, it not only prevents plantarflexion during swing but also prevents excessive rotation of the tibia over the fixed foot during stance. For this reason it is typically used for patients with paralysis of the dorsiflexor and plantarflexor muscles. In order to stabilize the ankle joint in this way the orthosis is made from heavy duty thermoplastic material which wraps anterior to the ankle joint.[101,110,112-114] The thickness of the plastic and the trimline of the orthosis around the ankle primarily determines its ability to resist collapse and excessive dorsiflexion during stance.[115] Often carbon composite inserts are used to reinforce the ankle.[116] Modifications to the base of shoes can be used to cushion heel strike and help move the weight from the back of the foot to the front of the foot during stance.[110,116]

Hinged solid plastic AFO
The hinged solid plastic AFO incorporates ankle joints (see Figure 6.17).[57] There are many different types of ankle joints. One type assists dorsiflexion. It incorporates steel springs which compress during stance but rebound during swing. In this way, it enables dorsiflexion during stance but prevents plantarflexion during swing. Other types of joints include plastic overlap joints and posterior stop joints.[14,57]

Toe-off AFO
The toe-off AFO is made from resin (see Figure 6.18).[117] It prevents foot-drop but also assists with the push-off phase of gait. It works on the principle of storing elastic energy for release at the end of stance. In this way, it is similar to the polyfibre feet of below-knee prostheses.[118]

Double metal upright AFO
The double metal upright AFO provides maximal control of the ankle. It is used in patients with paralysis of the dorsiflexor muscles and severe spasticity or contracture

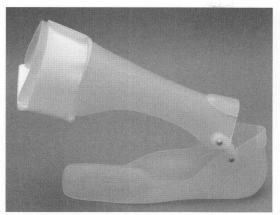

Figure 6.17 A hinged solid ankle–foot orthosis which allows dorsiflexion but limits plantarflexion. It is appropriate for paralysis of the dorsiflexor muscles.

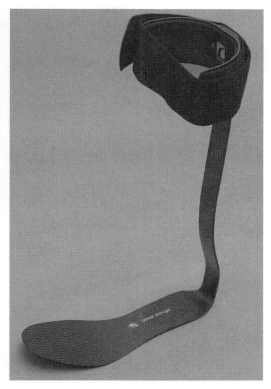

Figure 6.18 A toe-off AFO appropriate for paralysis of the dorsiflexor muscles. It also assists with the push-off phase of gait.

pulling the foot into plantarflexion and/or inversion (see Figure 6.19). It consists of metal uprights which are attached into lace-up shoes. Different types of joints are used to prevent plantarflexion and/or assist dorsiflexion. The need for lace-up shoes and its poor cosmesis prevents its wider use. However, the double metal stirrup AFO better accommodates oedema and is associated with less risk of skin breakdown than a thermoplastic orthosis.[58]

Implications of an AFO on gait and gait-related activities

All types of ankle–foot orthoses, even a light leaf spring AFO for isolated paralysis of the dorsiflexor muscles, affect gait.

An AFO which blocks plantarflexion necessitates additional knee flexion at heel strike to get the foot flat on the ground. This requires large knee extensor torques to prevent knee collapse.[59,93,116,119] The effect of an AFO on the knee at heel strike is exacerbated when walking up or down slopes (see Figure 6.20). Placing an AFO in a less dorsiflexed position reduces knee flexion at heel strike. Occasionally the ankle joint is intentionally positioned in some plantarflexion (this type of AFO is called a floor reaction AFO). This helps stabilize the knee in extension and is used for

Figure 6.19   A double metal upright AFO appropriate for paralysis of the dorsiflexor muscles and severe spasticity or contracture pulling the foot into plantarflexion and/or inversion.

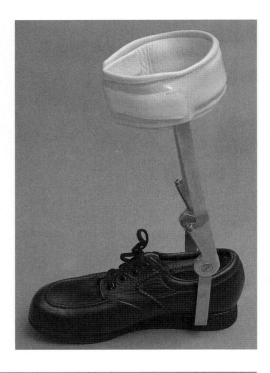

patients with weakness of the quadriceps muscles.[57,120–122] However, the more plantarflexed the ankle the more difficulty patients have with clearing the toes during swing.[101,116] Foot clearance can be helped by a heel raise on the opposite side, although clearly bilateral heel raises will not alleviate a bilateral problem with foot clearance.[58,123]

An AFO which blocks dorsiflexion has important implications for performance of gait-related tasks which rely on placing the foot in a fully dorsiflexed position. For example, moving from sit to stand relies on positioning the feet under the body with the ankles dorsiflexed. If the ankles are fixed at 90°, the only way to get the feet flat on the ground is by placing them further away from the body. This makes it difficult to get the centre of mass over the feet, a biomechanical prerequisite for standing up.[124] Patients therefore need to push down through the hands to initially shift weight over the feet.

Paralysis around the knee

Paralysis of the quadriceps muscles (L2, L3, L4)

The role of the quadriceps muscles during gait is clear.[61,91,94] These muscles prevent flexion of the knee during stance. After initial heel contact and during the early stages of weight acceptance, they work eccentrically to allow some knee flexion (yield).[92] Once maximal yield is attained, they contract concentrically to straighten the knee. The quadriceps muscles need to generate large extensor torques in order to resist the tendency for knee collapse. Generally, patients unable to stand one-legged through a flexed knee have insufficient quadriceps strength to prevent knee collapse during the stance phase of gait. Consequently, they adopt a compensatory strategy.

Figure 6.20 Walking down a slope with a plastic solid AFO blocking plantarflexion. Considerable knee flexion is required to get the foot flat on the ground.

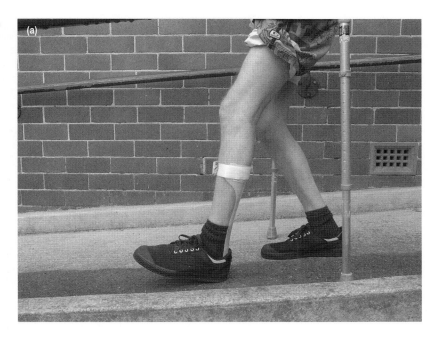

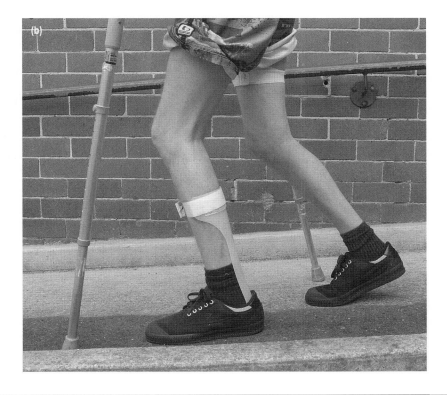

Either they push through their hands onto crutches or parallel bars, or they position the knee in hyper-extension. Knee hyper-extension necessitates ankle plantarflexion and hip flexion (see Figure 6.14).[61,68,92] Importantly, knee hyper-extension positions the centre of mass of the upper leg and body anterior to the knee joint, stabilizing the knee in extension. The more hyper-extended the knee, the more stable the joint will be. Knee hyper-extension can compensate for insufficient strength of the quadriceps muscles, so efforts to prevent hyper-extension without increasing strength of the quadriceps will be of little avail.

Isolated paralysis of the quadriceps muscles is rarely seen in patients with spinal cord injury, and usually patients with paralysis in the quadriceps muscles also have paralysis around the ankles (see Appendix). Knee–ankle–foot orthoses are therefore required to stabilize the knee in extension and fixate the ankle (see Figure 6.4).

Paralysis of hamstrings (L5, S1, S2)

The effects of paralysis of the hamstring muscles on gait are often underestimated and overlooked. The hamstring muscles primarily act eccentrically to prevent the knee from accelerating into uncontrolled hyper-extension at the end of swing and again at mid-terminal stance.[26,61,91] They also act concentrically at the end of stance to move the knee into flexion in preparation for swing. The hamstring muscles contribute little to knee flexion during swing provided patients walk at a reasonable speed.[68] Instead, knee flexion is primarily the result of inertia and the rapid movement of the hip into flexion at the beginning of swing.[26,125–129]

A common indication of hamstring weakness (or paralysis) is knee hyper-extension at the beginning or end of stance.[68,102,130] The gastrocnemius muscles can substitute for the action of the hamstring muscles about the knee but generally patients with poor hamstring strength also have poor strength in the gastrocnemius muscles. Instructing patients to avoid knee hyper-extension without addressing the underlying problem of hamstring muscle weakness will merely encourage patients to walk in a crouched position with increased knee and hip flexion (see Figure 6.13). This strategy avoids the need to recruit the hamstring muscles. Alternatively, knee hyper-extension can be prevented by exerting more force through the hands.

Knee splints to prevent hyper-extension

Patients with paralysis of the hamstring muscles may experience rapid and forceful hyper-extension in mid to late stance phase. If this is repeated often over many years it produces genu recurvatum (a knee hyper-extension deformity). Genu recurvatum is undesirable because it is unsightly and may be associated with chronic knee pain.[130–133] However, the cause–effect relationship between genu recurvatum and knee pain has been questioned.[130]

Various splints mechanically block knee hyper-extension (see Figure 6.21).[58] Some of these splints have been developed for orthopaedic problems but they are being increasingly used in patients with paralysis of the hamstring muscles. It is also possible to prevent knee hyper-extension with an AFO which fixes the foot in 5° dorsiflexion.[133,134] This prevents the tibia from rotating backwards on the fixed foot, thereby helping to hold the knee in a slightly flexed position.

Paralysis around the hip

Paralysis of hip flexors (L1, **L2**, L3)

The hip flexor muscles flex the hip during swing. They are particularly important for initiating swing[91] when walking at slow speeds. Without adequate hip flexion during

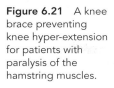

Figure 6.21 A knee brace preventing knee hyper-extension for patients with paralysis of the hamstring muscles.

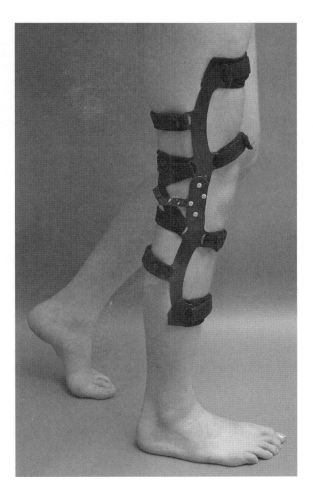

swing, knee flexion is more dependent on hamstring muscle activity.[59] Patients with paralysis of the hip flexor muscles attempt to advance the swing leg by either externally rotating the hip and using hip adductor muscles as hip flexors or by circumducting the leg.[59,61] The effects of hip flexor muscle paralysis on gait are particularly evident when walking up stairs or slopes, which requires lifting the leg.

There is no simple orthosis for the management of isolated paralysis of the hip flexor muscles. While the hip guidance and reciprocating gait orthoses mechanically assist hip flexion (see p. 115), neither is prescribed solely for this purpose. Rather they are prescribed for patients with extensive bilateral lower limb paralysis who also require orthotic support around the knees and ankles.

Paralysis of hip extensors (L5, S1, S2)

The hip extensor muscles are primarily active during the beginning of stance and are used to prevent hip flexion.[61,91,92] Patients with paralysis of the hip extensor muscles avoid the need to actively generate hip extensor torques by hyper-extending the hips.

Hip hyper-extension is achieved by dorsiflexing the ankle, extending the knee and hyper-extending the lumbar spine (see Figure 6.6).[61,92] This body position places the trunk's centre of mass behind the hip joint and generates a passive hip extension torque. If patients are unable to attain this position, they push down through the hands to prevent hip flexion.

There is no simple orthosis for the management of isolated paralysis of the hip extensor muscles. While the hip guidance and reciprocating gait orthoses mechanically prevent hip flexion, neither is used solely for this purpose. Instead they are used for patients with extensive bilateral lower limb paralysis (see p. 115).

Paralysis of hip abductors (L4, L5, S1, S1, S2)

Paralysis of the hip abductor muscles is evident during stance on the affected leg. The hip abductor muscles are responsible for controlling lateral translation of the pelvis and keeping the pelvis horizontal during single-leg support.[61,92] Without adequate hip abductor strength, the pelvis tilts down on the side of the swing leg. Tilting of the pelvis can be avoided by pushing down through walking aids on the swing side or leaning laterally over the standing (and affected) leg.[92,102,107,135]

There is no simple orthosis for the management of isolated paralysis of the hip abductor muscles. Hip–knee–ankle–foot orthoses substitute for paralysis of the hip abductor muscles; however, they are primarily prescribed for patients with extensive bilateral lower limb paralysis (see p. 115).

Electrical stimulation

Over the last 20 years, attention has been directed at the use of lower limb electrical stimulation to facilitate gait in people with complete or partial paralysis of the lower limbs. Electrical stimulation is used either alone or in combination with orthoses.[6,8,9,34,83] Typically, key muscles, such as the quadriceps, hip extensors, dorsiflexor or hamstring muscles are stimulated.[6,8,35,67,82,136] Simpler systems which solely stimulate the peroneal nerve to initiate mass flexion of the limb during swing are also used.[6,137–139] Alternatively, electrical stimulation is used to specifically target foot-drop in patients with paralysis of the dorsiflexor muscles.[140] Sometimes electrical stimulation is solely used to help patients get from sit to stand.

Electrical stimulation can be applied cutaneously[141,142] but with advanced technology the electrodes are being increasingly applied percutaneously (i.e. the electrodes are surgically implanted and directly attached to either nerves or muscles; the leads exit through the skin).[143–145] More recently entire electrical stimulation systems have been implanted, although these systems have only been used in a small number of patients.[6,143,146]

There are several technical limitations which make widespread use of electrical stimulation difficult. One of the biggest problems of electrical stimulation for gait is muscle fatigue. Fatigue occurs both because the paralysed muscles are deconditioned and because stimulation preferentially activates fatigable motor units. Fatigue can be substantially reduced with training and with sophisticated programming of the stimulation parameters which incorporates cyclic switching between key postural muscles. However, fatigue remains a problem.[137,147] There are also challenges ensuring the gait systems can adjust and respond to different environmental circumstances[142] and are sufficiently versatile to cope with everyday activities.[13,136] For these reasons gait driven by electrical stimulation is still primarily used for research purposes.[6,148]

References

1. Burke DC, Burley HT, Ungar GH: Data on spinal injuries — part II. Outcome of the treatment of 352 consecutive admissions. Aust N Z J Surg 1985; 55:377–382.
2. Tang SF, Tuel SM, McKay WB et al: Correlation of motor control in the supine position and assistive device used for ambulation in chronic incomplete spinal cord-injured persons. Am J Phys Med Rehabil 1994; 73:268–274.
3. Field-Fote EC, Fluet GG, Schafer SD et al: The Spinal Cord Injury Functional Ambulation Inventory (SCI-FAI). J Rehabil Med 2001; 33:177–181.
4. Hussey RW, Stauffer ES: Spinal cord injury: requirements for ambulation. Arch Phys Med Rehabil 1973; 54:544–547.
5. Hoffer MM, Feiwell E, Walker JM et al: Functional ambulation in patients with myelomeningocele. J Bone Joint Surg (Am) 1973; 55:137–148.
6. Nene AV, Hermens HJ, Zilvold G: Paraplegic locomotion: a review. Paraplegia 1996; 34:507–524.
7. Franceschini M, Baratta S, Zampolini M et al: Reciprocating gait orthoses: a multicenter study of their use by spinal cord injured patients. Arch Phys Med Rehabil 1997; 78:582–586.
8. Solomonow M, Aguilar E, Reisin E et al: Reciprocating gait orthosis powered with electrical muscle stimulation (RGO II) Part 1: Performance evaluation of 70 paraplegic patients. Orthopaedics 1997; 20:315–324.
9. Hirokawa S, Grimm M, Le T et al: Energy consumption in paraplegic ambulation using the reciprocating gait orthosis and electric stimulation of the thigh muscles. Arch Phys Med Rehabil 1990; 71:687–694.
10. Bowker P, Messenger N, Ogilvie C et al: Energetics of paraplegic walking. J Biomed Eng 1992; 14:344–350.
11. Saitoh E, Suzuki T, Sonoda S et al: Clinical experience with a new hip–knee–foot orthotic system using a medial single hip joint for paraplegic standing and walking. Am J Phys Med Rehabil 1996; 75:198–203.
12. Summers BN, McClelland MR, el Masri WS: A clinical review of the Adult Hip Guidance Orthosis (Parawalker) in traumatic paraplegics. Paraplegia 1988; 26:19–26.
13. Stallard J, Major RE, Patrick JH: A review of the fundamental design problems of providing ambulation for paraplegic patients. Paraplegia 1989; 27:70–75.
14. Hawran S, Biering-Sorensen F: The use of long leg calipers for paraplegic patients; a follow-up study of patients discharged 1973–82. Spinal Cord 1996; 34:666–668.
15. Noreau L, Richards CL, Comeau F et al: Biomechanical analysis of swing-through gait in paraplegic and non-disabled individuals. J Biomech 1995; 28:689–700.
16. Hong C, San Luise EB, Chung S: Follow-up study on the use of leg braces issued to spinal cord injury patients. Paraplegia 1990; 28:172–177.
17. Jaeger RJ, Yarkony GM, Roth EJ: Rehabilitation technology for standing and walking after spinal cord injury. Am J Phys Med Rehabil 1989; 68:128–133.
18. Heinemann AW, Magiera-Planey R, Schiro-Geist C et al: Mobility for persons with spinal cord injury: an evaluation of two systems. Arch Phys Med Rehabil 1987; 68:90–93.
19. Waters RL, Lunsford BR: Energy cost of paraplegic locomotion. J Bone Joint Surg (Am) 1985; 67:1245–1250.
20. Moore P, Stallard J: A clinical review of adult paraplegic patients with complete lesions using the ORLAU ParaWalker. Paraplegia 1991; 29:191–196.
21. Hahn HR: Lower extremity bracing in paraplegics with usage follow-up. Paraplegia 1970; 8:147–153.
22. Nativig H, McAdam R: Ambulation without wheelchairs for paraplegics with complete lesions. Paraplegia 1978; 16:142–146.
23. Sykes L, Edwards J, Powell E et al: The reciprocating gait orthosis: long-term usage patterns. Arch Phys Med Rehabil 1995; 76:779–783.
24. Lotta S, Fiocchi A, Giovannini R et al: Restoration of gait with orthoses in thoracic paraplegia: a multicentric investigation. Paraplegia 1994; 32:608–615.
25. Waters RL, Yakura JS, Adkins R et al: Determinants of gait performance following spinal cord injury. Arch Phys Med Rehabil 1989; 70:811–818.
26. Waters RL, Mulroy S: The energy expenditure of normal and pathologic gait. Gait Posture 1999; 9:207–231.
27. Waters RL, Adkins R, Yakura J et al: Prediction of ambulatory performance based on motor scores derived from standards of the American Spinal Injury Association. Arch Phys Med Rehabil 1994; 75:756–760.
28. Cerny D, Walters R, Hislop H et al: Walking and wheelchair energetics in persons with paraplegia. Phys Ther 1980; 60:1133–1139.
29. Burns SP, Golding DG, Rolle WA et al: Recovery of ambulation in motor incomplete tetraplegia. Arch Phys Med Rehabil 1997; 78:1169–1172.
30. Merriam WF, Taylor TK, Ruff SJ et al: A reappraisal of acute traumatic central cord syndrome. J Bone Joint Surg (Br) 1986; 68B:708–713.

31. Lajoie Y, Barbeau H, Hamelin M: Attentional requirements of walking in spinal cord injured patients compared to normal subjects. Spinal Cord 1999; 37:245–250.
32. Paul SS, Ada L, Canning CG: Automaticity of walking — implications for physiotherapy practice. Phy Ther Reviews 2005; 10:15–23.
33. Lapointe R, Lajoie Y, Serresse O et al: Functional community ambulation requirements in incomplete spinal cord injured patients. Spinal Cord 2001; 39:327–335.
34. Stallard J, Major RE: The influence of orthosis stiffness on paraplegics ambulation and its implications for functional electrical stimulation (FES) walking systems. Prosthet Orthot Int 1995; 19:108–114.
35. Nene AV, Major RE: Dynamics of reciprocal gait of adult paraplegics using the parawalker (hip guidance orthoses). Prosthet Orthot Int 1987; 11:124–127.
36. Edelstein JE: Orthotic assessment and management. In O'Sullivan SB, Schmitz TJ (eds): Physical Rehabilitation: Assessment and Treatment, 4th edn. Philadelphia, FA Davis Company, 2000:1025–1059.
37. Kreutz D: Standing frames and standing wheelchairs: Implications for standing. Top Spinal Cord Inj Rehabil 2000; 5:24–38.
38. Shields RK, Dudley-Javoroski S: Monitoring standing wheelchair use after spinal cord injury: a case report. Disabil Rehabil 2005; 27:142–146.
39. Kunkel CF, Scremin E, Eisenberg B et al: Effect of standing on spasticity, contracture, and osteoporosis in paralyzed males. Arch Phys Med Rehabil 1993; 74:73–78.
40. Guest RS, Klose KJ, Needham-Shropshir BM et al: Evaluation of a training program for persons with SCI paraplegia using the Parastep 1 ambulation system: part 4. Effect on physical self-concept and depression. Arch Phys Med Rehabil 1997; 78:804–807.
41. Ragnarsson KT, Krebs M, Naftchi NE et al: Head-up tilt effect on glomerular filtration rate, renal plasma flow, and mean arterial pressure in spinal man. Arch Phys Med Rehabil 1981; 62:306–310.
42. Kaplan PE, Gannhavadi B, Richards L et al: Calcium balance in paraplegic patients: influence of injury duration and ambulation. Arch Phys Med Rehabil 1978; 59:447–450.
43. Goemaere S, Van Laere M, De Neve P et al: Bone mineral status in paraplegic patients who do or do not perform standing. Osteoporisis Int 1994; 4:138–143.
44. Dunn RB, Walter JS, Lucero Y et al: Follow-up assessment of standing mobility device users. Assist Technol 1998; 10:84–93.
45. Frey-Rindova P, de Bruin ED, Stussi E et al: Bone mineral density in upper and lower extremities during 12 months after spinal cord injury measured by peripheral quantitative computed tomography. Spinal Cord 2000; 38:26–32.
46. de Bruin ED, Frey-Rindova P, Herzog RE et al: Changes of tibia bone properties after spinal cord injury: effects of early intervention. Arch Phys Med Rehabil 1999; 80:214–220.
47. Odeen I, Knutsson E: Evaluation of the effects of muscle stretch and weight load in patients with spastic paraplegia. Scand J Rehabil Med 1981; 13:117–121.
48. Bohannon RW: Tilt table standing for reducing spasticity after spinal cord injury. Arch Phys Med Rehabil 1993; 74:1121–1122.
49. Figoni SF: Cardiovascular and haemodynamic responses to tilting and to standing in tetraplegic patients: a review. Paraplegia 1984; 22:99–109.
50. Henshaw JT: Walking appliances for paraplegics and tetraplegics. Paraplegia 1979; 17:163–169.
51. Cybulski GR, Jaeger RT: Standing performance of persons with paraplegia. Arch Phys Med Rehabil 1986; 67:103–108.
52. Eng JJ, Levins SM, Townson AF et al: Use of prolonged standing for individuals with spinal cord injuries. Phys Ther 2001; 81:1392–1399.
53. Needham-Shropshire BM, Broton JG, Klose K et al: Evaluation of a training program for persons with SCI paraplegia using the Parastep 1 Ambulation System: part 3. Lack of effect on bone mineral density. Arch Phys Med Rehabil 1997; 78:799–803.
54. Caulton JM, Ward KA, Alsop CW et al: A randomised controlled trial of standing programme on bone mineral density in non-ambulant children with cerebral palsy. Arch Dis Child 2004; 89:131–135.
55. Thoumie P, Le Claire G, Beillot J et al: Restoration of functional gait in paraplegic patients with the RGO-II hybrid orthosis A multicenter controlled study. II: Physiological evaluation. Paraplegia 1995; 33:654–659.
56. Ben M, Harvey L, Denis S et al: Does 12 weeks of regular standing prevent loss of ankle mobility and bone mineral density in people with recent spinal cord injuries? Aust J Physiother 2005; 51:251–256.
57. Trautman P: Lower limb orthoses. In Redford JB, Basmajian JV, Trautman P (eds): Orthotics: Clinical Practice and Rehabilitation Technology. New York, Churchill Livingstone, 1995:13–39.
58. Racette WL: Orthotics: evaluation, prognosis, and intervention. In Umphred DA (ed): Neurological Rehabilitation. St Louis, MO, Mosby, 2001.
59. Perry J: Gait analysis. Normal and Pathological function. SLACK Incorporated, Thorofare, NJ, 1992.
60. Crosbie WJ, Nicol AC: Biomechanical comparison of two paraplegic gait patterns. Clin Biomech 1990; 5:97–107.

61. Lehmann J, De Lateur B: Gait analysis: diagnosis and management. In Kottke JF, Lehmann JF (eds): Krusen's Handbook of Physical Medicine and Rehabilitation. Philadelphia, WB Saunders, 1990:108–125.

62. Williams LO, Anderson AD, Campbell J et al: Energy costs of walking and of wheelchair propulsion by children with myelodysplasia: comparison with normal children. Dev Med Child Neurol 1983; 25:617–624.

63. Somers MF: Spinal Cord Injury: Functional Rehabilitation, 2nd edn. Upper Saddle River, NJ, Prentice Hall, 2001.

64. Chafetz RS, Johnston TE, Calhoun CL: Outcomes in upright mobility in individuals with a spinal cord injury. Top Spinal Cord Inj Rehabil 2005; 10:94–108.

65. Jefferson RJ, Whittle MW: Performance of three walking orthoses for the paralysed: a case study using gait analysis. Prosthet Orthot Int 1990; 14:103–110.

66. Ferrarin M, Stallard J, Palieri R et al: Estimation of deformation in a walking orthosis for paraplegic patients. Clin Biomech 1993; 8:255–261.

67. McClelland M, Andrews BJ, Patrick JH et al: Augmentation of the Oswestry Parawalker orthosis by means of surface electrical stimulation: gait analysis of three patients. Paraplegia 1987; 25:32–38.

68. Whittle MW, Cochrane GM, Chase AP et al: A comparative trial of two walking systems for paralysed people. Paraplegia 1991; 29:97–102.

69. Whittle MW, Cochrane GM: A comparative evaluation of the hip guidance orthosis (HGO) and the reciprocating gait orthosis (RGO). In Herrington C (ed): Health Equipment Information No. 192. London, NHS Procurement Directorate, 1989.

70. Harvey LA, Smith MB, Davis GM et al: Functional outcomes attained by T9–12 paraplegic patients with the walkabout and the isocentric reciprocal gait orthoses. Arch Phys Med Rehabil 1997; 78:706–711.

71. Harvey LA, Newton-John T, Davis G et al: A comparison of the attitude of paraplegic individuals to the Walkabout Orthosis and the Isocentric Reciprocal Gait Orthosis. Spinal Cord 1997; 35:580–584.

72. Harvey L, Davis G, Smith M et al: Energy expenditure during gait using the Walkabout and Isocentric Reciprocal Gait orthoses in person with paraplegia. Arch Phys Med Rehabil 1998; 79:945–949.

73. Winchester PK, Carollo JJ, Parekh RN et al: A comparison of paraplegic gait performance using two types of reciprocating gait orthoses. Prosthet Orthot Int 1993; 17:101–106.

74. Beckman J: The Louisiana State University reciprocating gait orthosis. Physiotherapy 1987; 73:386–392.

75. Nene AV, Patrick JH: Energy cost of paraplegic locomotion with the ORLAU ParaWalker. Paraplegia 1989; 27:5–18.

76. Carroll NC: The orthotic management of spina bifida children. Present status — future goals. Prosthet Orthot Int 1977; 1:39–42.

77. Butler PB, Farmer IR, Poiner R et al: Use of the ORLAU swivel walker for the severely handicapped patient. Physiotherapy 1982; 68:324–326.

78. Griffiths JC, Henshaw JT, Haywood OB: Clinical applications of the paraplegic swivel walker. J Biomed Eng 1980; 2:250–256.

79. Rose GK: The principles and practice of hip guidance articulations. Prosthet Orthot Int 1979; 3:37–43.

80. Molnar GE: Orthotic management of children. In Redford JB, Basmajian JV, Trautman P (eds): Orthotics. Clinical Practice and Rehabilitation Technology. New York, Churchill Livingstone, 1995:137–165.

81. Dall PM, Muller B, Stallard I et al: The functional use of the reciprocal hip mechanism during gait for paraplegic patients walking in the Louisiana State University reciprocating gait orthosis. Prosthet Orthot Int 1999; 23:152–162.

82. Phillips CA: Electrical muscle stimulation in combination with a reciprocating gait orthosis for ambulation by paraplegics. J Biomed Eng 1989; 11:338–344.

83. Isakov E, Douglas R, Berns P: Ambulation using the reciprocating gait orthosis and functional electrical stimulation. Paraplegia 1992; 30:239–245.

84. Douglas R, Larson PF, D'Ambrosia R et al: The LSU reciprocating gait orthosis. Orthopaedics 1983; 6:834–839.

85. Motlock W: Principles of orthotic management for child and adult paraplegia and clinical experience with the isocentric RGO. In Proceeding of the 7th World Congress of the International Society for Prosthetics and Orthotics, Chicago. Copenhagen, 1992.

86. Kirtley C: Principles and practice of paraplegic locomotion: experience with the walkabout walking system. Aust Orthot Prosthet Mag 1992; 7:4–7.

87. Middleton JW, Yeo JD, Blanch L, Vare V et al: Clinical evaluation of a new orthosis, the 'Walkabout,' for restoration of functional standing and short distance mobility in spinal paralysed individuals. Spinal Cord 1997; 35:574–579.

88. Major RE, Stallard J, Rose GK: The dynamics of walking using the hip guidance orthosis (HGO) with crutches. Prosthet Orthot Int 1981; 5:19–22.

89. Ferrarin M, Pedotti A, Boccardi S et al: Biomechanical assessment of paraplegic locomotion with hip guidance orthosis (HGO). Clin Rehabil 1993; 7:303–308.

90. IJzerman MJ, Baardman G, Hermens HJ et al: The influence of the reciprocal cable linkage in the advanced reciprocating gait orthosis on paraplegic gait performance. Prosthet Orthot Int 1997:52–61.

91. Inman VT, Ralston HJ, Todd F: Human Walking. Baltimore, Williams & Wilkins, 1981.

92. Norkin CC: Gait analysis. In O'Sullivan SB, Schmitz TJ (eds): Physical Rehabilitation: Assessment and Treatment. Philadelphia, FA Davis Company, 2000:257–307.

93. Lehmann JF, Condon SM, de Lateur BJ et al: Gait abnormalities in peroneal nerve paralysis and their corrections by orthoses: a biomechanical study. Arch Phys Med Rehabil 1986; 67:380–386.

94. DeVita P: The selection of a standard convention for analyzing gait data based on the analysis of relevant biomechanical factors. J Biomech 1994; 27:501–508.

95. Lehmann JF, Condon SM, de Lateur BJ et al: Gait abnormalities in tibial nerve paralysis: a biomechanical study. Arch Phys Med Rehabil 1985; 66:80–85.

96. Murray MP, Guten GN, Sepic SB et al: Function of the triceps surae during gait. Compensatory mechanisms for unilateral loss. J Bone Joint Surg (Am) 1978; 60:473–476.

97. Simon SR, Mann RA, Hagy JL et al: Role of the posterior calf muscles in normal gait. J Bone Joint Surg (Am) 1978; 60:465–472.

98. Sutherland DH, Cooper L, Daniel D: The role of the ankle plantar flexors in normal walking. J Bone Joint Surg (Am) 1980; 62:354–363.

99. Hof A, Geelen BA, Van Den Gerg JW: Calf muscle moment; work and efficiency in level walking; role of series elasticity. J Biomech 1983; 16:523–537.

100. Gage JR: Gait analysis. An essential tool in the treatment of Cerebral Palsy. Clin Orthop Relat Res 1993; 288:126–134.

101. Hullin MG, Robb JE, Loudon IR: Ankle–foot orthosis function in low-level myelomeningocele. J Pediatr Orthop 1992; 12:518–521.

102. The Pathokinesiology Department & The Physical Therapy Department Rancho Los Amigos Medical Center: Observational Gait Analysis Handbook. Amigos Medical Center, CA, The Professional Staff Association Ranchos Los Amigos Medical Center, 1989.

103. Vankoski SJ, Sarwark JF, Moore C et al: Characteristic pelvic, hip, and knee kinematic patterns in children with lumbosacral myelomeningocele. Gait Posture 1995; 3:51–57.

104. Perry J, Mulroy SJ, Renwick SE: The relationship of lower extremity strength and gait parameters in patients with post-polio syndrome. Arch Phys Med Rehabil 1993; 74:165–169.

105. Perry J, Antonelli D, Ford W: Analysis of knee-joint forces during flexed-knee stance. J Bone Joint Surg (Am) 1975; 57:961–967.

106. Hsu AT, Perry J, Gronley JK et al: Quadriceps force and myoelectric activity during flexed knee stance. Clin Orthop Relat Res 1993; 288:254–262.

107. Duffy CM, Hill AE, Cosgrove AP et al: Three-dimensional gait analysis in spina bifida. J Pediatr Orthop 1996; 16:786–791.

108. Winter TF, Gage JR, Hicks R: Gait patterns in spastic hemiplegia in children and young adults. J Bone Joint Surg (Am) 1987; 69:437–441.

109. Yamamoto S, Ebina M, Iwasaki M et al: Comparative study of mechanical characteristics of plastic AFOs. J Prosth Orth 1993; 5:59–64.

110. Rubin G, Cohen E: Prostheses and orthoses for the foot and ankle. Clin Podiatr Med Surg 1988; 5:692–719.

111. Lehmann JF: Biomechanics of ankle–foot orthoses: prescription and design. Arch Phys Med Rehabil 1979; 60:200–207.

112. Bowker P: Applied mechanics: Biomechanics of orthoses. Physiotherapy 1987; 73:270–275.

113. Lehmann JF, Esselman PC, Ko MJ et al: Plastic ankle–foot orthoses: evaluation of function. Arch Phys Med Rehabil 1983; 64:402–407.

114. Edelstein JE: Orthotic options for standing and walking. Top Spinal Cord Inj Rehabil 2000; 5:11–23.

115. Sumiya T, Suzuki Y, Kasahara T: Stiffness control in posterior-type plastic ankle–foot orthoses; effect of ankle trimline. Part 2: Orthosis characteristics and orthosis/patient matching. Prosthet Orthot Int 1996; 20:132–137.

116. Lehmann JF: Lower limb orthotics. In Redford JB (ed): Orthotics Etcetera. Baltimore, Williams & Wilkins, 1986:278–351.

117. Lehneis HR: New developments in lower-limb orthotics through bioengineering. Arch Phys Med Rehabil 1972; 53:303–353.

118. Ehara Y, Beppu M, Nomura S et al: Energy storing property of so-called energy-storing prosthetic feet. Arch Phys Med Rehabil 1993; 74:68–72.

119. Brodlke DS, Skinner SR, Lamoreux LW et al: Effects of ankle–foot orthoses on the gait of children. J Pediatr Orthop 1989; 9:702–708.

120. Perry J: Kinesiology of lower extremity bracing. Clin Orthop Relat Res 1974; 102:18–31.

121. Lyles M, Munday J: Report of the evaluation of the Vannini-Rizzoli Stabilizing Limb Orthosis. J Rehabil Res Dev 1992; 29:77–104.

122. Stallard J: Assessment of the mechanical function of orthoses by force vector visualisation. Physiotherapy 1987; 73:398–402.

123. Abdulhadi HM, Kerrigan DC, LaRaia PJ: Contralateral shoe-lift: effect on oxygen cost of walking with an immobilized knee. Arch Phys Med Rehabil 1996; 77:670–672.

124. Cattaneo D, Marazzini F, Crippa A et al: Do static or dynamic AFOs improve balance? Clin Rehabil 2002; 16:894–899.

125. Hoy MG, Zernicke RF: The role of intersegmental dynamics during rapid limb oscillations. J Biomech 1986; 19:867–877.

126. Robertson DG, Winter DA: Mechanical energy generation, absorption and transfer amongst segments during walking. J Biomech 1980; 13:845–854.

127. Wisleder D, Zernicke RF, Smith JL: Speed-related changes in hindlimb intersegmental dynamics during the swing phase of cat locomotion. Exp Brain Res 1990; 79:651–660.

128. Herbert R, Moore S, Moseley A et al: Making inferences about muscle forces from clinical observations. Aust J Physiother 1993; 39:195–201.

129. Zernicke RF, Schneider K, Bufort JA: Intersegmental dynamics during gait: implications for control. In Patla AE (ed): Adaptability of Human Gait: Implications for the Control of Locomotion. Amsterdam, Elsevier Science, 1991.

130. Kerrigan DC, Deming LC, Holden MK: Knee recurvatum in gait: a study of associated knee biomechanics. Arch Phys Med Rehabil 1996; 77:645–650.

131. Williams J, Graham GP, Dunne KB et al: Late knee problems in myelomeningocele. J Pediatr Orthop 1993; 13:701–703.

132. Hogue RE, McCandless S: Genu recurvatum: auditory biofeedback treatment for adult patients with stroke or head injuries. Arch Phys Med Rehabil 1983; 64:368–370.

133. Morris ME, Matyas TA, Bach T et al: The effect of electrogoniometric feedback on knee hyperextension following stroke. In Proceedings of World Congress of Physiotherapy. London, 1991.

134. Rosenthal RK, Deutsch SD, Miller W et al: A fixed-ankle, below-the-knee orthosis for the management of genu recurvatum in spastic cerebral palsy. J Bone Joint Surg (Am) 1975; 57:545–547.

135. Duffy CM, Hill A, Cosgrove AP et al: The influence of abductor weakness on gait in spina bifida. Gait Posture 1996; 4:34–38.

136. Phillips CA, Hendershot DM: A systems approach to medically prescribed functional electrical stimulation. Ambulation after spinal cord injury. Paraplegia 1991; 29:505–513.

137. Barbenel JC, Paul JP: Bioengineering developments for paraplegic patients. Paraplegia 1992; 30:61–64.

138. Ladouceur M, Barbeau H: Functional electrical stimulation-assisted walking for persons with incomplete spinal injuries: longitudinal changes in maximal overground walking speed. Scand J Rehabil Med 2000; 32:28–36.

139. Kralj A, Bajd T, Turk R: Enhancement of gait restoration in spinal injured patients by functional electrical stimulation. Clin Orthop 1988; Aug:34–43.

140. Kim CM, Eng JJ, Whittaker MW: Effects of a simple functional electric system and/or a hinged ankle–foot orthosis on walking in person with incomplete spinal cord injury. Arch Phys Med Rehabil 2004; 85:1718–1723.

141. Klose KL, Jacobs PL, Broton JG et al: Evaluation of a training program for persons with SCI paraplegia using the Parastep ambulation system: part 1: ambulation performance and anthropometric measures. Arch Phys Med Rehabil 1997; 78:780–793.

142. Brissot R, Gallien P, Le Bot M et al: Clinical experience with functional electrical stimulation-assisted gait with Parastep in spinal cord-injured patients. Spine 2000; 25:501–508.

143. Johnston TE, Betz RR, Smith BT et al: Implanted functional electrical stimulation: an alternative for standing and walking in pediatric spinal cord injury. Spinal Cord 2003; 41:144–152.

144. Shimada Y, Sato K, Kagaya H et al: Clinical use of percutaneous intramuscular electrodes for functional electrical stimulation. Arch Phys Med Rehabil 1996; 77:1014–1018.

145. Mulcahery MJ, Betz RR: Upper and lower extremity applications of functional electrical stimulation: a decade of research with children and adolescents with spinal injuries. Pediatr Phys Ther 1997; 9:113–122.

146. Kobetic R, Triolo RJ, Marsolais EB: Muscle selection and walking performance of multichannel FES system for ambulation in paraplegia. IEEE Trans Rehabil Eng 1997; 5:23–29.

147. Krajl A, Bajd T, Turk R et al: Posture switching for prolonging functional electrical stimulation standing in paraplegic patients. Paraplegia 1986; 24:221–230.

148. Sykes L, Ross E, Powell E et al: Objective measurement of use of the reciprocating gait orthosis (RGO) and the electrically augmented RGO in adult patients with spinal cord lesions. Prosthet Orthot Int 1996; 20:182–190.

Management of impairments

CHAPTER 7
Training motor tasks
137

CHAPTER 8
Strength training
155

CHAPTER 9
Contracture management
177

CHAPTER 10
Pain management
193

CHAPTER 11
Respiratory management
205

CHAPTER 12
Cardiovascular fitness training
227

Contents

Motor control and
motor learning 137

Principles of effective
motor task training 138

Treadmill training with
body weight support.
A way of providing
intensive practice 149

Training motor tasks

Often patients with spinal cord injury are unable to perform motor tasks because they lack skill. That is, they do not know how to move optimally with their newly acquired paralysis. For example, rolling in bed is initially difficult for a patient with high-level paraplegia. An inability to roll is rarely due to lack of upper limb strength or poor joint range of motion; more often it is due to an inability to swing the arms rapidly across the body while lifting the head.[1] The task is novel and must be learnt. Some motor tasks are within themselves novel, such as performing a wheelstand.[2,3] They also must be learnt.

The learning of novel motor tasks by patients with spinal cord injury is analogous to an able-bodied person learning an unfamiliar sport such as tennis, golf or swimming. The patient, like the sports person, is unable to roll in bed or perform a wheelstand because the task requires novel patterns of muscle activation. Physiotherapists can help patients master novel motor tasks in much the same way as sports coaches can help athletes learn new sporting skills.

Motor control and motor learning

The importance of training motor tasks for patients with neurological disabilities was first advocated by Carr and Shepherd as part of their 'Motor Relearning Approach',[4–7] and later by Shumway-Cook and Woollacott in their 'Task-Oriented Approach' (also called the 'Systems Approach').[8] These approaches are based on theories about motor control and motor learning and primarily developed for the physical rehabilitation of patients with stroke and brain impairments.[5–7,9–14]

The mechanisms underlying motor control and the acquisition of motor tasks are complex and not fully understood. A range of paradigms, each with their own theories, have been used to explain motor control and motor learning.[6,8,15–18] Two key theories which have influenced neurological physiotherapy are Bernstein's 'motor schema theory'[19] and Fitts and Posner's three key stages of motor learning.[20] These theories have primarily evolved from research with able-bodied individuals and athletes, but arguably are equally applicable to patients with spinal cord injury. They are important because they help explain how patients with spinal cord injury learn motor tasks and how physiotherapists can best facilitate the learning process.

The 'motor schema theory' is based on the premise that control strategies are matched to the specific context of motor tasks. There are an infinite number of contexts for the performance of motor tasks, so it is not possible to learn separate motor strategies for all the possible contexts. Instead, it is proposed that motor tasks are largely controlled by motor schemas.[16–18] Motor schemas provide a background programme or code which dictates the timing, order and force of muscle contractions. They are like basic building blocks which dictate the general rules for movement. Once motor schemas are set down, motor tasks can be performed with a certain degree of automaticity.[21] This enables people to perform motor tasks while concentrating on other mental or physical activities. It also explains the skilled performer's ability to perform a motor task very rapidly when there is little time to rely on feedback mechanisms. Motor schemas can be modulated to accommodate variations in speed or the precise way motor tasks are performed. Patients with spinal cord injury are initially unable to perform novel motor tasks because they do not have the necessary motor schemas. New motor schemas are required to code how, when and in what way non-paralysed muscles need to contract for purposeful movement.

Fitts and Posner[20] proposed that motor tasks are learnt in three key stages. These are:

1. *Cognitive stage.* During this time people attain a general understanding and 'cognitive' map of the overall motor task. People use trial and error to gain an approximation of the motor sequencing. Attempts at movement are associated with excessive effort and unnecessary muscle contractions. Visual feedback and other sensory cues are particularly important during this stage.
2. *Associative stage.* Refinement of the motor task occurs at this point.
   The movement is performed in a more consistent way and unnecessary movements are progressively eliminated. People are increasingly attentive to proprioceptive cues which refine how movements are performed
3. *Autonomous stage.* In this stage movement becomes more automated, requiring less effort and concentration. There is little error and little unnecessary associated movements. The skill can now be successfully performed in varied environments and does not require ongoing practice to maintain competency.

Principles of effective motor task training

The training of motor tasks in patients with spinal cord injury relies on physiotherapists' problem-solving skills and their understanding of how patients with different patterns of paralysis move (see Chapters 3–6). Initially, physiotherapists need to identify the motor tasks which patients can hope to master (such as rolling, sitting unsupported, moving from lying to sitting, transferring or walking; see Chapter 2). This is formally done through the goal planning process. Patients are asked to perform these tasks and their attempts at each motor task are then analysed. The aim of the analysis is to identify which sub-tasks patients can and cannot perform, and determine the reason why patients cannot perform specific sub-tasks. The reason for failure to perform a sub-task needs to be expressed in terms of one or more impairments (usually lack of skill, strength, joint mobility or fitness). When lack of skill is the primary impairment, physiotherapists need to teach patients appropriate movement strategies. This chapter focuses on how physiotherapists can train important motor tasks which need to be learned by patients with spinal cord injury.

The importance of practice

A key feature of learning motor tasks is intense, well structured and active practice which is task- and context-specific.[4–8] Task- and context-specific practice implies practise of precisely the task which needs to be learned. For example, patients with the potential to stand need to actively and intensely practise standing[6] and patients with the potential to transfer need to practise transferring.

The practice of motor tasks, such as walking or transferring, can be difficult for patients who are at the early stages of rehabilitation and are unable to successfully perform any aspect of the task. There are two solutions. One is to provide sufficient manual assistance, supports or aids to make completion of the task possible. For example, a patient with insufficient strength in the knee extensor muscles can practise walking with overhead suspension, robotics, electrical stimulation or orthoses. Alternatively, a physiotherapist can manually support the knee in extension during stance. The second solution is to devise training drills which are 'similar but simpler'.

The 'similar but simpler' approach

The 'similar but simpler' approach requires breaking complex motor tasks into sub-tasks and practising each individually, if necessary in a simplified way.[6] Sub-tasks are progressively made more difficult as patients master them. Sub-tasks are then practised in an appropriate sequence until the whole task is mastered.

For example, a patient with C6 tetraplegia may be unable to move from lying to sitting because of an inability to bear and shift weight through the elbows in an awkward side-lying position: an essential sub-task of moving from lying to sitting (see Figure 7.1a). The patient may benefit from practising bearing and shifting weight in the same awkward position but with the elbows supported on a higher adjacent bed (see Figure 7.1b). Alternatively the patient may benefit from practising bearing and shifting weight in a prone position (see Figure 7.1c). In both instances the patient practises a motor task which is similar but simpler to the original sub-task. If patients are in the very early days of rehabilitation and unable to do either of these exercises, they might practise an even simpler variation, such as sitting in a wheelchair leaning through elbows placed on high adjacent beds (see Figure 7.2b). The

Figure 7.1 A patient with C6 tetraplegia unable to move from lying to sitting (a) may benefit from practising a 'similar but simpler' task, as seen in (b) or (c).

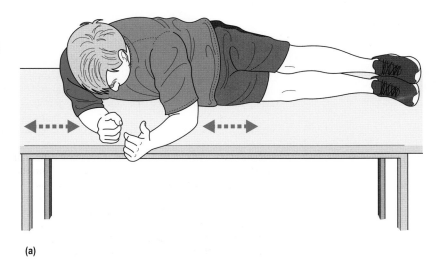

(a)

Figure 7.1 Continued

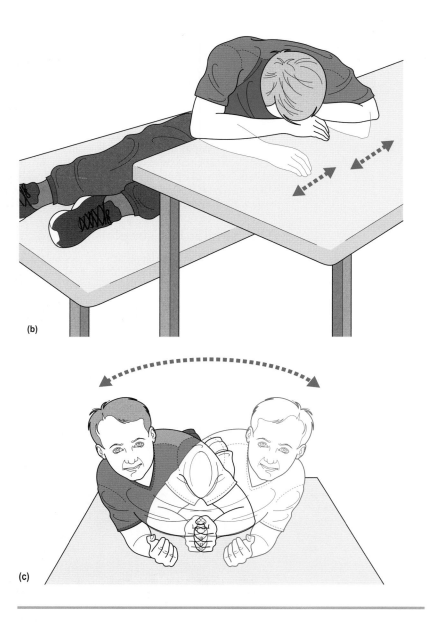

(b)

(c)

height of the bed can be adjusted to increase difficulty. These exercises are directed at improving patients' ability to bear weight through the elbows because this is an essential sub-task of moving from lying to sitting.

If the same patient was unable to transfer due to an inability to lift and shift weight forwards and laterally (see Figure 7.2a), therapy would consist of simplified drills and exercises to address this specific sub-task of transferring. For instance, the patient could practise lifting through fully extended elbows while sitting on a plinth. Small blocks could be placed under the hands if this made the task easier for the

Figure 7.2 A patient with C6 tetraplegia unable to transfer between a wheelchair and bed (a) may benefit from practising a 'similar but simpler' task, as seen in (b) and (c).

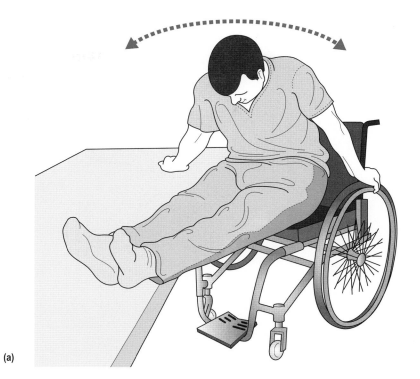

(a)

(b)

Figure 7.2   Continued

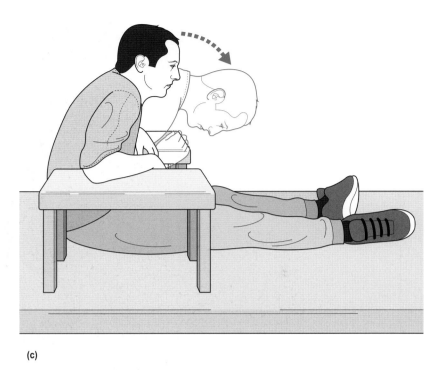

(c)

patient (see Figure 7.6). A slippery board or sheet could be placed under the legs to promote a forward slide. The patient could practise with the knees extended to minimize the likelihood of a backwards fall but then progress to lifting with the knees flexed (i.e. sitting over the edge of the plinth). Initially the patient may require trunk support but with progress this can be withdrawn. Some patients may be unable to do any of these exercises, and instead may benefit from practising something as simple as lifting body weight through flexed elbows while either sitting in a wheelchair (see Figure 7.2b) or sitting on a plinth (see Figure 7.2c).

A similar process is followed for patients with more advanced skills. For instance, a patient with thoracic paraplegia unable to perform difficult transfers in community settings might benefit from practising a similar but easier transfer between two physiotherapy plinths (see Figure 7.3). The transfer training concentrates on the particular sub-task which the patient is having difficulty with.

The principles are the same for training other motor tasks such as gait, moving from sitting to standing, or upper limb function for patients with different types of spinal cord injuries. For instance, a patient learning to walk with a reciprocating gait orthosis who is unable to swing the leg may benefit from practising the swing motion while standing one-legged on a block with the swing leg free to move. A patient learning to get from sitting to standing may benefit from initially learning to stand from a higher chair. Training of tenodesis grip might start with lifting and holding large light objects, and then progress to lifting and manipulating small heavy objects.

Regardless of what task is being trained, physiotherapists need to work backwards from the functional goal. Physiotherapists must identify the sub-tasks which patients are unable to perform and then devise similar but simpler ways of practising these sub-tasks.

Experienced physiotherapists have a large repertoire of appropriate drills and exercises for all the sub-tasks comprising the various motor tasks patients need to

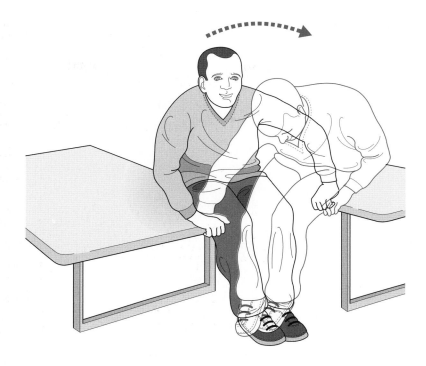

Figure 7.3 A patient with thoracic paraplegia having difficulty with horizontal transfers may benefit from practising this sub-task in a simplified way.

learn. They draw on this repertoire to provide patients with varied, interesting and effective training programmes appropriate for patients' stages of learning and rehabilitation. Examples of ways to simplify sub-tasks for training can be found throughout the tables in Chapter 3. Readers are also directed to a website developed by the author and her colleagues: www.physiotherapyexercises.com. This website describes hundreds of ways to simplify motor tasks. Alternatively, with a little imagination, physiotherapists can devise their own unique training drills.

Progression

Training needs to be appropriately progressed. This is achieved by articulating goals for each therapy session (see Chapter 2). The goals may be for very modest increments in performance, but nonetheless must be clearly defined. As soon as a goal is consistently attained, a new goal is set. The new goal may be to perform the same task in a slightly different situation, at a slightly faster pace, or while performing concurrent tasks.[21,22] Concurrent tasks might be physical or cognitive. For instance, gait training could progress to walking while carrying shopping bags or reciting numbers.[21] Initially, the patient might practise in the fairly constrained and close environment of the physiotherapy gymnasium then progress to practising in a more complex and changing community environment with its inherent distractions. Goals should be written and their achievement recorded.

Practice outside formal therapy sessions

Complex motor tasks cannot be learnt without repetitious practice.[6,23,24] Surprisingly, however, only two randomized controlled trials have looked at the effectiveness of

Figure 7.4 A training booklet to encourage and monitor practice. Booklets like this can be compiled using freely available software at www.physiotherapyexercises.com.

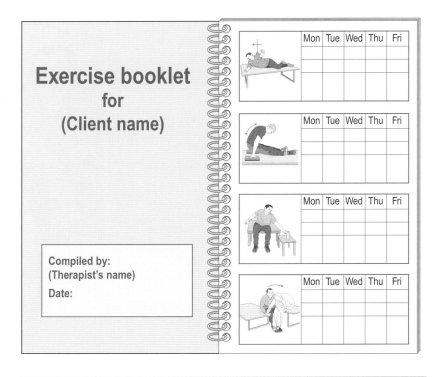

practice and training in people with spinal cord injury. Both studies looked at the effectiveness of a wheelchair skills training programme, and demonstrated the effectiveness of structured and repetitious practice for the acquisition of wheelchair skills.[25,26]

Practice needs to be performed during therapy sessions but also, wherever possible, practice should be performed in patients' own time. Practice out of therapy time should be structured with the same care as practice in therapy time. Importantly, practice outside formal therapy needs to be monitored. For example, an ambulating patient who is asked to practise stepping outside therapy should be required to record either the number of steps or the time spent on this activity. Commercially available step counters can be used for this purpose. Physiotherapists need to review written records of practice, and provide feedback on the quantity and quality of practice to reinforce the belief that practice is important. Personalized exercise booklets provide an excellent way of structuring and monitoring practice, both within and outside formal therapy sessions (see Figure 7.4). The website at www.physiotherapyexercises.com can be used to generate professional looking customized exercise booklets.

One of the biggest challenges in designing effective training programmes is ensuring they maintain interest and motivation. This can be achieved by providing a variety of exercises, setting clear and attainable goals, and progressing task difficulty as performance improves. A particularly useful strategy for maximizing interest and motivation is to provide group sessions in which patients of similar ability practise together.[11] This also serves to reduce demands on physiotherapists' time.

Other members of the rehabilitation team can encourage and promote practice outside formal therapy sessions. For instance, patients capable of transferring into bed can practise this transfer with nursing staff when getting in and out of bed each day. Patients capable of walking can walk to the bathroom and dining room as part of their daily routines. Such reinforcement of practice outside formal therapy sessions relies on good team communication, an effective goal planning process and an appreciation by all team members of the importance of a coordinated and consistent approach to rehabilitation. It also depends on good staffing levels and staff who are well trained in appropriate manual handling skills to ensure their own as well as their patients' safety.

Effective training methods

Motor learning can be enhanced by effective use of instructions, demonstrations and feedback.

Instructions

Instructions need to be tailored to the stage of learning and the patients' cognitive abilities. During the early stages of learning, instructions need to be general and targeted at the overall goal. For example, instructions appropriate for a patient's initial attempts at transferring might outline the overall purpose of the task and one or two key strategies to prevent skin damage and injury (see Chapter 3). As some overall ability to transfer is developed, instructions can become more specific. Instructions might include suggestions for positioning of the hands or for timing of the lift. Instructions need to be articulated according to patients' education and understanding of the task. Some will benefit from understanding the intricacies of movement and being cued to increase their awareness of internal feedback systems. For example, they might find it helpful to think about the position of the head in relation to the hips, or the amount of shoulder depression and trunk forward lean associated with a successful transfer. Others will be better served by the provision of external cues based on vision. For example, they might look down between their legs to ensure they have moved far enough forward in the wheelchair prior to transferring. (If the patient has moved far enough forward they should not be able to see the seat between their thighs.)

Demonstration

A demonstration of the task can provide patients with a clear idea of what they are trying to achieve. Sometimes the demonstration can be performed by the physiotherapist. Alternatively, video footage may be helpful, especially footage showing skilled performers' early attempts at movement, and their improvements over time. As patients develop competency they may benefit from viewing video footage played in slow motion. They can be cued to look at specific aspects of the movement. Patients may also benefit from seeing footage of motor tasks performed in slightly different ways. This, with appropriate guidance from a physiotherapist, may prompt them to experiment with different movement strategies. Video footage of people with spinal cord injury performing a range of motor tasks can be found at www.physiotherapyexercises.com. Physiotherapists may find it useful to compile their own video libraries for demonstration purposes.

Feedback

If practice is to be effective, the learner must receive feedback. Feedback may comprise details about the success of task performance (*knowledge of results*) or details about how well the movement is performed (*knowledge of performance*).[7] Often knowledge of results is readily available: patients will know whether they have or have not succeeded in their overall attempts at task performance provided it is clear to them what constitutes success and failure. For example, the success of transferring may be evident from the ability to get from a chair to a bed. However, knowledge of performance may be less readily available: when the task is not performed successfully patients might not know why they failed. Knowledge of performance helps patients develop strategies to correct errors and improve subsequent attempts at task performance. Patients learn to move by making and then correcting errors.[7]

The role of the physiotherapist is to provide both knowledge of results and knowledge of performance. The feedback needs to be well timed, accurate and in appropriate detail for the stage of learning. It can be provided in various ways, including with the use of video footage, mirrors, electromyography,[27–29] scales and positional feedback displays,[30,31] but most commonly it is provided in the form of verbal feedback from the physiotherapist.

Initially, verbal feedback needs to be directed at ensuring patients have knowledge of results. That is, awareness of when attempts at movement are and are not successful. With progress, feedback can become more specific. Feedback can be directed at knowledge of performance and, specifically, at the critical aspects of the movement which need to change.[7] However, feedback which is too detailed merely serves to confuse patients. Novice learners of motor tasks have difficulties concentrating on more than one aspect of performance at a time. For this reason physiotherapists need to determine the key problem and restrict feedback to this issue. Invariably this means ignoring other less critical problems for a later stage. Feedback needs to be provided soon after attempts at movement and followed up with immediate practice. Patients should be encouraged to reflect on why attempts at movement either succeeded or failed.

It is important to distinguish between verbal feedback aimed at improving performance and verbal encouragement aimed at motivating patients to persist with practice. Clearly, verbal encouragement is important and patients should be supported in their efforts. However, encouragement should not be confused with feedback. If the performance was not good, then patients should not be misled by praise for effort. Patients quickly learn to ignore repeated, effusive praise which becomes meaningless and does little to improve performance. On the other hand, constant criticism based on unrealistic expectations will undermine motivation.[32] An appropriate balance between the two extremes can be more easily achieved by setting realistic goals for each treatment session. Goals should be challenging yet achievable. During the early stages of learning, when successful task performance may be very difficult, goals can be set in terms of frequencies. For example, an appropriate goal for the early stage of learning might be to perform 10% of all attempts correctly. Alternatively, a goal may be to perform one small aspect of the whole task in a particular way.

Feedback can be provided with video footage. In this way, patients can view their own attempts at movement. Alternatively, more simple ways of providing feedback can be used. For example, a patient with C6 tetraplegia who is learning to shift and bear weight through one shoulder while prone can be given feedback by reaching for an object with one hand (see Figure 7.5). Instant feedback about ability to shift weight is provided by success in reaching for the object. For patients unable to lift their body weight in sitting, feedback can be provided with scales or an inflated blood pressure cuff under the hands (see Figure 7.6). Alternatively, a biofeedback device which generates noise or light with weight can be used. In all scenarios the patient receives instant feedback about the ability to shift body weight.

Electrical stimulation can also be used as a means of providing feedback and helping patients to learn appropriate muscle recruitment patterns.[33–36] The stimulation of specific muscles at the appropriate phase of movement provides feedback and additional

Figure 7.5 A patient with C6 tetraplegia learning to shift and bear weight through one shoulder while prone will receive instant feedback about success by attempting to reach for a target. Bathroom scales or a blood pressure cuff positioned under the weight-bearing arm can also be used to provide immediate feedback.

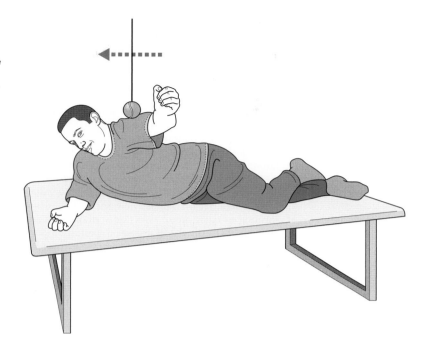

Figure 7.6 A pair of bathroom scales placed under the hands can provide feedback about success of lifting.

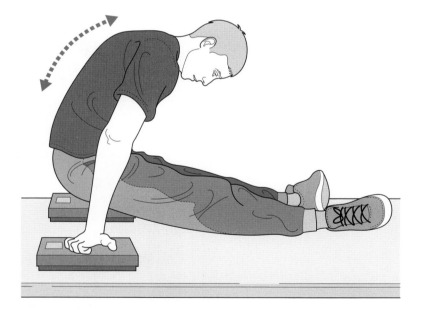

cues for successful performance. For instance, stimulation of the dorsiflexor muscles during swing can help a patient learn to recruit these muscles actively during this phase of gait. Similarly, electromyographic biofeedback can be used to encourage appropriate activation of muscles.[28] Alternatively, specific devices which provide auditory feedback about the position of joints can be used.[31] In all scenarios, the patient receives some type of feedback to improve the ability to appropriately recruit muscles for purposeful movement.

Balance

Effective movement requires the body's centre of mass to remain over the base of support. This is achieved by activating specific muscles at the right time, both before and during task performance. The postural adjustments required during particular motor tasks are specific to that task.[6,7,37] Appropriate postural adjustments prevent falling. When a task is performed without falling we say the patient is balanced.

Balance is a particular problem for patients with spinal cord injury because paralysis can render the usual postural adjustments impossible. Patients with spinal cord injury need to learn to make new postural adjustments to prevent falling while performing everyday motor tasks. Much of the training of motor tasks involves learning appropriate postural adjustments to perform motor tasks without falling.

The use of the term 'balance' is, however, problematic because it implies that balance is a discrete motor task. Yet it is not possible to separate balance from the successful performance of motor tasks. They are one and the same thing.[6,7,37] This has important implications for training. It suggests that balance should not be taught out of context of functional motor tasks. For example, if a patient with thoracic paraplegia has difficulty staying upright when repositioning the hands during a transfer manoeuvre then the patient needs to practise staying upright while transferring (see Figure 7.7). There may be little value in practising 'sitting balance' outside of the

Figure 7.7 A patient with T4 paraplegia having difficulty maintaining an upright position while repositioning the hands during transfers may benefit from practising repositioning the hands in a 'similar but simpler' task while sitting on the edge of a plinth.

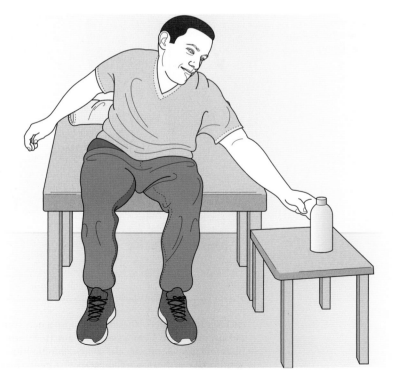

context of transfers, for example by catching and throwing a ball in sitting. Throwing and catching a ball may require quite different postural adjustments to those required while transferring.

Treadmill training with body weight support. A way of providing intensive practice

It is difficult to provide task- and context-specific practice of stepping and walking for patients with the potential to walk but with extensive lower limb weakness. Ideally, practice needs to involve stepping and walking in an upright and weight-bearing position. However, this may be difficult for patients with significant lower limb paralysis because often they require extensive physical assistance to remain upright and move their legs. Providing this assistance can be strenuous for physiotherapists and can cause injury to patients and therapists.

One relatively simple way to reduce the effort and risk of practice is to use orthoses or walking aids. For example, if a patient with an incomplete lesion is having difficulty walking because of knee collapse during stance, a knee extension orthosis can be used (see Chapter 6). However, walking with an orthosis does not require the use of the same muscles as walking without an orthosis. It would therefore be better if patients could practise without an orthosis in a way which does not depend on excessive manual assistance from physiotherapists.

Overhead suspension with partial body weight support can be used to avoid orthoses and provide a more normal walking pattern without the need for physiotherapists to physically hold patients upright. It provides a way of enabling very disabled patients to engage in intensive gait practice using a relatively normal walking pattern.[38,39] Electrical stimulation[40] and robotics[41,42] can be used to drive the legs. Alternatively, there are gait training devices incorporating motor-driven footplates which move the legs backwards and forwards on the spot in standing.[43-46] The relative effectiveness of these different interventions is unclear, although presumably interventions which closely mimic gait and encourage active recruitment of muscles are more likely to have lasting therapeutic effects than interventions which do not.

Walking with partial body weight support can be done overground or on a treadmill (see Figure 7.8).[47-51] Overground walking is achieved with a mobile suspension system which moves as the patient walks. These systems generally provide less stability because the entire apparatus moves with the patient in any direction. Some patients will be unable to walk in a straight line with overground suspension unless a physiotherapist guides the apparatus. In contrast, the treadmill suspension system is fixed in place over the belt of the treadmill so there is usually no need to control the direction in which the patient walks. The speed and incline of the treadmill can be changed to accommodate a patient's skill level.

There are advantages and disadvantages of treadmill and overground walking but one clear difference is the opportunity for practice. Treadmill walking reduces reliance of more independent walkers on physiotherapists, thus increasing the opportunity for practice.[52] It also provides a means of encouraging patients to walk faster and with a more appropriate inter-limb coordination.[53] Some argue that treadmill walking helps ensure that patients fully extend the hips at the end of stance,[48] although others argue that the hip extension provided by the treadmill is passive and does not encourage active recruitment of the hip extensor muscles.[54]

Treadmill walking may have an additional and important benefit over other types of gait training devices. Accumulating evidence indicates that some sensory aspect associated with stepping on a treadmill triggers a spinal cord-mediated stepping

Figure 7.8 A patient with incomplete tetraplegia walking on a treadmill with overhead suspension and manual assistance from a physiotherapist.

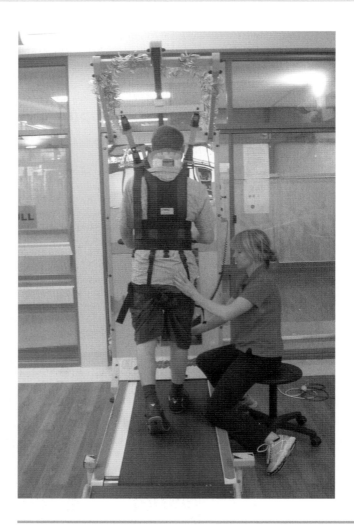

response[54-57] and that this response is trainable.[39,58-63] Some believe that treadmill walking can improve neurological recovery in people with spinal cord injury.[47,48,54,59,61,63-65]

There is little doubt that, in animals, stepping is orchestrated within the spinal cord. The spinal cord networks which control stepping have been referred to as central pattern generators. As early as 1906, Sherrington was able to elicit coordinated rhythmic movements in the hind limbs of animals with complete transections of the spinal cord.[66] Since this time, similar types of cyclical motor response, such as scratching and paw shaking, have been demonstrated in animals with transections of the spinal cord.[67,68] Central pattern generators for walking have also been demonstrated in infants and people with spinal cord injury.[56,57] Technically, these cannot be called reflexes as they are too complex and involve rhythmic and reciprocal activation of many muscles. However, in other respects, they are similar to reflexes because once triggered they can be generated without input from higher centres. Central pattern generators provide spinal cord integrated coding for certain complex but repetitive motor behaviours. This coding is normally modulated by input from higher centres and sensory feedback from muscle and cutaneous receptors.[57]

In animals, central pattern generators can be trained with treadmill walking. Studies of cats have shown that they can regain the ability to step independently with their hind limbs on a treadmill even if the spinal cord is completely transected.[69] The ability to step is, however, only regained after intensive stepping on a treadmill, initially with body weight support and maximal assistance but ultimately without support or assistance. It is believed that some aspect of cyclic walking provides a sufficiently strong sensory stimulus to the spinal cord to stimulate neural rearrangement within the spared spinal networks. This enables the cat to ultimately step independently with the hind limbs on the treadmill, even though there is no input from higher centres. These findings in animals underpin the current intense interest in the potential therapeutic role of gait training with treadmills in people with spinal cord injury.[69–71] Perhaps the same neural adaptations demonstrated in cats in response to cyclic walking on a treadmill can also be triggered in people with spinal cord injury. At this stage, attention has primarily been directed at using treadmill training for people with incomplete lesions and some potential to walk, not for people with complete spinal cord injury.

Single case studies and uncontrolled clinical trials in people with incomplete spinal cord injury provide some evidence of physiological benefits of intense treadmill walking with overhead suspension.[48,54,72–82] However, the results of these studies need to be interpreted with caution, both because they lack the rigorous control of randomized trials and because it is not clear what mechanisms cause the observed outcomes.[83] These studies do not necessarily indicate that central pattern generators have been trained[39,58,61] because it is possible that treadmill training has a peripheral strengthening effect on already innervated muscle fibres.[84] The benefits of treadmill walking on neural growth and regeneration of the damaged spinal cord are yet to be demonstrated.[58]

Studies of the physiological effects of treadmill training are interesting but they do not tell us whether the intervention is of clinical benefit. Proof of clinical benefit requires rigorously designed clinical trials to tell us if treadmill training improves the ability of people with spinal cord injury to walk more than simpler methods of gait training. One large randomized controlled trial involving 146 patients with recent but incomplete spinal cord injury compared treadmill training with conventional gait training methods. Conventional gait training consisted of standing and stepping practice with orthoses, aids, manual assistance and, if necessary, parallel bars.[60] Importantly, all patients in both groups received the same overall time on gait-related activities. Treadmill training did not produce consistently better outcomes than conventional training. These results are in keeping with a Cochrane systematic review which summarized the results of randomized controlled trials in people following stroke.[85] Similar conclusions have been drawn by others.[86,87] These results imply there is nothing therapeutically unique about treadmill gait training.[88] Treadmill training is probably no more or less effective than other ways of providing intensive task- and context-specific practice to patients with the potential to walk.[39,83]

References

1. Tanaka S, Yoshimura O, Kobayashi R et al: Three-dimensional measurement of rolling in tetraplegia patients. Spinal Cord 2000; 38:683–686.
2. Kirby RL, Dupuis DJ, MacPhee AH et al: The Wheelchair Skills Test (version 2.4): measurement properties. Arch Phys Med Rehabil 2004; 85:794–804.
3. Kirby RL, Swuste J, Dupuis DJ et al: The wheelchair skills test: a pilot study of a new outcome measure. Arch Phys Med Rehabil 2002; 83:10–18.
4. Carr JH, Shepherd RB: A Motor Relearning Programme for Stroke. London, Heinemann Medical, 1982.

5. Carr JH, Shepherd RB: A Motor Relearning Programme for Stroke, 2nd edn. Oxford, Heinemann Physiotherapy, 1987.

6. Carr J, Shepherd RB: A motor learning model for rehabilitation of the movement disabled. In Ada L, Canning C (eds): Key Issues in Neurological Physiotherapy. Oxford, Butterworth Heinemann, 1990.

7. Carr JH, Shepherd RB: A motor relearning model for rehabilitation. In Carr JH, Shepherd RB (eds): Movement Science: Foundations for Physical Therapy in Rehabilitation. Rockville, MD, Aspen, 2000:33–110.

8. Shumway-Cook A, Woollacott MH: Motor control: Issues and theories. In Shumway-Cook A, Woollacott MH (eds): Motor Control. Theory and Practical Applications. Philadelphia, Lippincott Williams & Wilkins, 2001:1–25.

9. Shumway-Cook A, Wollacott MH: A conceptual framework for clinical practice. In Shumway-Cook A, Woollacott MH (eds): Motor Control: Translating Research into Clinical Practice. Philadelphia, Lippincott Williams & Wilkins, 2001:110–126.

10. Richards CL, Malouin F, Wood-Dauphinee S et al: Task-specific physical therapy for optimization of gait recovery in acute stroke patients. Arch Phys Med Rehabil 1993; 74:612–620.

11. Dean CM, Richards CL, Malouin F: Task-related circuit training improves performance of locomotor tasks in chronic stroke: a randomized, controlled pilot trial. Arch Phys Med Rehabil 2000; 81:409–417.

12. Chan DYL, Chan CCH, Au KS: Motor relearning programme for stroke patients: a randomized controlled trial. Clin Rehabil 2006; 20:191–200.

13. Dean C, Shepherd R: Task-related training improves performance of seated reaching tasks after stroke. A randomized controlled trial. Stroke 1997; 28:722–728.

14. Langhammer B, Stranghelle JK: Bobath or motor relearning programme? A comparison of two different approaches of physiotherapy in stroke rehabilitation: a randomized controlled study. Clin Rehabil 2000; 14:361–369.

15. Gentile AM: Skill acquisition: action, movement, and neuromotor processes. In Carr JH, Shepherd RB (eds): Movement Science: Foundations for Physical Therapy in Rehabilitation. Rockville, MD, Aspen, 2000:111–187.

16. Schmidt RA: Motor Control and learning: A Behavioral Emphasis, 3rd edn. Champaign, IL, Human Kinetics, 1999.

17. Tremblay L, Welsh TN, Elliott D: Specificity versus variability: effects of practice conditions on the use of afferent information for manual aiming. Motor Control 2001; 5:347–360.

18. O'Sullivan SB: Strategies to Improve Motor Control and Motor Learning. Philadelphia, FA Davis, 2000.

19. Bernstein N: The Coordination and Regulation of Movement. London, Pergamon Press, 1967.

20. Fitts P, Posner MI: Human Performance. Belmont, CA, Brooks/Cole, 1967.

21. Paul SS, Ada L, Canning CG: Automaticity of walking — implications for physiotherapy practice. Phy Ther Reviews 2005; 10:15–23.

22. Orrell AJ, Eves FF, Masters RS: Motor learning of a dynamic balancing task after stroke: implicit implications for stroke rehabilitation. Phys Ther 2006; 86:369–380.

23. Johnson P: The acquisition of skill. In Smyth MM, Wind AM (eds): The Psychology of Human Movement. London, Academic Press, 1984:215–240.

24. Newell A, Rosenbloom PS: Mechanisms of skill acquisition and the law of practice. In Anderson JE (ed): Cognitive Skills and their Acquisition. Hillsdale, NJ, Lawrence Erlbaum, 1981:1–55.

25. MacPhee AH, Kirby RL, Coolen AL et al: Wheelchair skills training program: a randomized clinical trial of wheelchair users undergoing initial rehabilitation. Arch Phys Med Rehabil 2004; 85:41–50.

26. Best KL, Kirby RL, Smith C et al: Wheelchair skills training for community–based manual wheelchair users: a randomized controlled trial. Arch Phys Med Rehabil 2005; 86:2316–2323.

27. Morris ME, Matyas TA, Bach T et al: Electrogoniometric feedback: its effect on genu recurvatum in stroke. Arch Phys Med Rehabil 1992; 73:1147–1154.

28. Intiso D, Santilli V, Grasso MG et al: Rehabilitation of walking with electromyographic biofeedback in foot-drop after stroke. Stroke 1994; 25:1189–1192.

29. Schleenbaker RE, Mainous AG: Electromyographic biofeedback for neuromuscular reeducation in the hemiplegic stroke patient: a meta-analysis. Arch Phys Med Rehabil 1993; 74:1301–1304.

30. Winchester P, Montgomery J, Bowman B et al: Effects of feedback stimulation training and cyclical electrical stimulation on knee extension in hemiparetic patients. Phys Ther 1983; 63:1096–1103.

31. Mandel AR, Nymark JR, Balmer SJ et al: Electromyographic versus rhythmic positional biofeedback in computerized gait retraining with stroke patients. Arch Phys Med Rehabil 1990; 71:649–654.

32. Parry R: A video analysis of how physiotherapists communicate with patients about errors of performance: insights for practice and policy. Physiotherapy 2005; 91:204–214.

33. Bogataj U, Gros N, Malezic M et al: Restoration of gait during two to three weeks of therapy with multichannel electrical stimulation. Phys Ther 1989; 69:319–327.

34. Klose KJ, Schmidt DL, Needham BM et al: Rehabilitation therapy for patients with long-term spinal cord injuries. Arch Phys Med Rehabil 1990; 71:659–662.
35. Chae J: Neuromuscular electrical stimulation for motor relearning in hemiparesis. Phys Med Rehabil Clin N Am 2003; 14:S92–S109.
36. Popovic MR, Thrasher TA, Adams ME et al: Functional electrical therapy: retraining grasping in spinal cord injury. Spinal Cord 2006; 44:143–151.
37. Horak FB, Henry SM, Shumway-Cook A: Postural perturbations: new insights for treatment of balance disorders. Phys Ther 1997; 77:517–533.
38. Edgerton VR, de Leon RD, Harkema SJ et al: Retraining the injured spinal cord. J Physiol 2001; 533:15–22.
39. Dobkin B: Recovery of locomotor control. Neurologist 1996; 2:239–224.
40. Postans NJ, Hasler JP, Granat MH et al: Functional electrical stimulation to augment partial weight-bearing supported treadmill training for patients with acute incomplete spinal cord injury: A pilot study. Arch Phys Med Rehabil 2004; 85:604–610.
41. Colombo G, Joerg M, Schreier R et al: Treadmill training of paraplegic patients using a robotic orthosis. J Rehabil Res Dev 2000; 37:693–700.
42. Wirz M, Zemon DH, Rupp R et al: Effectiveness of automated locomotor training in patients with chronic incomplete spinal cord injury: a multicenter trial. Arch Phys Med Rehabil 2005; 86:672–680.
43. Hesse S, Uhlenbrock D, Werner C et al: A mechanized gait trainer for restoring gait in nonambulatory subjects. Arch Phys Med Rehabil 2000; 81:1158–1161.
44. Hesse S, Uhlenbrock D, Sarkodie-Gyan T: Gait pattern of severely disabled hemiparetic subjects on a new controlled gait trainer as compared to assisted treadmill walking with partial body weight support. Clin Rehabil 1999; 13:401–410.
45. Hesse S, Uhlenbrock D: A mechanized gait trainer for restoration of gait. J Rehabil Res Dev 2000; 37:701–708.
46. Werner C, Von Frankenberg S, Treig T et al: Treadmill training with partial body weight support and an electromechanical gait trainer for restoration of gait in subacute stroke patients: a randomized crossover study. Stroke 2002; 33:2895–2901.
47. Field-Fote EC: Spinal cord control of movement: implications for locomotor rehabilitation following spinal cord injury. Phys Ther 2000; 80:477–484.
48. Field-Fote E: Combined use of body weight support, functional electrical stimulation, and treadmill training to improve walking ability in individuals with chronic incomplete spinal cord injury. Arch Phys Med Rehabil 2001; 82:818–824.
49. Barbeau H, Visintin M: Optimal outcomes obtained with body-weight support combined with treadmill training in stroke subjects. Arch Phys Med Rehabil 2003; 84:1458–1465.
50. Visintin M, Barbeau H, Korner-Bitensky N et al: A new approach to retrain gait in stroke patients through body weight support and treadmill stimulation. Stroke 1998; 29:1122–1128.
51. Barbeau H, Ladouceur M, Normam KR et al: Walking after spinal cord injury: evaluation, treatment and functional recovery. Arch Phys Med Rehabil 1999; 80:225–235.
52. Hesse S, Werner C: Poststroke motor dysfunction and spasticity: novel pharmacological and physical treatment strategies. CNS Drugs 2003; 17:1093–1107.
53. Ada L, Dean CM, Hall JM et al: A treadmill and overground walking program improves walking in persons residing in the community after stroke: a placebo-controlled, randomised trial. Arch Phys Med Rehabil 2003; 84:1486–1491.
54. Behrman AL, Harkema SJ: Locomotor training after human spinal cord injury: a series of case studies. Phys Ther 2000; 80:688–700.
55. Edgerton VR, de Leon RD, Tillakaratne NJ et al: Use-dependent plasticity in spinal stepping and standing. Adv Neurol 1997; 72:233–247.
56. Lamb T, Yang JF: Could different directions of infant stepping be controlled by the same locomotor central pattern generator? J Neurophysiol 2000; 183:2814–2824.
57. Yang JF, Gorassini M: Spinal and brain control of human walking: implications for retraining of walking. Neuroscientist 2006; 12:379–389.
58. Fouad K, Pearson K: Restoring walking after spinal cord injury. Prog Neurobiol 2004; 73: 107–126.
59. Dobkin BH: Neuroplasticity: key to recovery after central nervous system injury. West J Med 1993; 159:56–60.
60. Dobkin B, Apple D, Barbeau H et al: Weight-supported treadmill vs over-ground training for walking after acute incomplete SCI. Neurology 2006; 66:484–493.
61. Dobkin BH, Apple D, Barbeau H et al: Methods for a randomized trial of weight-supported treadmill training versus conventional training for walking during inpatient rehabilitation after incomplete traumatic spinal cord injury. Neurorehabil Neural Repair 2003; 17:153–157.
62. Dobkin BH, Harkema SJ, Requejo P et al: Modulation of locomotor-like EMG activity in subjects with complete and incomplete spinal cord injury. J Neurol Rehabil 1995; 9:183–190.
63. Harkema SJ: Neural plasticity after human spinal cord injury: application of locomotor training to the rehabilitation of walking. Neuroscientist 2001;7:455–468.

64. Edgerton VR, Roy RR, Hodgson JA et al: A physiological basis for the development of rehabilitative strategies for spinally injured patients. J Am Paraplegia Soc 1991; 14:150–157.

65. Muir GD, Steven JD: Sensorimotor stimulation to improve locomotor recovery after spinal cord injury. Trends Neurosci 1997; 20:72–77.

66. Sherrington CS: Observations on the scratch-reflex in the spinal dog. J Physiol 1906; 34:1–50.

67. Koshland GF, Smith JL: Mutable and immutable features of paw-shake responses after hindlimb deafferentation in the cat. J Neurophysiol 1989; 62:162–173.

68. Pearson KG, Rossignol S: Fictive motor patterns in chronic spinal cats. J Neurophysiol 1991; 66:1874–1887.

69. Barbeau H, Rossignol S: Recovery of locomotion after chronic spinalization in the adult cat. Brain Res 1987; 412:84–95.

70. Lovely RG, Gregor RJ, Roy RR et al: Effects of training on the recovery of full-weight-bearing stepping in the adult spinal cat. Exp Neurol 1986; 92:421–435.

71. de Leon RD, Hodgson JA, Roy RR et al: Locomotor capacity attributable to step training versus spontaneous recovery after spinalization in adult cats. J Neurophysiol 1998; 79:1329–1340.

72. Harkema SJ, Hurley SL, Patel UK et al: Human lumbosacral spinal cord interprets loading during stepping. J Neurophysiol 1997; 77:797–811.

73. Visintin M, Barbeau H: The effects of parallel bars, body weight support and speed on the modulation of the locomotor pattern of spastic paretic gait. A preliminary communication. Paraplegia 1994; 32:540–553.

74. Stewart JE, Barbeau H, Gauthier S: Modulation of locomotor patterns and spasticity with clonidine in spinal cord injured patients. Can J Neurol Sci 1991; 18:321–332.

75. Wernig A, Muller S: Laufband locomotion with body weight support improved walking in persons with severe spinal cord injuries. Paraplegia 1992; 30:229–238.

76. Wernig A, Nanassy A, Muller S: Laufband (treadmill) therapy in incomplete paraplegia and tetraplegia. J Neurotrauma 1999; 16:719–726.

77. Dietz V, Colombo G, Jensen L: Locomotor activity in spinal man. Lancet 1994; 334:1260–1263.

78. Fung J, Stewart JE, Barbeau H: The combined effects of clonidine and cyproheptadine with interactive training on the modulation of locomotion in spinal cord injured subjects. J Neurol Sci 1990; 100:85–93.

79. Wernig A, Muller S, Nanassy A et al: Laufband therapy based on 'rules of spinal locomotion' is effective in spinal cord injured persons. Eur J Neurol 1995; 7:823–829.

80. Gardnes MB, Holden MK, Leikauskas JM et al: Partial body weight support with treadmill locomotion to improve gait after incomplete spinal cord injury: a single-subject experimental design. Phys Ther 1998; 78:361–374.

81. Wernig A, Nanassy A, Muller S: Maintenance of locomotor abilities following Laufband (treadmill) therapy in para- and tetraplegic persons: follow-up studies. Spinal Cord 1998; 36:744–749.

82. Protas EJ, Holmes SA, Qureshy H et al: Supported treadmill ambulation training after spinal cord injury: a pilot study. Arch Phys Med Rehabil 2001; 82:825–831.

83. Dobkin BH: An overview of treadmill locomotor training with partial body weight support: a neurophysiologically sound approach whose time has come for randomized clinical trials. Neurorehabil Neural Repair 1999; 13:157–165.

84. Pearson KG: Could enhanced reflex function contribute to improving locomotion after spinal cord repair? J Physiol 2001; 533:75–81.

85. Moseley AM, Stark A, Cameron ID et al: Treadmill training and body weight support for walking after stroke. The Cochrane Database of Systematic Reviews 2005: Issue 4. Art. No.: CD002840. DOI: 10.1002/14651858.CD002840.pub2.

86. Manning CD, Pomeroy VM: Effectiveness of treadmill retraining on gait of hemiparetic stroke patients: systematic review of current evidence. Physiotherapy 2003; 89:337–349.

87. Sipski ML, Richards JS: Spinal cord injury rehabilitation: State of the science. Am J Phys Med Rehabil 2006; 85:310–342.

88. Wolpaw JR: Treadmill training after spinal cord injury: good but not better. Neurology 2006; 66:466–467.

Contents

Assessment of strength 157

Neurally intact muscles 163

Strength training for
partially paralysed
muscles 166

Avoiding injury and
other complications 170

Strength training for
general well-being 171

Strength training

Poor strength is the first impairment which comes to mind when people think of spinal cord injury. This reflects the importance of strength for mobility and independence.

In people with spinal cord injury, the performance of motor tasks can be limited by the strength of *completely paralysed, partially paralysed or non-paralysed* muscles. For example, a patient with thoracic paraplegia may be unable to transfer from floor to wheelchair because of complete paralysis of the lower limbs and poor strength in the upper limbs (see Figure 8.1). The obvious impairment in this case is paralysis of the lower limbs. However, paradoxically paralysis of lower limb muscles is of little immediate interest to physiotherapists because strengthening programmes cannot induce neurological repair following complete spinal cord injury. Instead, physiotherapists are primarily interested in the strength of the neurally intact upper limb muscles, notably the triceps and latissimus dorsi muscles. These upper limb muscles are not directly affected by spinal cord injury nor are they necessarily any weaker than the upper limb muscles of most able-bodied individuals. However, 'normal' upper limb strength is typically not sufficient to lift the entire body weight off the floor. To master this motor task, patients need to develop strength over and above that typically required by able-bodied individuals. Upper limb strength may be an even greater problem in patients who are deconditioned from extended periods of prior bedrest or who are overweight. The appropriate intervention is a strengthening programme which specifically targets the ability of the triceps and latissimus dorsi muscles to generate force.

Often the performance of motor tasks is limited by strength of partially paralysed muscles.[1] For example, a patient with C6 tetraplegia may have partial paralysis of the pectoralis muscles due to damage of some, but not all, motor neurons innervating the pectoralis muscles. Weakness of the pectoralis muscles may limit shoulder horizontal adduction and hence prevent rolling in bed (see Chapter 3). Likewise, a patient with incomplete paraplegia may have partial paralysis of the tibialis anterior muscles, and therefore may be unable to hold the ankle dorsiflexed during the swing phase of gait. In these examples, the appropriate intervention is a strengthening programme for the partially paralysed muscles.

Figure 8.1 Transfer from floor to wheelchair for a patient with thoracic paraplegia. Patients are often unable to perform this task because of insufficient strength in the triceps and latissimus dorsi muscles.

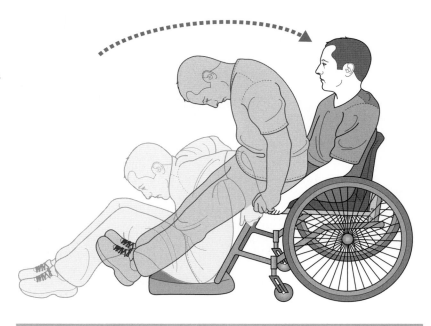

The performance of motor tasks can also be limited by *muscle power*. Power refers to the amount of work done over a specified period of time.[2] For example, lifting a set weight rapidly requires more muscle power than lifting the same weight slowly. Muscle power is important for motor tasks which need to be done at high speed. In the able-bodied population, the vertical jump is commonly provided as a good example of a task requiring high levels of lower limb power.[3] There are comparable tasks for patients with spinal cord injury where large forces need to be generated at high speeds.[2] For instance, pushing a manual wheelchair up a slope or jumping up steps with bilateral knee–ankle–foot orthoses requires upper limb power.

Motor tasks can also be limited by muscle endurance. *Muscle endurance* refers to the ability of muscles to generate force over extended periods of time. For example, a patient with incomplete paraplegia may have sufficient lower limb strength to walk about the physiotherapy gymnasium but insufficient muscle endurance to walk about a shopping centre.

Small changes in strength, power and endurance can have important implications for the ability to perform motor tasks, particularly in patients with tetraplegia. For example, a small increase in the strength of the shoulder flexor muscles of a patient with C5 tetraplegia can make the difference between attaining and not attaining independence with feeding (see Chapter 5, Figure 5.3). A subtle increase in wrist extensor strength of a patient with C6 tetraplegia can make the difference between useful and very limited hand function.[4] Similarly, small changes in lower limb strength can have implications even for very weak patients unable to walk. The ability to move the legs even slightly can make it easier to transfer.

The broad aims and approaches to physiotherapy are similar regardless of whether the problem is one of strength, power or endurance and regardless of whether the problem is with partially paralysed or non-paralysed muscles. In all cases, the focus of training is driven by an analysis of task performance (see Chapter 2). This determines which muscles are targeted and how training is best structured.

Assessment of strength

Strength can be measured in several ways. Some methods are quick and easy while others are more time-consuming and require elaborate equipment. All reflect the ability of muscles to maximally generate force and all have differing levels of reliability, sensitivity and validity. Brief discussions of the most common ways to assess strength are provided below. The appropriate type of assessment depends on the purpose of the assessment as well as the strength and mobility of the patient.

Manual muscle test

Manual muscle tests have traditionally been used by physiotherapists to measure strength of patients with spinal cord injury. There are numerous variations in the way manual muscles tests are performed.[5] One type of manual muscle test rates strength of individual muscles (e.g. the brachioradialis and brachialis)[6] and another rates strength of muscle groups (e.g. the elbow flexor muscles).[7] Strength is usually assessed on either a six-point[8] or 11-point scoring system, although there are variations on these systems.[6] For example, the original six-point scoring system is sometimes used with transitional grades ('plus' and 'minus' grades). Some physiotherapists replace the numeric scales with descriptors such as 'trace', 'poor', 'fair', 'good' and 'normal' (see Table 8.1). To add further confusion, sometimes grade 4/5 and 5/5 strength is tested with resistance applied as patients move through full range of motion,[8] and at other times these higher grades are tested with resistance applied during an isometric contraction.[6] A range of testing positions are used, and these are documented in several classic texts which describe manual muscle test protocols.[8,9] The manual muscle test used as part of the ASIA assessment is yet another variation. The ASIA assessment uses the six-point scale but all testing is conducted with the patient in the supine position.[10] In the ASIA assessment only 10 muscles representing the C5 to T1 and L2 to S1 myotomes are tested (see Chapter 1 for details).

The results of manual muscle tests correlate broadly with more objective measures of strength.[11,12] For example, patients with grade 4/5 strength attain higher dynamometric measures of isometric strength than patients with grade 3/5 strength. However, this conceals an important limitation of manual muscle tests identified over 50 years ago,[13] namely their poor sensitivity. This is particularly apparent with grade 4/5 and 5/5 strength.[4,14–20] Grades 4/5 and 5/5 encompass a much wider range of strengths than that encompassed by grades 0/5 to 3/5. Consequently, two patients with grade 4/5 strength can have clinically important differences in strength. As a result, manual muscle tests are of limited use for testing strength of stronger patients.[17] Manual muscle tests also have limited use in patients with marked spasticity.[19] It is often difficult to distinguish between voluntary strength and spasticity, especially if spasticity is elicited with attempts at movement during testing.

Despite some of the inherent problems of manual muscle tests, they are still useful for broadly identifying neurological weakness and detecting marked neurological deterioration or improvement. This is particularly important for acutely-injured patients when it is important to monitor the effects of interventions such as surgical decompressions. Manual muscle tests are also useful because the results are readily interpretable by all, including patients.

The frequency with which manual muscle tests are performed is often determined by hospital protocols. Muscle tests may need to be done daily, or sometimes even several times a day if a patient's neurological status is rapidly changing. However, once neurological status has stabilized manual muscle tests can be done less frequently.

TABLE 8.1   Different ways of scoring results of manual muscle test

Descriptive scoring system		6-point scoring system	11-point scoring system	Definition
Normal	N	5	10	Full available ROM, against gravity, strong manual resistance
Good plus	G+	4+	9	Full available ROM, against gravity, nearly strong manual resistance
Good	G	4	8	Full available ROM, against gravity, moderate manual resistance
Good minus	G−	4−	7	Full available ROM, against gravity, nearly moderate manual resistance
Fair plus	F+	3+	6	Full available ROM, against gravity, slight manual resistance
Fair	F	3	5	Full available ROM, against gravity, no resistance
Fair minus	F−	3−	4	At least 50% ROM, against gravity, no resistance
Poor plus	P+	2+	3	Full available ROM, gravity eliminated, slight manual resistance
Poor	P	2	2	Full available ROM, gravity eliminated, no resistance
Poor minus	P−	2−	1	At least 50% ROM, gravity eliminated, no resistance
Trace plus	T+	1+		Minimal observable motion (less than 50% ROM), gravity minimized, no resistance
Trace	T	1	T	No observable motion, palpable muscle contraction, no resistance
Zero	0	0	0	No observable or palpable muscle contraction

From White DJ: Musculoskeletal assessment. In O'Sullivan SB, Schmitz TJ (eds): Physical Rehabilitation: Assessment and Treatment, 5th edition. Philadelphia, FA Davis, 2007, Table 6.6, p. 181, with permission.

For example, after the acute phase, it may be appropriate to perform manual muscle tests every 3–4 weeks and thereafter every 3–4 months. Once patients have been discharged from rehabilitation, manual muscle tests are performed less frequently and primarily used to monitor neurological status and detect neurological complications such as syringomyelia.[21] Syringomyelia can occur many years after injury and lead to loss of strength, typically in the myotomes immediately above the level of the injury.

One repetition maximum

Strength can by assessed by determining the 'one repetition maximum' (1 RM).[22,23] This test is appropriate for muscle groups with grade 4/5 and 5/5 strength. One repetition maximum refers to the maximum weight a patient can lift through an entire range of motion against gravity. The physiotherapist initially estimates a weight which the patient will only just be able to lift. The patient attempts to lift that weight. If the weight can be lifted two or more times it is less than the true 1 RM. If it cannot be lifted at all with a maximum effort it is greater than the 1 RM. Testing involves adjusting the weight until it can be lifted but not more than once. This weight is the 1 RM. It is important that patients receive sufficient rest between each attempt to avoid fatigue.[23,24] Testing the 1 RM of multiple muscles can be time-consuming and may need to be done over two or more occasions.

To determine the 1 RM of most upper and lower limb muscles, the weight is secured to the wrist or ankle, commonly with wrap-around velcro weights (see Figure 8.2a). For the upper limbs, a dumbbell can be held in the hand if patients have sufficient grasp (see Figure 8.2b). Alternatively, a weight and pulley system can be used (see Figure 8.2c). When using a weight and pulley system to assess 1 RM it is important to ensure the line of pull is reproducible on subsequent tests; this is best done by ensuring that the line of pull is perpendicular to the limb when halfway through range of motion. The weight a patient can lift using a weight and pulley system does not correspond with the weight a patient can lift using a dumbbell because the same weight generates a different torque when lifted in the two ways.

A 'modified' 1 RM can be used to measure strength in muscles with grade 3/5 or less strength. Instead of lifting a weight against gravity, the patient moves a weight horizontally. The limb is supported using slideboards or overhead suspension (see Figure 8.6). Alternatively, devices can be used which counteract the weight of limbs, enabling very weak patients to move in anti-gravity positions (see Figure 8.7).

Hand-held myometers

Strength can also be measured with hand-held myometers. Myometers are small portable devices used to test isometric strength (see Figure 8.3).[4,14,15,25,26] There are mechanical and electronic versions. All provide measures of force, not torque. Reliability is dependent on replicating the position of the patient, the position of the myometer and the angle at which the force is directed through the myometer.[25–31] Myometers are more difficult to use in stronger patients because physiotherapists cannot always provide adequate resistance and stabilization especially when testing the larger lower limb muscles.[16,30,32] Hand-held myometers are useful for testing strength in patients confined to bed, although it is not always possible to test all

Figure 8.2 Examples of ways to test and train strength for the hamstring muscles using a velcro wrap-around sandbag weight (a), the shoulder flexors using a dumbbell weight (b), the shoulder adductor muscles using weights and pulleys (c), the shoulder abductor muscles using equipment (d), and the shoulder adductor and elbow extensor muscles using a high bed (e).

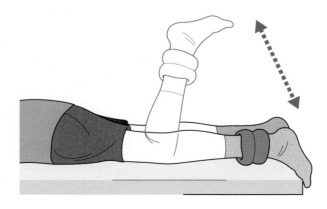

(a)

Figure 8.2 Continued

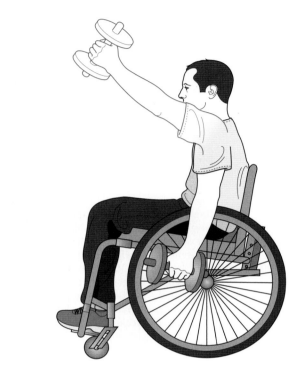

(b)

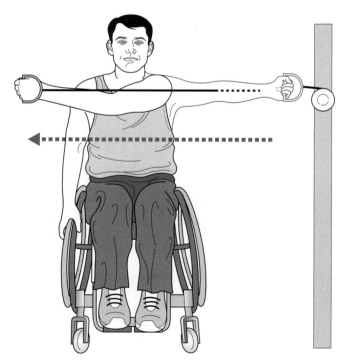

(c)

Figure 8.2 Continued

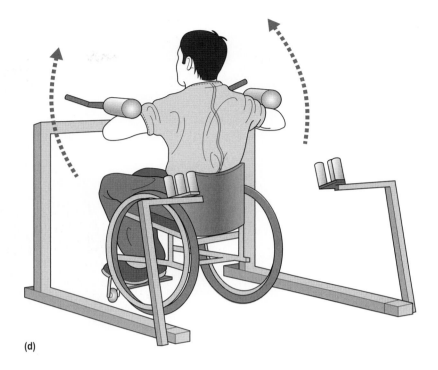

(d)

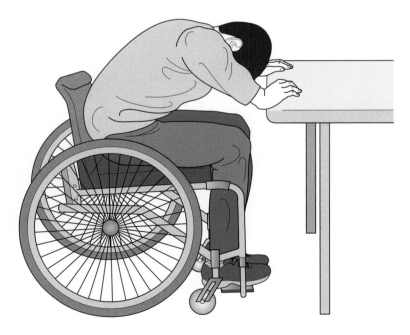

(e)

Figure 8.3 Use of an electronic hand-held myometer to test isometric strength of the elbow flexor muscles.

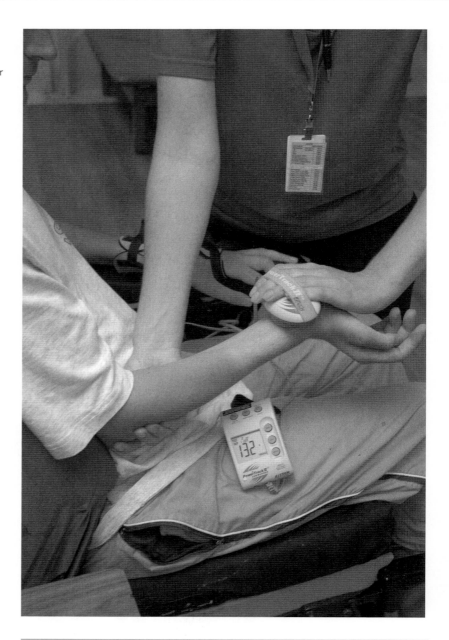

muscles. For example, it is not possible to test the strength of the hip extensor muscles in patients restricted to the supine position.

Isokinetic dynamometers

Isokinetic dynamometers measure torque during dynamic (concentric or eccentric) contractions at a constant angular velocity.[16,32,33] They are not commonly used in spinal cord injury units because the equipment is expensive, not easy to adjust when testing many muscle groups, and not appropriate for patients with profound weakness or patients restricted to bed.[2,16]

Neurally intact muscles

Most of what is known about strength training of neurally intact muscles comes from studies in healthy able-bodied individuals. These studies indicate that training typically increases strength by approximately 2% per week.[34,35] Gains in strength are greater during the early stages of training, especially in previously deconditioned individuals. However, strength continues to improve over extended periods of time if training is sustained. Males and females of all ages benefit in a similar way from strength training.[34,36,37]

Training increases muscle fibre cross-sectional area and leads to muscle hypertrophy. These changes are well correlated with increases in strength. Training also induces other morphological and histochemical changes. For example, it changes the protein content of muscles, increases the density of capillaries and prompts fibre type conversion.[22,38–40] Improvements in strength with training may also be due to better motor unit synchronization, firing and recruitment.[41–51] Evidence to support these types of neural adaptations come from studies demonstrating increases in strength of untrained limbs in response to imagined training[49] or training of contralateral limbs.[44–46,52] At least with short-term training it is thought that increases in strength are not due primarily to muscle hypertrophy. Instead increases in strength have been attributed to improvements in synchronization, firing and recruitment of motor units.[46] These neural adaptations may be due to changes within the spinal and supraspinal sensorimotor networks.[43,45,46,52]

Progressive resistance training

Strength is best improved with progressive resistance training. The key aspects of progressive resistance training are resistance, repetition and progression.[53] The optimal resistance is equivalent to an 8–12 repetition maximum (RM). This means that if training involves lifting dead weights the weight needs to be adjusted so that after 8–12 lifts the patient cannot possibly lift the weight again.[54,55] This weight is normally equivalent to about 60–80% of a 1 RM.[41,55,56] In a training session the patient should repeatedly lift this weight 8–12 times. Typically, the patient would then rest for 1–3 minutes before repeating the process a second and third time. The whole process should be repeated two to three times a week.[41,57] As the patient gets stronger the weight is increased (that is, training is 'progressed'). The patient should not be able to lift the weight more than 8–12 times.

These principles of progressive resistance training can be applied to most types of strengthening programmes, regardless of whether the exercise involves lifting weights, using isokinetic strengthening equipment, pulling on theraband[22] or practising motor tasks (see Figure 8.2).

There is considerable debate and research around subtle questions relating to optimal protocols for progressive resistance training.[22,53–55,58–61] For instance, while most advocate multiple sets within a training session, one review argues that there is now sufficient evidence to indicate that one set is equally effective.[61] Some evidence suggests that training with long rests between sets (3 minutes) is superior to training with shorter rests (40 seconds), that eccentric strengthening is superior to concentric strengthening[41,62,63] and that varying the load between sessions is better than fixing the load.[64,65] Similarly, there is some evidence that the speed at which the weight is lifted may be important.[53,60,66,67] These controversies have not yet been resolved, but there remains broad agreement that regular, progressive high-resistance exercise is needed to increase strength. Such programmes continue to be recommended by the American College of Sports Medicine.[57]

Specificity of training

The effects of progressive resistance training are specific to the way training is performed. That is, strength training will be most effective when it closely mimics the way muscles are required to generate torque. This includes mimicking factors such as the need for co-contraction, the position of the joint, the type (i.e. eccentric, concentric or isometric) and speed of contraction.[41,68] For this reason strength training for a particular functional task is best done as far as possible within the context of that specific motor task. For instance, upper limb strength training aimed at increasing the ability of patients with paraplegia to get from the floor into a wheelchair could involve lifting upwards and backwards from a small stool positioned in front of the wheelchair or lifting sideways between two stools (see Figure 8.4a,b). Weaker patients can practise lifting their body weight in long-sitting, with or without externally applied resistance.[69] As the patient becomes stronger strength training can be performed during practice of the whole task. That is, by moving between the floor and wheelchair. Strengthening in this way helps ensure that training targets the right muscles and involves muscle contractions at the speeds and muscle lengths required for the motor task.[41,68] For example, it strengthens muscles used for stabilization which might otherwise be neglected in a training programme consisting solely of lifting weights.

It is important that training done within the context of motor tasks involves contracting muscles against sufficient resistance to induce a training effect. For example, if training involves lifting from blocks, the height of the blocks should be adjusted so that the patient can perform between 8 and 12 repetitions of the lift but no more. Sometimes it is difficult to adhere to these principles because patients are limited by factors such as their ability to maintain an upright position. If it is not possible to control training intensity within the context of motor tasks, strength training is probably best done using strengthening equipment such as dead weights.

Training muscle power and endurance

Progressive resistance strength training has carry-over effects on muscle power and endurance.[40] All are closely related. However, to further target power, training needs to involve speed with an emphasis on 'explosive' power rather than just generation of high forces. To achieve speed, lighter loads are required (i.e. 30–60% 1 RM). Power training can also be done within the context of motor tasks. For example, a programme aimed at increasing upper limb power for wheelchair propulsion might consist of pushing up inclines as quickly as possible with extra weight placed on the wheelchair.[2] Similarly a programme to improve a patient's ability to lift themselves upstairs with knee–ankle–foot orthoses might consist of repeated rapid shoulder depression exercises in standing within the parallel bars (see Figure 8.5). Resistance can be applied by attaching weights to the ankles. Alternatively, arm ergometers can be used to train general upper limb power (see Chapter 12, Figure 12.1). For example, patients can cycle against a fixed load as fast as possible in 30-second bouts.[70]

Progressive resistance training also has carry-over effects on endurance.[22] However, to further target endurance, training needs to place a sustained demand on muscles. This requires low to moderate resistance with high repetitions (20 or more) and minimal time for recovery between sets (less than 1 minute if doing 10–15 repetitions,

Figure 8.4 Two different ways of performing strength training to improve the ability to move between floor and wheelchair: lifting up backwards from a stool positioned in front of the wheelchair (a), and lifting between two low stools (b). It is important that the tasks provide resistance equivalent to 8–12 RM.

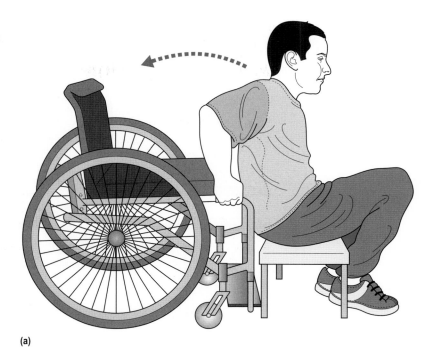

(a)

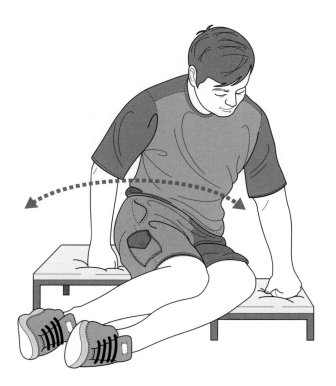

(b)

Figure 8.5 Muscle power of the upper limbs can be increased by practising repeated lifts in quick succession within parallel bars. Weights can be attached to the ankles to add resistance.

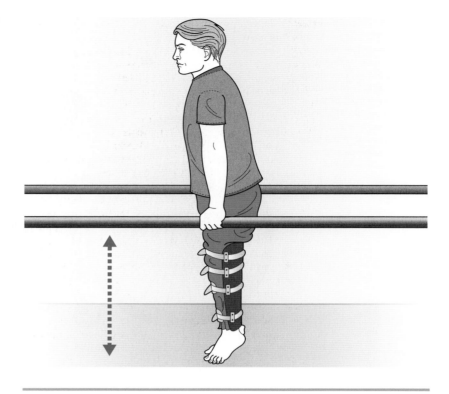

and 1–3 minutes if doing 15–20 repetitions). The repetitions are done at high training velocities (i.e. 180° per sec).[22] In general, endurance exercise is likely to be most effective when the exercise closely resembles the task which is to be trained.

Effective strength, endurance and power training requires considerable exertion and discomfort. It cannot be easily done by patients without supervision unless patients have had prior strength training experience. The challenge for physiotherapists is to motivate patients to exercise against sufficient resistance to optimize the training effect. Patients are most likely to maintain motivation if training is varied and has an enjoyable and social aspect. Strength training within group settings is particularly useful for this purpose. Motivation is also improved by setting SMART goals and ensuring progress is monitored and recorded (see Chapter 2).

Sometimes it may be necessary to compromise the quality of strength-training programmes to ensure adherence.[54,71,72] Programmes with a few carefully selected exercises which are continued will achieve a better outcome than more comprehensive and demanding programmes which are abandoned. Patients may also reap some benefit if they train less frequently than three times a week[73] or with fewer than three sets,[53,71] or perhaps even if they train with lighter loads.[41,53,58,71,74,75] However, the *optimal* strengthening programmes involve multiple sets of regular high-resistance exercise.

Strength training for partially paralysed muscles

While a lot is known about strength training for non-paralysed muscles, the same cannot be said for training of partially paralysed muscles following spinal cord injury.

There are few clinical trials in this area,[73,76–79] and few involving patients with other neurological disabilities.[18,80–94] Evidence about the carry-over effects of strength training on mobility are as yet inconclusive.[18,94,95]

It is generally assumed that the most effective way to increase strength in partially paralysed muscles is by adopting the same principles of progressive resistance training which are recommended for non-paralysed muscles. Exercises for muscles with grade 2/5 strength are done in gravity-eliminated positions. The easiest way to do this is to exercise in a horizontal plane. For example, the biceps muscles can be trained in side-lying with slings to support the arm (see Figure 8.6a). From this position patients flex the elbow horizontally through range. Similarly, patients with grade 2/5 strength in their hamstring muscles can flex the knee while lying on their sides with a slideboard between their legs (see Figure 8.6b). In these examples the only resistance to movement is provided by the passive properties of the joints and the friction of the slideboard. As soon as patients can move through range 8–12 times with gravity eliminated then patient position is changed and the limb is lifted against gravity. The resistance can be gradually increased by progressively rotating the plane of the movement away from the horizontal. Alternatively, it is possible to use specifically designed devices which enable strength training for the very weak in anti-gravity positions (see Figure 8.7). However, in practice it is difficult, with very weak muscles, to set the resistance to an 8–12 RM training load. The closest possible approximations need to be used.

Strength training for patients with partial paralysis can also be done within the context of motor tasks. For example, patients with partial paralysis of the lower limbs and difficulty standing can perform squats while standing on a sliding tilt

Figure 8.6 Strengthening exercises for the elbow flexor muscles using an overhead cage and slings (a) and for the knee flexor muscles using a slideboard (b) appropriate for patients with grade 2/5 or less strength.

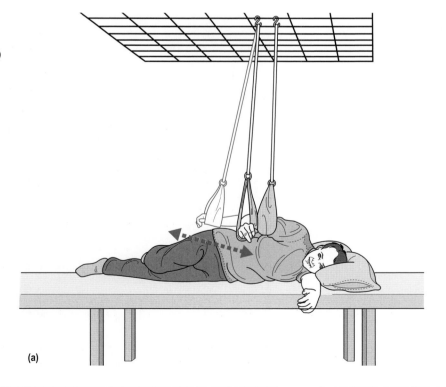

(a)

Figure 8.6 Continued

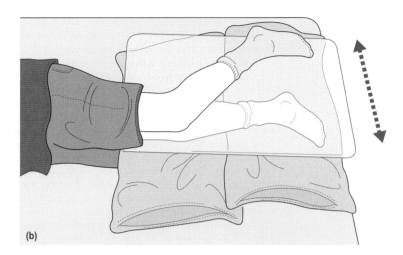

(b)

Figure 8.7 A simple wheel device can be used to test and train strength of the wrist extensor muscles in patients with less than grade 3/5 strength. Weights (B) are hung from a wheel (A) to apply a resistive torque. A counterweight (C) is used to eliminate the torque due to the mass of the wrist and hand device. These devices are not commercially available but can be readily made at hospital-based workshops.

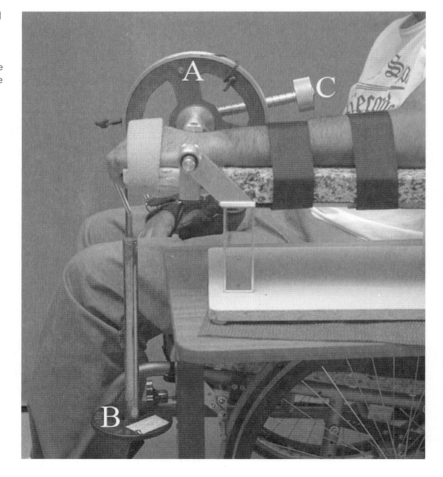

Figure 8.8 Strength training for patients with partial paralysis of the lower limbs can be carried out using sliding tilt tables. Patients perform squats with the tilt of the table adjusted so they can only just perform 8–12 repetitions before requiring a rest. The resistance can be adjusted by varying the tilt of the table or adding weights to the sliding mechanism.

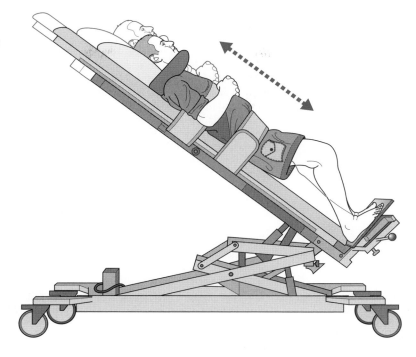

table (see Figure 8.8). Resistance can be changed by adjusting the tilt of the table or adding weights to the sliding mechanism. In this way, most of the muscles responsible for upright standing are trained at the one time.

Strength training for patients with flickers of movement

Strength training is more difficult in patients who are extremely weak (less than grade 2/5) with little or no ability to move through range. Assistive devices need to be used to help patients move through range or strength training needs to be restricted to isometric contractions. For these patients, EMG feedback can be used to provide patients and physiotherapists with feedback and encouragement. Some commercially available EMG feedback devices can be used to structure training sessions with timed phases of effort and relaxation. These devices can also be used to ensure patients contract to a pre-selected minimum effort with auditory feedback about success.

Alternatively, there may be merit in encouraging patients to use mental practice and motor imagery.[96] The two are slightly different, involving systematic and repeated cognitive practice or imagery of an activity without movement.[96–99] The benefits for people with spinal cord injury are speculative but there is strong evidence that repeated and intense mental rehearsal improves task performance in high-level athletes and possibly also in patients with various types of neurological disabilities.[96,99–102] Patients with profound weakness following spinal cord injury probably adopt cognitive strategies without prompting in an attempt to encourage neurological recovery. It is not clear whether this type of practice is of therapeutic benefit.

The use of electrical stimulation to increase voluntary strength

Electrical stimulation has long been advocated as a way of inducing hypertrophy in paralysed muscles and increasing stimulated strength.[103-105] Increasing 'strength' in fully paralysed muscles may be beneficial if electrical stimulation can subsequently be used for purposeful tasks. For example, electrical stimulation can be used to provide crude hand function to patients with tetraplegia (see Chapter 5).[106-110] Similarly, electrical stimulation continues to be used to develop sophisticated ways of enabling people with full lower limb paralysis to walk[111] and cycle.[105] Electrical stimulation is sometimes used to induce hypertrophy and improve blood flow.[105,112-114] Improved blood flow, particularly in the gluteal area, may reduce the incidence of pressure ulcers.[115,116]

Electrical stimulation is also used as a means of increasing voluntary strength of partially paralysed muscles.[117] Despite the widespread use of electrical stimulation for this purpose, few clinical trials have been directed at ascertaining whether electrical stimulation alone or in combination with any type of progressive resistance training increases voluntary strength of partially paralysed muscles more than voluntary exercise alone.[117-120] A recent systematic review identified just three clinical trials in people with spinal cord injury[117-119] but none were of sufficient quality to guide clinical practice.[121] A few clinical trials in people following stroke[122-126] demonstrate small increases in strength with electrical stimulation but it is unclear whether these results can be extrapolated to people with spinal cord injury. In the absence of clear evidence, and given the time-consuming nature of administering electrical stimulation, it is probably prudent to concentrate therapeutic effort on voluntary strength training interventions alone. If electrical stimulation is to be used, then it is probably best if it is applied in conjunction with voluntary strength training and appropriate resistance to ensure patients adhere to the principles of progressive resistance training.[104,127]

Avoiding injury and other complications

For a long time progressive resistance training was avoided in patients with neurologically-induced weakness and concurrent spasticity. It was believed that performing exercises against resistance increased spasticity.[128] This concern primarily arose from the work of Bobath in the area of stroke rehabilitation.[83,129] She believed strengthening exercises reinforced abnormal 'movement patterns'. While this issue has not been specifically investigated in patients with spasticity following spinal cord injury, there is evidence from patients with other types of neurological disabilities to indicate that initial concerns about possible deleterious effects of progressive resistance training on spasticity are probably unfounded.[18,33,83,92,94,95]

Strengthening programmes may need to be modified, at least initially, for frail and elderly patients or patients with little prior exposure to physical activity and exercise. It may be necessary to gradually increase the intensity of training to an optimal level in order to provide a period of gradual adjustment and to avoid injuries.[55] However, studies in untrained able-bodied individuals indicate that progressive resistance training is not associated with a high incidence of injuries, so the gradual exposure to high-resistance training may be unnecessarily conservative.[36,37]

A possible cause for concern arises when training muscles whose antagonists are completely paralysed, as is a common scenario in the shoulder muscles of people with tetraplegia (see Appendix). Some physiotherapists believe that extreme imbalances in the strength of agonist and antagonist muscles predispose patients to injury. If there are clear differences in strength of agonists and antagonists it is advisable to increase training intensity over a more prolonged period of time and to closely monitor patients for the development of pain (see Chapter 10).

Training programmes that include unaccustomed eccentric contractions will usually induce muscle soreness in the first couple of weeks of training. Patients are more likely to tolerate this soreness if they have been informed that this is a normal response to strength training prior to commencement.

Strength training for general well-being

This chapter has considered how strength training can improve performance of motor tasks. This is consistent with the problem-solving approach advocated throughout this book. During the initial rehabilitation of patients with spinal cord injury it is appropriate to concentrate on identifying the impairments preventing purposeful movement. However, progressive resistance training may also have important benefits for the sense of general well-being and quality of life, irrespective of any changes in mobility or independence. Long-term progressive resistance training programmes performed in group settings may be particularly beneficial. It has been shown that 9 months of a community-based progressive resistance training for people with spinal cord injury reduced pain and increased quality of life, perceived health, and satisfaction with physical function.[73] The particularly interesting aspect of this study was that the participants only trained twice a week. More generic evidence comes from studies of strength-training programmes for other populations, including the frail and elderly.[84,130–133] Studies in these populations indicate that strengthening programmes have beneficial effects on mood, pain and life satisfaction. There is no reason to believe that people with spinal cord injury would not attain similar benefits. It is on this basis that strengthening programmes for community patients with spinal cord injury are advocated.

Some of the barriers which prevent people with spinal cord injury engaging in community strengthening programmes include limited time, access to appropriate equipment, assistance from appropriately qualified staff and transport to and from facilities, as well as limited access to ongoing programme advice and support.[134,135] Physiotherapists should advocate for the removal of these barriers and encourage community-based strengthening programmes (see Chapter 12, p. 237).

References

1. Thomas CK, Zaidner EY, Calancie B et al: Muscle weakness, paralysis, and atrophy after human cervical spinal cord injury. Exp Neurol 1997; 148:414–423.
2. Jacobs PL, Beekhuizen KS: Appraisal of physiological fitness in persons with spinal cord injury. Top Spinal Cord Inj Rehabil 2005; 10:32–50.
3. Adams K, O'Shea JP, O'Shea KL et al: The effect of six weeks of squat, plyometric and squat-plyometric training on power production. J Appl Sport Sci Res 1992; 6:36–41.
4. Marciello MA, Herbison GJ, Ditunno JF et al: Wrist strength measured by myometry as an indicator of functional independence. J Neurotrauma 1995; 12:99–106.
5. White DJ: Musculoskeletal assessment. In O'Sullivan SB, Schmitz TJ (eds): Physical Rehabilitation: Assessment and Treatment. Philadelphia, FA Davis, 2000:101–132.
6. Kendall FP, Kendall McCreary E, Provance PG: Muscles, Testing and Function: with Posture and Pain, 4th edn. Baltimore, Williams & Wilkins, 1993.
7. Hislop HJ, Montgomery J: Daniels and Worthingham's Muscle Testing: Techniques of Manual Examination, 7th edn. Philadelphia, WB Saunders, 2002.
8. Daniels L, Worthingham C: Muscle Testing: Techniques of Manual Examination, 5th edn. Philadelphia, WB Saunders, 1986.
9. Kendall FP, McCreary E: Muscles, Testing and Function, 3rd edn. Baltimore, Williams & Wilkins, 1983.

10. American Spinal Injury Association: Reference Manual for the International Standards for Neurological Classification of Spinal Cord Injury. Chicago, ASIA, 2002.

11. Aitkens S, Lord J, Bernauer R et al: Relationship of manual muscle testing to objective strength measurements. Muscle Nerve 1989; 12:173–177.

12. Laing BA, Mastaglia FL, Lo SK et al: Comparative assessment of knee strength using hand-held myometry and isometric dynamometry in patients with inflammatory myopathy. Physiother Theory Pract 1995; 11:151–156.

13. Beasley WC: Influence of method on estimates of normal knee extensor force among normal and post polio children. Phy Ther Reviews 1956; 36:21–41.

14. Schwartz S, Cohen ME, Herbison GJ et al: Relationship between two measures of upper extremity strength; manual muscle test compared to hand-held myometry. Arch Phys Med Rehabil 1992; 73:1063–1068.

15. Herbison GJ, Isaac Z, Cohen ME et al: Strength post-spinal cord injury: myometer vs manual muscle test. Spinal Cord 1996; 34:534–538.

16. Scott DA, Bond EQ, Sisto SA et al: The intra- and interrater reliability of hip muscle strength assessments using a handheld versus a portable dynamometer anchoring station. Arch Phys Med Rehabil 2004; 85:598–603.

17. Dvir Z: Grade 4 in manual muscle testing: the problem with submaximal strength assessment. Clin Rehabil 1997; 11:36–41.

18. Eng JJ: Strength training in individuals with stroke. Physiother Can 2004; 56:189–201.

19. Frese E, Brown M, Norton BJ: Clinical reliability of manual muscle testing. Middle trapezius and gluteus medius muscles. Phys Ther 1987; 67:1072–1076.

20. Griffin JW, McClure MH, Bertorini TE: Sequential isokinetic and manual muscle testing in patients with neuromuscular disease. A pilot study. Phys Ther 1986; 66:32–35.

21. Schurch B, Wichmann W, Rossier AB: Post-traumatic syringomyelia (cystic myelopathy): a prospective study of 449 patients with spinal cord injury. J Neurol Neurosurg Psychiatry 1996; 60:61–67.

22. Campos GE, Luecke TJ, Wendeln HK et al: Muscular adaptations in response to three different resistance-training regimens: specificity of repetition maximum training zones. Eur J Appl Physiol 2002; 88:50–60.

23. Phillips WT, Batterham AM, Valenzuela JE et al: Reliability of maximal strength testing in older adults. Arch Phys Med Rehabil 2004; 85:329–334.

24. Staron RS, Malicky ES, Leonardi MJ et al: Muscle hypertrophy and fast fiber type conversions in heavy resistance-trained women. Eur J Appl Physiol Occup Physiol 1990; 60:71–79.

25. Agre JC, Magness JL, Hull SZ et al: Strength testing with a portable dynamometer: reliability for upper and lower extremities. Arch Phys Med Rehabil 1987; 68:454–458.

26. Bohannon RW, Andrews AW: Interrater reliability of hand-held dynamometry. Phys Ther 1987; 67:931–933.

27. Bohannon RW: Test–retest reliability of hand-held dynamometry during a single session of strength assessment. Phys Ther 1986; 66:206–209.

28. van Langeveld SHB, Aufdemkampe G, van Asbeck FWA: Reliability of force measurement with a hand-held dynamometer in healthy subjects and force measurements in patients with poliomyelitis anterior acuta. J Rehabil Sci 1996; 9:2–10.

29. Goonetilleke A, Modarres-Sadeghi H, Guiloff RJ: Accuracy, reproducibility, and variability of hand-held dynamometry in motor neuron disease. J Neurol Neurosurg Psychiatry 1994; 57:326–332.

30. Riddle DL, Finucane SD, Rothstein JM et al: Intrasession and intersession reliability of hand-held dynamometer measurements taken on brain-damaged patients. Phys Ther 1989; 69:182–194.

31. Kramer JF, Vaz MD, Vandervoort AA: Reliability of isometric hip abductor torques during examiner- and belt-resisted tests. J Gerontol 1991; 46:M47–M51.

32. Kramer JF, Nusca D, Bisbee L et al: Isometric and isokinetic torques of the forearm pronators and supinators: reliability and interrelationships. Isokinet Exerc Sci 1993; 3:195–201.

33. Eng JJ, Kim CM, MacIntyre DL: Reliability of lower extremity strength measures in persons with chronic stroke. Arch Phys Med Rehabil 2002; 83:322–328.

34. Hubal MJ, Gordish-Dressman H, Thompson PD et al: Variability in muscle size and strength gain after unilateral resistance training. Med Sci Sports Exerc 2005; 37:964–972.

35. Herbert R: Human strength adaptations. Implications for therapy. In Crosbie WJ, McConnell J (eds): Key Issues in Musculoskeletal Physiotherapy. London, Butterworth Heinemann, 1993: 142–171.

36. Ivey FM, Roth SM, Ferrell RE et al: Effects of age, gender, and myostatin genotype on the hypertrophic response to heavy resistance strength training. J Gerontol 2000; 55:M641–M648.

37. Petrella JK, Kim JS, Cross JM et al: Efficacy of myonuclear addition may explain differential myofiber growth among resistance-trained young and older men and women. Am J Physiol Endocrinol Metab 2006; 291:E937–E946.

38. McCall GE, Byrnes WC, Dickinson A et al: Muscle fiber hypertrophy, hyperplasia, and capillary density in college men after resistance training. J Appl Physiol 1996; 81:2004–2012.
39. Staron RS, Karapondo DL, Kraemer WJ et al: Skeletal muscle adaptations during early phase of heavy-resistance training in men and women. J Appl Physiol 1994; 76:1247–1255.
40. Widrick JJ, Stelzer JE, Shoepe TC et al: Functional properties of human muscle fibers after short-term resistance exercise training. Am J Physiol Regul Integr Comp Physiol 2002; 283:R408–R416.
41. Kraemer WJ, Ratamess NA: Fundamentals of resistance training: progression and exercise prescription. Med Sci Sports Exerc 2004; 36:674–688.
42. Sale DG: Neural adaptation to strength training. In Komi PV (ed): Strength and Power in Sport. Oxford, Blackwell Scientific, 1992:249–265.
43. Gandevia SC: Spinal and supraspinal factors in human muscle fatigue. Physiol Rev 2001; 81: 1725–1789.
44. Enoka RM: Muscle strength and its development. New perspectives. Sports Med 1988; 6:146–168.
45. Zhou S: Chronic neural adaptations to unilateral exercise: mechanisms of cross education. Exerc Sport Sci Rev 2000; 28:177–184.
46. Munn J, Herbert RD, Hancock MJ et al: Training with unilateral resistance exercise increases contralateral strength. J Appl Physiol 2005; 99:1880–1884.
47. Herbert RD, Dean C, Gandevia SC: Effects of real and imagined training on voluntary muscle activation during maximal isometric contractions. Acta Orthop Scand 1998; 163:361–368.
48. Sale DG: Neural adaptation to resistance training. Med Sci Sports Exerc 1988; 20:S135–145.
49. Yue G, Cole KJ: Strength increases from the motor program: comparison of training with maximal voluntary and imagined muscle contraction. J Neurophysiol 1992; 67:1114–1123.
50. Patten C, Kamen G: Adaptations in motor unit discharge activity with force control training in young and older human adults. Eur J Appl Physiol 2000; 83:128–143.
51. Rutherford OM, Jones DA: The role of learning and coordination in strength training. Eur J Appl Physiol Occup Physiol 1986; 55:100–105.
52. Munn J, Herbert RD, Gandevia SC: Contralateral effects of unilateral resistance training: a meta-analysis. J Appl Physiol 2004; 96:1861–1866.
53. Munn J, Herbert RD, Hancock MJ et al: Resistance training for strength: effect of number of sets and contraction speed. Med Sci Sports Exerc 2005; 37:1622–1626.
54. Feigenbaum MS, Pollock ML: Prescription of resistance training for health and disease. Med Sci Sports Exerc 1999; 31:38–45.
55. Rhea MR, Alvar BA, Burkett LN et al: A meta-analysis to determine the dose response for strength development. Med Sci Sports Exerc 2003; 35:456–464.
56. Hoeger WW, Barette SL, Hale DF et al: Relationship between repetitions and selected percentages of one repetition maximum. J Appl Sport Sci Res 1987; 1:11–13.
57. Kraemer WJ, Adams K, Cafarelli E et al: American College of Sports Medicine. American College of Sports Medicine position stand. Progression models in resistance training for healthy adults. Med Sci Sports Exerc 2002; 34:364–380.
58. Rhea MR, Alvar BA, Burkett LN: Single versus multiple sets for strength: a meta-analysis to address the controversy. Res Q Exerc Sport 2002; 73:485–488.
59. Carpinelli RN: Berger in retrospect: effect of varied weight training programmes on strength. Br J Sports Med 2002; 36:319–324.
60. Pereira MI, Gomes PS: Movement velocity in resistance training. Sports Med 2003; 33:427–438.
61. Carpinelli RN, Otto RM: Strength training single versus multiple sets. Sports Med 1998; 26:73–84.
62. Dudley GA, Tesch PA, Miller BJ et al: Importance of eccentric actions in performance adaptations to resistance training. Aviat Space Environ Med 1991; 62:543–550.
63. Keogh JWL, Qilson GJ, Weatherby RP: A cross-sectional comparison of different resistance training techniques in the bench press. J Strength Cond Res 1999; 13:247–258.
64. Fleck SJ: Periodized strength training: a critical review. J Strength Cond Res 1999; 13:82–89.
65. Kraemer WJ: A series of studies — the physiological basis for strength training in American football: fact over philosophy. J Strength Cond Res 1997; 11:131–142.
66. Farthing JP, Chilibeck PD: The effect of eccentric training at different velocities on cross-education. Eur J Appl Physiol 2003; 89:570–577.
67. Paddon-Jones D, Leveritt M, Lonergan A et al: Adaptation to chronic eccentric exercise in humans: The influence of contraction velocity. Eur J Appl Physiol 2001; 85:466–471.
68. Sale D, MacDougall D: Specificity in strength training: a review for the coach and athlete. Can J Appl Sport Sci 1981; 6:87–92.
69. Nilsson S, Staff PH, Pruett ED: Physical work capacity and the effect of training on subjects with long-standing paraplegia. Scand J Rehabil Med 1975; 7:51–56.
70. Bar-Or O: The Wingate anaerobic test. An update on methodology, reliability and validity. Sports Med 1987; 4:381–394.
71. Hass CJ, Garzarella L, De Hoyos D et al: Single versus multiple sets in long-term recreational weightlifters. Med Sci Sports Exerc 2000; 32:235–242.

72. Henry KD, Rosemond C, Eckert LB: Effect of number of home exercises on compliance and performance in adults over 65 years of age. Phys Ther 1999; 79:270–277.

73. Hicks AL, Martin KA, Ditor DS et al: Long-term exercise training in persons with spinal cord injury: effects on strength, arm ergometry performance and psychological well-being. Spinal Cord 2003; 41:34–43.

74. Sale DG, Jacobs I, MacDougall JD et al: Comparison of two regimens of concurrent strength and endurance training. Med Sci Sports Exerc 1990; 22:348–356.

75. Stone WJ, Coulter SP: Strength/endurance effects from three resistance training protocols with women. J Strength Cond Res 1994; 8:231–234.

76. Jacobs PL, Nash MS: Exercise recommendations for individuals with spinal cord injury. Sports Med 2004; 34:727–751.

77. Taylor NF, Dodd KJ, Damiano DL: Progressive resistance exercise in physical therapy: a summary of systematic reviews. Phys Ther 2005; 85:1208–1223.

78. Nash MS, Jacobs PL, Woods JM et al: A comparison of 2 circuit exercise training techniques for eliciting matched metabolic responses in persons with paraplegia. Arch Phys Med Rehabil 2002; 83:201–209.

79. Davis GM, Shephard RJ: Strength training for wheelchair users. Br J Sports Med 1990; 24:25–30.

80. Bourbonnais D, Bilodeau S, Lepage Y et al: Effect of force-feedback treatments in patients with chronic motor deficits after a stroke. Am J Phys Med Rehabil 2002; 81:890–897.

81. Engardt M, Knutsson E, Jonsson M et al: Dynamic muscle strength training in stroke patients: effects on knee extension torque, electromyographic activity, and motor function. Arch Phys Med Rehabil 1995; 76:419–425.

82. Saunders DH, Greig CA, Young A et al: Physical fitness training for stroke patients. The Cochrane Database of Systematic Reviews 2004: Issue 1. Art. No.: CD003316. DOI: 10.1002/14651858.CD003316.pub2.

83. Patten C, Lexell J, Brown HE: Weakness and strength training in persons with poststroke hemiplegia: rationale, method, and efficacy. J Rehabil Res Dev 2004; 41:293–312.

84. Morris SL, Dobb KL, Morris ME: Outcomes of progressive resistance strength training following stroke: a systematic review. Clin Rehabil 2004; 18:27–39.

85. Dodd KJ, Taylor NF, Damiano DL: A systematic review of the effectiveness of strength-training programs for people with cerebral palsy. Arch Phys Med Rehabil 2002; 83:1157–1164.

86. Darrah J, Fan JSW, Chen LC et al: Review of the effects of progressive resisted muscle strengthening in children with cerebral palsy: a clinical consensus exercise. Pediatr Phys Ther 1997; 9:12–17.

87. White CM, Pritchard J, Turner-Stokes L: Exercise for people with peripheral neuropathy. The Cochrane Database of Systematic Reviews 2004: Issue 4. Art. No.: CD003904. DOI: 10.1002/14651858.CD003904.pub2.

88. Winstein CJ, Rose DK, Tan SM et al: A randomized controlled comparison of upper-extremity rehabilitation strategies in acute stroke: A pilot study of immediate and long-term outcomes. Arch Phys Med Rehabil 2004; 85:620–628.

89. Kim CM, Eng JJ, MacIntyre DL et al: Effects of isokinetic strength training on walking in persons with stroke: a double-blind controlled pilot study. J Stroke Cerebrovasc Dis 2001; 10:265–273.

90. McCubbin JA, Shasby G: Effects of isokinetic exercise on adolescents with cerebral palsy. Adapt Phys Act Q 1985; 2:56–64.

91. Dodd KJ, Taylor NF, Graham HK: A randomized clinical trial of strength training in young people with cerebral palsy. Dev Med Child Neurol 2003; 45:652–657.

92. Andersson C, Grooten W, Hellsten M et al: Adults with cerebral palsy: walking ability after progressive strength training. Dev Med Child Neurol 2003; 45:220–228.

93. Lindeman E, Leffers P, Spaans F et al: Strength training in patients with myotonic dystrophy and hereditary motor and sensory neuropathy: A randomized clinical trial. Arch Phys Med Rehabil 1995; 76:612–620.

94. Ada L, Dorsch S, Canning C: Strengthening interventions increase strength and improve activity after stroke: a systematic review. Aust J Physiother 2006; 52:242–248.

95. Moreland JD, Goldsmith CH, Huijbregts MP et al: Progressive resistance strengthening exercises after stroke: a single-blind randomized controlled trial. Arch Phys Med Rehabil 2003; 84:1433–1440.

96. Malouin F, Richards CL, Doyon J et al: Training mobility tasks after stroke with combined mental and physical practice: a feasibility study. Neurorehabil Neural Repair 2004; 18:66–75.

97. Decety J, Biosson D: Effect of brain and spinal cord injuries on motor imagery. Eur Arch Psychiatry Clin Neurosci 1990; 240:39–43.

98. Denis M: Visual imagery and the use of mental practice in the development of motor skills. Can J Appl Sport Sci 1985; 10:4S–16S.

99. Feltz DL, Landers DM: The effects of mental practice on motor skill learning and performance: a meta analysis. J Sport Psych 1983; 5:27–57.

100. Hinshaw KE: The effects of mental practice on motor skill performance: critical evaluation and meta-analysis. Imagin Cogn Personality 1991; 11:3–35.

101. Driskell JE, Copper C, Moran A: Does mental practice enhance performance? J Appl Psychol 1994; 79:481–492.
102. Jackson PL, Doyon J, Richards CL et al: The efficacy of combined physical and mental practice in learning of a foot-sequence task after stroke: a case report. Neurorehabil Neural Repair 2004; 18:106–111.
103. Belanger M, Stein RB, Wheeler GD et al: Electrical stimulation: can it increase muscle strength and reverse osteopenia in spinal cord injured individuals? Arch Phys Med Rehabil 2000; 81: 1090–1098.
104. Hartkopp A, Harridge SD, Mizuno M et al: Effect of training on contractile and metabolic properties of wrist extensors in spinal cord-injured individuals. Muscle Nerve 2003; 27:72–80.
105. Baldi JC, Jackson RD, Moraille R et al: Muscle atrophy is prevented in patients with acute spinal cord injury using functional electrical stimulation. Spinal Cord 1998; 36:463–469.
106. Bryden AM, Sinnott KA, Mulcahey MJ: Innovative strategies for improving upper extremity function in tetraplegia and considerations in measuring functional outcomes. Top Spinal Cord Inj Rehabil 2005; 10:75–93.
107. JIjzerman MJ, Stoffers TS, Groen FAC et al: The NESS handmaster orthosis: restoration of hand function in C5 and stroke patients by means of electrical stimulation. J Rehabil Sci 1996; 9:86–89.
108. Kilgore KL, Peckham PH, Keith MW et al: An implanted upper-extremity neuroprosthesis. Follow-up of five patients. J Bone Joint Surg (Am) 1997; 79:533–541.
109. Prochazka A, Gauthier M, Wieler M et al: The bionic glove; an electrical stimulator garment that provides controlled grasp and hand opening in quadriplegia. Arch Phys Med Rehabil 1997; 78:608–614.
110. Peckham PH, Keith MW, Freehafer AA: Restoration of functional control by electrical stimulation in the upper extremity of the quadriplegic patient. J Bone Joint Surg (Am) 1988; 70:144–148.
111. Marsolais EB, Kobetic R: Functional walking in paralyzed patients by means of electrical stimulation. Clin Orthop Relat Res 1983; May:30–36.
112. Bogataj U, Gros N, Kljajic M et al: The rehabilitation of gait in patients with hemiplegia: a comparison between conventional therapy and multichannel functional electrical stimulation therapy. Phys Ther 1995; 75:490–502.
113. Sabatier MJ, Stoner L, Mahoney ET et al: Electrically stimulated resistance training in SCI individuals increases muscle fatigue resistance but not femoral artery size or blood flow. Spinal Cord 2006; 44:227–233.
114. Stoner L, Sabatier MJ, Mahoney ET et al: Electrical stimulation-evoked resistance exercise therapy improves arterial health after chronic spinal cord injury. Spinal Cord 2007; 49:49–56.
115. Regan M, Teasell RW, Keast D et al: Pressure ulcers following spinal cord injury. In Eng JJ, Teasell RW, Miller WC et al (eds): Spinal Cord Injury Rehabilitation Evidence. Vancouver, SCIRE, 2006:20.1–20.26.
116. Bogie KM, Triolo RJ: Effects of regular use of neuromuscular electrical stimulation on tissue health. J Rehabil Res Dev 2003; 40:469–475.
117. Klose KJ, Schmidt DL, Needham BM et al: Rehabilitation therapy for patients with long-term spinal cord injuries. Arch Phys Med Rehabil 1990; 71:659–662.
118. Kohlmeyer KM, Hill JP, Yarkony GM et al: Electrical stimulation and biofeedback effect on recovery of tenodesis grasp: a controlled study. Arch Phys Med Rehabil 1996; 77:701–706.
119. Needham-Shropshire BM, Broton JG, Klose K et al: Evaluation of a training program for persons with SCI paraplegia using the Parastep 1 Ambulation System: part 3. Lack of effect on bone mineral density. Arch Phys Med Rehabil 1997; 78:799–803.
120. Callaghan MJ, Oldham JA: A critical review of electrical stimulation of the quadriceps muscles. Crit Rev Phys Rehabil Med 1997; 9:301–314.
121. Glinsky J, Harvey L, Gandevia SC: Efficacy of electrical stimulation to increase muscle strength in people with neurological conditions: A systematic review. Phys Res Int (in press). Published online at Wiley Interscience (www.interscience.wiley.com) DOI: 10.1002/pri. 375.
122. Powell J, Pandyan AD, Granat M et al: Electrical stimulation of wrist extensors in poststroke hemiplegia. Stroke 1999; 30:1384–1389.
123. Winchester P, Montgomery J, Bowman B et al: Effects of feedback stimulation training and cyclical electrical stimulation on knee extension in hemiparetic patients. Phys Ther 1983; 63:1096–1103.
124. Yan T, Hui-Chan CW, Li LS: Functional electrical stimulation improves motor recovery of the lower extremity and walking ability of subjects with first acute stroke: A randomized placebo-controlled trial. Stroke 2005; 36:80–85.
125. Glanz M, Klawansky S, Stason W et al: Functional electrostimulation in poststroke rehabilitation: a meta-analysis of the randomized controlled trials. Arch Phys Med Rehabil 1996; 77:549–553.
126. Heckmann J, Mokrusch T, Krockel A et al: EMG-triggered electrical muscle stimulation in the treatment of central hemiparesis after a stroke. J Phys Med Rehabil 1997; 7:138–141.

127. Bax L, Staes F, Verhagen A: Does neuromuscular electrical stimulation strengthen the quadriceps femoris? A systematic review of randomised controlled trials. Sports Med 2005; 35:191–212.

128. Barry MJ: Physical therapy interventions for patients with movement disorders due to cerebral palsy. J Child Neurol 1996; 11:S51–S60.

129. Bobath B: Adult Hemiplegia: Evaluation and Treatment, 3rd edn. Oxford, Heinemann Medical, 1990.

130. Buchner DM, Beresfod SA, Larson EB et al: Effects of physical activity on health status in older patients. II. Interventions studies. Ann Rev Public Health 1992; 13:469–488.

131. Netz Y, Wu MJ, Becker BJ et al: Physical activity and psychological well-being in advanced age: a meta-analysis of intervention studies. Psychol Aging 2005; 20:272–284.

132. Latham NK, Bennett DA, Stretton CM et al: Systematic review of progressive resistance strength training in older adults. J Gerontol A Biol Sci Med Sci 2004; 59:48–61.

133. Latham N, Anderson C, Bennett D et al: Progressive resistance strength training for physical disability in older people. The Cochrane Database of Systematic Reviews 2003: Issue 2. Art. No.: CD002759. DOI: 10.1002/14651858.CD002759.

134. Laskin JJ, James SA, Cantwell BM: A fitness and wellness program for people with spinal cord injury. Top Spinal Cord Inj Rehabil 1997; 3:16–33.

135. Rimmer JH, Braddock D, Pitetti KH: Research on physical activity and disability: an emerging national priority. Med Sci Sports Exerc 1996; 28:1366–1372.

Contracture management

Contents

Assessment 178

Treatment and prevention
of contractures 179

Preventing and anticipating
contractures 185

Prioritizing treatments: a
touch of reality 188

Reducing muscle
extensibility 189

Contractures, or loss of joint mobility, are a common complication of spinal cord injury (see Figures 9.1 and 9.2).[1–5] Neurally mediated contractures are due to spasticity (see Chapter 1)[6–11] and non-neurally mediated contractures are due to structural changes in soft tissues overlying joints.

Contractures are undesirable for several reasons but primarily because they prevent the performance of motor tasks.[2,12–14] For example, hip flexor contractures can impede walking in patients with paraplegia (see Figure 9.1). However, contractures also create unsightly deformities and are thought to predispose patients to pressure ulcers, pain and sleep disturbances.[1–3,13,15–17]

Subtle losses of extensibility in muscles acting across two joints are common sequelae of spinal cord injury but do not always result in disfiguring and obvious contracture. Such losses of extensibility can, however, have important implications for function. For example, even a modest loss of extensibility in the hamstring muscles

Figure 9.1 A hip flexion contracture in the left leg of a patient with paraplegia. This type of contracture can impede walking, especially if the patient also has paralysis of the hip extensor muscles.

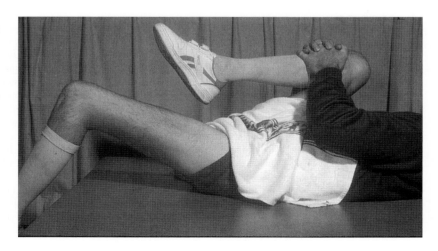

Figure 9.2 Patients with C6 tetraplegia can develop contractures of elbow flexors, wrist extensors and thumb adductor muscles. These types of contractures limit function and are unsightly.

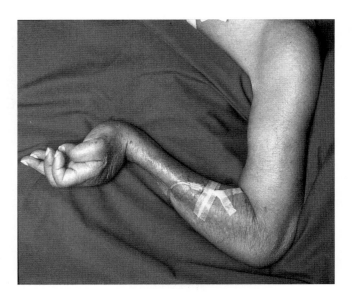

can prevent a patient with C6 tetraplegia from sitting unsupported on a bed with the knees extended (see Figure 3.2, p. 59). Similarly, a small loss of extensibility in the gastrocnemius muscles can limit the gait of a patient with the potential to walk.

Contractures, like other impairments, need to be linked to activity and participation goals during the goal planning process (see Chapter 2). In the above examples, hip flexor contractures would be linked to walking-related goals and loss of hamstring muscle extensibility would be linked to sitting-related goals. The linking of contractures to activity and participation goals ensures that interventions are concentrated where they really matter. It is also important during the goal planning process to anticipate contractures which may develop in the future, and which may ultimately limit activity and participation, so strategies can be put in place to prevent them.

Assessment

Measurements of passive joint range of motion are used to quantify the severity of contractures. A baseline assessment of all joints is required to identify existing problems and monitor change over time. These measurements are typically done with a goniometer. To identify the loss of extensibility in muscles crossing two joints, it is important to ensure appropriate positioning of the second joint. For example, measurements of hip flexion with the knee flexed reflect the extensibility of the tissues on the extensor aspect of the hip and measurements of hip flexion with the knee extended specifically reflect the extensibility of the hamstring muscles. Similarly, measurements of wrist extension with the fingers extended reflect the extensibility of the extrinsic finger flexor muscles.[18]

Joint angle is a direct function of the torque applied to a joint (usually through the hands of therapists, and sometimes from the weight of a limb). Joint range of motion measured with a larger torque will be greater than joint range of motion measured with a smaller one.[19] Consequently, if comparisons are to be made of repeated measures, it is important that the same torque is applied on each occasion. It is often difficult for therapists to manually apply a consistent torque when testing joint range of motion, especially when measurements are taken weeks or months apart. In this situation, changes in joint range of motion are not necessarily indicative of underlying changes in tissue extensibility. There are various devices which can be used to standardize torque to overcome this problem.[18,20-22] The use of these devices is warranted when accurate measurements are important (e.g. to determine the effectiveness of costly, time-consuming, inconvenient or surgical interventions).

It is useful to try and distinguish between neurally mediated and non-neurally mediated contractures because treatment may differ.[23] For example, anti-spasticity medication is appropriate for management of neurally but not non-neurally mediated contractures. In practice, however, contractures are often due to both factors and a distinction between the relative importance of each factor is difficult. A contracture is likely to have a neurally mediated component if there are signs of spasticity such as clonus or a velocity-dependent increase in resistance to stretch. Measurements of joint range of motion are more reproducible when spasticity is not a key feature. Spasticity can be dampened by measuring joint range of motion after a sustained 2- or 3-minute stretch. However, the only definite way to determine the contribution of neurally mediated factors to a contracture is to measure passive joint range of motion when spasticity is pharmacologically blocked (e.g. when patients are anaesthetized). There are standardized measures of spasticity, although their clinical usefulness is disputed (see Chapter 1).

Treatment and prevention of contractures

Stretch and passive movements

Stretch and passive movements have become the cornerstone of physiotherapy management directed at the treatment and prevention of contractures in patients with spinal cord injury.[24-28] In many spinal cord injury units it has become accepted practice for therapists to routinely administer between 2 and 10 minutes of passive movements and stretch a day to each affected joint of each patient, particularly patients confined to bed in the period immediately following injury.[25,29] These types of interventions are labour intensive and can equate to an hour of treatment per patient per day.

While clinical lore supports the efficacy of passive movements and stretch, the science is less convincing. There is still much uncertainty about whether these interventions are truly effective and, if they are, how long stretches need to be maintained and how frequently passive movements need to be administered. The optimal stretch torque is also unknown although one study, at least, indicates that therapists have differing ideas of what constitutes a therapeutic stretch.[30] Some therapists apply stretches to the hamstring muscles of patients with spinal cord injury well in excess of that which would be tolerated by able-bodied people with normal sensation. It is also unclear whether passive movements and stretch primarily target the neurally mediated or non-neurally mediated determinants of contractures. Definitive answers to these questions are unknown but some of the current controversies are outlined in the next section.

Evidence from animal studies

The use of passive movements and stretch-based interventions to treat and prevent contractures is usually justified by animal studies.[31-33] Animal studies indicate that soft tissues undergo deleterious changes in response to prolonged immobilization, especially immobilization in shortened positions.[34-36] For example, 10 days immobilization of the ankles of rabbits in a plantarflexed position (the shortened position of the plantarflexor muscles) results in approximately a 10% reduction in resting length of soleus muscle–tendon units,[36] which produces functionally significant loss of ankle joint mobility. Muscle shortening is associated with decreases in the number of sarcomeres,[34,35,37] changes in the extent and arrangement of collagen[38,39] and concentration of glycosaminoglycans,[40] and decreases in tendon resting length.[5,31,34-36,38,41-50] These deleterious structural and morphological changes associated with immobilization can be prevented[36]or reversed[34] by prolonged and uninterrupted stretch. In animals, prolonged stretch is typically applied with plaster casts for many days. Stretch is believed to provide a sufficiently strong stimulus to trigger appropriate remodelling of soft tissues. Similar findings have been found in denervated muscles, although the response appears to be slower.[51-53]

While animal studies show that continuous and uninterrupted stretch can prevent or reverse deleterious soft tissue adaptations associated with immobilization, the effectiveness of short periods of stretch are less clear.[43,54] Most of what is known about the effects of short periods of stretch comes from one important study in mice, which found that just 15 minutes of stretch each day partly prevented loss of sarcomeres in the plantarflexor muscles of ankles immobilized in a shortened position, and 30 minutes of stretch were sufficient to completely prevent loss of sarcomeres.[54] The effectiveness of less than 15 minutes of stretch a day, such as typically administered in the clinical setting, is unknown. The results of animal studies need to be interpreted with caution because animal muscles respond to stimuli such as stretch more rapidly than human muscles. A 15-minute stretch which prevents loss of sarcomeres in the plantarflexor muscles of small animals will not necessarily produce the same effects in humans with spinal cord injury.

Evidence from clinical trials

A large number of trials have examined the effects of stretch on tissue extensibility in various populations. Most of these trials have been carried out in able-bodied individuals.[55,56] Two methodological issues limit the usefulness of many trials. First, most trials measure the effects of stretch soon after the last stretch intervention. Measurements at this time reflect the transient effects of stretch due to viscous deformation.[57-61] They do not provide good evidence of the lasting effects of stretch on tissue extensibility and remodelling[31] essential for the treatment and prevention of contracture. A second limitation is that most trials do not standardize the torque used to measure joint range of motion. They are therefore unable to differentiate between underlying changes in tissue extensibility and changes in patients' tolerance to uncomfortable stretch when sensation is present.[62,63]

A few randomized trials of the effects of stretch have been conducted in patients with spinal cord injury.[27,64-67] All involved the application of 30 minutes of stretch three to five times a week over a 4-week or 3-month period to either the plantarflexor,[64,66] shoulder[27], thumb[67] or hamstring muscles[65] of patients with spinal cord injury. In four of the five studies outcomes were measured using standardized torques at least 1 day after the application of the last stretch. All five studies showed that regular stretch had little or no effect on joint range of motion. These results are consistent with randomized controlled trials in patients with other types of neurological disabilities[68-73] and indicate that therapists' confidence about the effectiveness of stretch is not yet justified.

One possible interpretation of the negative findings is that stretches administered by physiotherapists offer no added benefits over good routine care typically involving anti-spasticity medication and regular change of position. Alternatively, it may be that the benefits of regular stretch are not seen until they have been applied for months if not years. Therefore it would be premature to suggest that stretches be abandoned. However, stretches administered for a few minutes a day are unlikely to be therapeutically worthwhile. Instead, stretches should be sustained for as long as practically feasible and for at least 20 minutes a day.

Ways of administering sustained stretches

If stretches are to be sustained for more than a few minutes a day, they cannot be applied manually by therapists. Instead, stretches need to be applied with positioning, splinting[74] and standing[75] programmes. These programmes should be incorporated into patients' daily routines and continued after discharge. Often only simple strategies are needed, especially if stretches are instigated before contractures have developed (see section below on Preventing and anticipating contractures). For example, the shoulder extensor, hamstring, hip internal and hip extensor muscles can all easily be stretched by placing the arms or legs on stools or tables (see Figures 9.3–9.6).

More sustained stretches can be applied with serial casts to immobilize joints in their stretched positions. The casts are reapplied every few days to maintain the stretch. Serial casts should only be considered for severe and disabling contractures because they can impede independence, be uncomfortable and are time-consuming to apply. They are also associated with a substantial risk of skin breakdown.[70,76]

Patients also need to be educated about methods of self-administering stretches. For example, the hip internal rotator muscles can be stretched by sitting with one foot on the opposite leg (see Figure 9.7). Patients with lower levels of tetraplegia can

Figure 9.3 Sitting with the arms supported on high tables is a way of applying a sustained stretch to the shoulder extensor muscles.

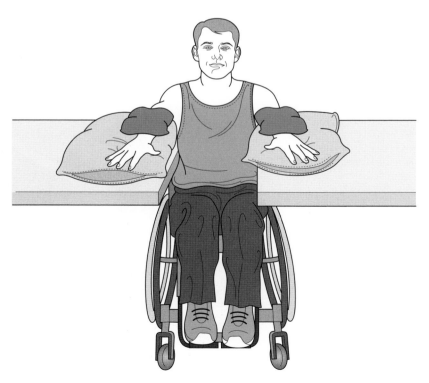

Figure 9.4 Sitting with the legs up on a chair and a strap around the feet is a way of applying a sustained stretch to the hamstring and plantarflexor muscles.

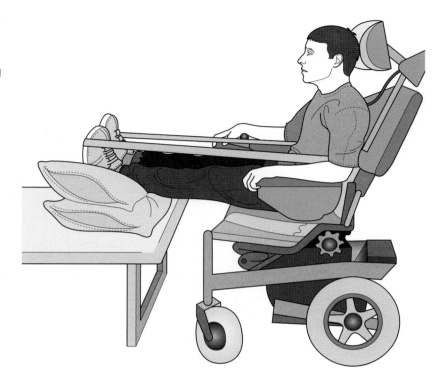

Figure 9.5 Sitting with the legs in a 'frog' position is a way of applying a sustained stretch to the adductor and internal rotator muscles of the hip.

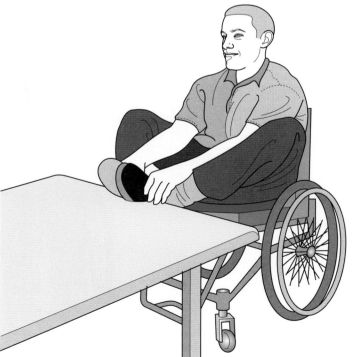

Figure 9.6 Sitting with the legs flexed up towards the chest is a way of applying a sustained stretch to the soleus and hip extensor muscles.

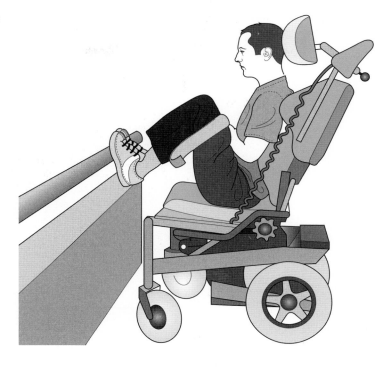

Figure 9.7 Sitting with one leg on the opposite knee is a way of self-administering sustained stretch to the hip internal rotator muscles.

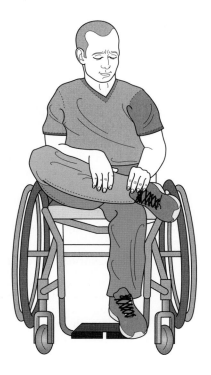

Figure 9.8 Patients can use the rim of the wheelchair to self-administer sustained stretch into extension of the interphalangeal joints of the fingers.

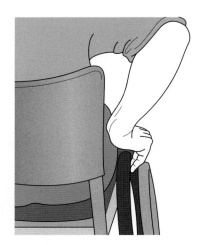

Figure 9.9 Patients can self-administer sustained stretch into flexion of the metacarpophalangeal joints of the fingers.

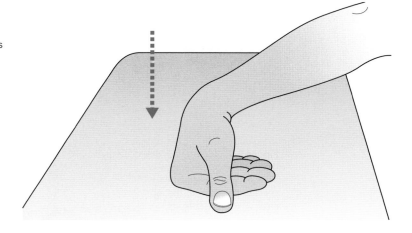

self-stretch the interphalangeal joints (IP) of the fingers into extension while sitting in a wheelchair by using the rim of the wheel as a pivot bar (see Figure 9.8). Similarly, they can stretch the metacarpophalangeal (MCP) joints of the hand into flexion by appropriately placing the hand on a hard surface (see Figure 9.9). All these types of strategies can be incorporated into patients' lives with minimal inconvenience and reliance on others. For similar stretch ideas, readers are referred to www.physiotherapyexercises.com.

Passive movements

It is not known whether passive movements confer additional benefits to stretches. Some have claimed that repetitive passive movements are important for preventing intra-articular adhesions and immobilization-induced deterioration of joint cartilage, although there is little support for this proposition from randomized trials in humans. Until further work is done in this area, it is probably prudent to administer as many passive movements as feasible to selected joints rather than a few passive movements to every joint. Precisely how many passive movements are required is not known but it would seem unlikely that less than 5 minutes of passive movements to a joint each day would be therapeutic. Physiotherapists must assess the effectiveness of the passive movements they provide to gain guidance on this issue.

Passive movements should be concentrated on joints most vulnerable to contracture and pain and most likely to influence future independence. These include the small joints of the hand, especially for those with C5 and below levels of tetraplegia and the complex joints of the shoulder and scapulo-thoracic girdle, especially in those vulnerable to shoulder pain (see Chapter 10). Elsewhere, therapeutic effort is probably better directed at prolonged stretches which can be administered for prolonged periods of time.

The touch and regular contact with empathetic therapists during the provision of passive movements may provide psychological comfort to patients in the early days after injury. This aspect of overall well-being should not be underestimated. The effectiveness of passive movements for other purposes, such as the treatment and prevention of oedema and poor circulation, is more contentious.[28,77]

Preventing and anticipating contractures

It is widely believed that contractures can be more readily prevented than treated, and that maintaining tissue extensibility requires a less intensive stretch programme than increasing extensibility. Although the validity of these beliefs has not yet been substantiated, therapists are well advised to concentrate on preventing contractures, especially if this can be done with positioning strategies which involve minimal inconvenience to patients. For example, sleeping and sitting with the feet supported at 90° discourages plantarflexor contractures and is easily implemented (see Figure 9.10).

Factors that predispose patients to contractures

The skill of preventing contractures lies largely in accurately predicting them.[78] At-risk soft tissues are those habitually held in shortened positions. Fortunately, it is possible to predict susceptible soft tissues by looking at factors such as the pattern of innervation, pain, oedema, and the position in which patients spend the majority of each day.[79] For example, patients with C5 and C6 tetraplegia are susceptible to elbow flexion contractures (see Figure 9.2).[4,15] These patients have paralysis of the triceps but not biceps muscles. Consequently, they tend to sit and lie with the elbows flexed. The problem is exacerbated if they are nursed in a supine position for extended periods of time. In this position it is difficult for patients with paralysis of the triceps muscles to extend the elbows passively once flexed. A simple positioning programme to prevent elbow flexion contractures may include placing a small weight on the wrist to hold the elbow in an extended position (see Figure 9.11).

Similarly, patients with C4 and above tetraplegia often develop pronation contractures. These patients commonly lie and sit with their forearms pronated, encouraging forearm contractures. Pronation contractures can be avoided by ensuring patients spend time with the forearms supinated (see Figure 9.12). Minor modifications to the armrests of wheelchairs may be required but otherwise this is a simple positioning and stretching protocol to implement provided it is started early. In contrast, once passive supination is lost it is difficult to effectively stretch the forearm and often cumbersome splints are required.[80]

Patients confined to bed tend to lose hip and shoulder passive abduction. This is simply avoided by ensuring the shoulders[1] and legs are abducted rather than

Figure 9.10 Lying with feet supported at 90° is a way of applying a sustained stretch to the plantarflexor muscles. The heels are free from the mattress to prevent pressure ulcers.

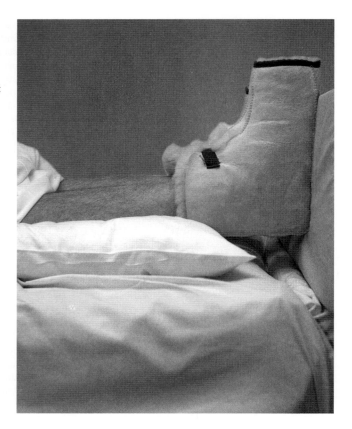

Figure 9.11 Placing a small weight on the wrist is a way of applying a sustained stretch to the elbow flexor muscles.

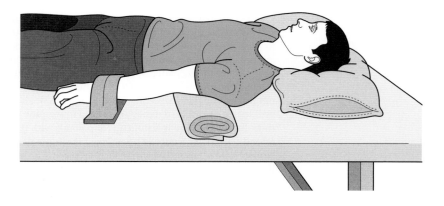

adducted for at least part of each day (see Figures 9.13 and 9.14). Similarly, ankles need to be supported to prevent plantarflexion contractures (see Figure 9.10). This requires staff education, but minimal equipment.

Patterns of paralysis and position are not the only factors determining susceptibility to contractures. Pain is also important. Pain increases the tendency to contract

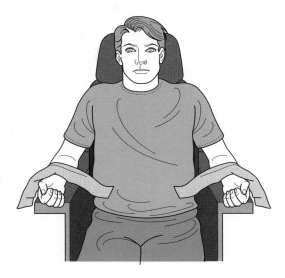

Figure 9.12 Sitting with the arms in supination is a way of applying a sustained stretch to the elbow pronator muscles.

Figure 9.13 Lying with the arms in abduction is a way of applying a sustained stretch to the shoulder adductor muscles.

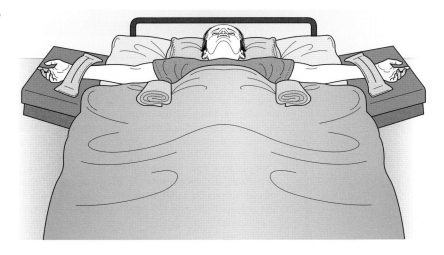

non-paralysed muscles which in turn increases the time muscles spend in shortened positions. This is particularly problematic if the antagonist muscles are paralysed. For example, patients with C5 tetraplegia and shoulder pain are more likely to hold their shoulders adducted and internally rotated. Prolonged immobilization in this position leads to contractures of the shoulder adductor and internal rotator muscles.

Independence with activities of daily living reduces susceptibility to contractures. For instance, a patient with C6 tetraplegia who transfers independently throughout the day extends the elbows while bearing weight through the upper limbs (see Chapter 3, Table 3.8)[14,15,81] and is therefore less likely to develop elbow flexion contractures than a more dependent patient with the same neurological loss.

The pattern and extent of spasticity also influences susceptibility to contractures.[11] Spasticity not only directly influences the extensibility of muscles (i.e. contributes to

Figure 9.14 Lying with an abduction wedge between the legs is a way of applying a sustained stretch to the hip adductor muscles.

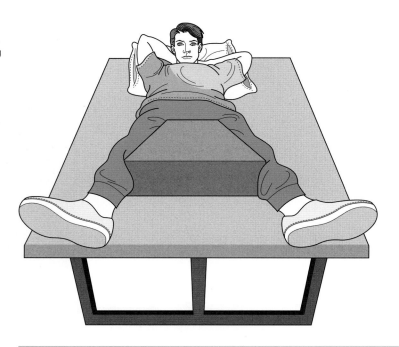

neurally mediated contractures, as discussed above), but it also increases the time which muscles and surrounding soft tissues spend in shortened positions.[6,9,82,83] For example, spasticity of elbow flexor muscles increases the time the elbow spends flexed so it predisposes patients to non-neurally mediated elbow flexion contractures. Paradoxically, spasticity can also prevent contractures. Patients otherwise susceptible to elbow flexion contractures can benefit from regular and strong elbow extensor spasticity because the spasticity can act to minimize the length of time the elbow spends in a flexed position (this pattern of spasticity is more common in patients with C5 than C6 tetraplegia; see p. 12 for explanation).

Prioritizing treatments: a touch of reality

Ideally, full passive range would be maintained in all joints of all patients throughout their lives. However, this is rarely achieved in patients with extensive paralysis. For example, often over the years and despite best intentions, those with lower limb paralysis lose passive dorsiflexion around the ankle and those with tetraplegia lose passive extension of the IP joints of the hand. The difficulty of maintaining full range of motion in all joints of all patients throughout their lives underpins the importance of prioritizing treatments so therapeutic attention is concentrated where it truly matters. Prioritization requires an understanding of the implications of losses of extensibility on function. The implications vary with the level and type of spinal cord injury. Thus, while almost all contractures are undesirable and would ideally be avoided, *slight* loss of extensibility has more deleterious implications in some soft tissues and for some patients than others. Clearly, this is where therapeutic attention should be concentrated.[79]

For example, slight loss of extensibility in the soft tissues spanning the flexor aspect of the elbow has few functional implications for patients with C5 tetraplegia because these patients are unable to bear weight through the upper limbs. However, the same loss can prevent patients with C6 tetraplegia from attaining independence with transfers (see Chapter 3).[4,14,15,81] Similarly, slight loss of extensibility in soft tissues spanning the plantar aspect of the ankle (e.g. the soleus muscle) has few functional implications for wheelchair-dependent patients with high levels of tetraplegia but marked implications for patients with the potential to walk. Likewise, hamstring extensibility is important for those who will sit unsupported on a bed with the legs in front of them while dressing and transferring, but less important for those who will not sit independently (see Chapter 3). Concentrated effort should be directed at preventing loss of extensibility where such loss will limit function and quality of life. Prioritization is easiest if contractures are linked to activity and participation goals.

Non-stretch-based modalities

A range of non-stretch-based modalities have been advocated for the treatment and prevention of contractures. These include manual pressure, joint compression, slow rolling or rocking, slow spinning, heat, cold, electrical stimulation, biofeedback, tone inhibitory casts, hydrotherapy, TENS and vibration, as well as therapeutic and Bobath exercise techniques. Some of these interventions may have transient effects on the neural and non-neural determinants of joint mobility, but none are likely to induce lasting changes in joint range of motion.[84,85]

Reducing muscle extensibility

Sometimes therapy is directed not at increasing extensibility but decreasing it. For example, excessive extensibility of the paralysed extrinsic finger and thumb flexor muscles is deleterious for the hand function of patients with C6 and C7 tetraplegia (see Chapter 5).[86–90] Similarly, excessive extensibility in the hamstring muscles is undesirable for wheelchair-dependent patients reliant on its passive tension to prevent a forwards fall when sitting (see Figure 3.3). In both scenarios, treatment is directed at reducing muscle extensibility. Reductions in extensibility are presumably best achieved by avoiding activities that place muscles in a stretched position. For example, to induce shortening in the hamstring muscles patients need to avoid sitting unsupported with the knees extended. Similarly, to induce shortening in the extrinsic finger flexor muscles patients should not sit weight bearing through an outstretched hand. The effectiveness of more aggressive interventions that immobilize muscles in shortened positions for prolonged periods of time is not known; however, at least one clinical trial suggests that it may be more difficult for therapists to induce shortening in muscles than commonly assumed.[91]

References

1. Scott JA, Donovan WH: The prevention of shoulder pain and contracture in the acute tetraplegia patient. Paraplegia 1981; 19:313–319.
2. Yarkony GM, Bass LM, Keenan V et al: Contractures complicating spinal cord injury: incidence and comparison between spinal cord centre and general hospital acute care. Paraplegia 1985; 23:265–271.

3. Dalyan M, Sherman A, Cardenas DD: Factors associated with contractures in acute spinal cord injury. Spinal Cord 1998; 36:405–408.

4. Bryden AM, Kilogre KL, Lind BB et al: Triceps denervation as a predictor of elbow flexion contractures in C5 and C6 tetraplegia. Arch Phys Med Rehabil 2004; 85:1880–1885.

5. McDonald MF, Garrison MK, Schmit BD: Length-tension properties of ankle muscles in chronic human spinal cord injury. J Biomech 2005; 8:2344–2353.

6. Sinkjaer T, Toft E, Larsen K et al: Non-reflex and reflex mediated ankle joint stiffness in multiple sclerosis patients with spasticity. Muscle Nerve 1993; 16:69–76.

7. Herman R: The myotatic reflex. Clinico-physiological aspects of spasticity and contracture. Brain 1970; 93:273–312.

8. Lamontagne A, Malouin F, Richards CL et al: Evaluation of reflex- and nonreflex-induced muscle resistance to stretch in adults with spinal cord injury using hand-held and isokinetic dynamometry. Phys Ther 1998; 78:964–978.

9. O'Dwyer NJ, Ada L: Reflex hyperexcitability and muscle contracture in relation to spastic hypertonia. Curr Opin Neurol 1996; 9:451–455.

10. Sinkjaer T, Magnussen I: Passive, intrinsic and reflex-mediated stiffness in the ankle extensors of hemiparetic patients. Brain 1994; 117:355–363.

11. Dietz V: Spastic movement disorder. Spinal Cord 2000; 38:389–393.

12. Moseley AM: The effect of casting combined with stretching on passive ankle dorsiflexion in adults with traumatic head injuries. Phys Ther 1997; 77:240–247.

13. Cooper JE, Shwedyk E, Quanbury AO et al: Elbow joint restriction: effect on functional upper limb motion during performance of three feeding activities. Arch Phys Med Rehabil 1993; 74:805–809.

14. Harvey LA, Crosbie J: Weight bearing through flexed upper limbs in quadriplegics with paralyzed triceps brachii muscles. Spinal Cord 1999; 37:780–785.

15. Grover J, Gellman H, Waters RL: The effect of a flexion contracture of the elbow on the ability to transfer in patients who have quadriplegia at the sixth cervical level. J Bone Joint Surg (Am) 1996; 78:1397–1400.

16. Freehafer AA: Flexion and supination deformities of the elbow in tetraplegics. Paraplegia 1977; 15:221–225.

17. Waring WP, Maynard FM: Shoulder pain in acute traumatic quadriplegia. Paraplegia 1991; 29:37–42.

18. Harvey L, King M, Herbert R: Reliability of a tool for measuring the length of long finger flexor muscles. J Hand Ther 1995; 7:251–254.

19. Flowers KR, Pheasant SD: The use of torque angle curves in the assessment of digital joint stiffness. J Hand Ther 1988; 1:69–74.

20. Moseley AM, Adams R: Measurement of passive ankle dorsiflexion: procedure and reliability. Aust J Physiother 1991; 37:175–181.

21. Harvey L, Byak A, Ostrovskaya M et al: Reliability of a device designed to measure ankle mobility. Spinal Cord 2003; 41:559–562.

22. Harvey L, Simpson D, Glinsky J et al: Quantifying the passive extensibility of the flexor pollicis longus muscle in people with tetraplegia. Spinal Cord 2005; 43:620–624.

23. Patrick E, Ada L: The Tardieu Scale differentiates contracture from spasticity whereas the Ashworth Scale is confounded by it. Clin Rehabil 2006; 20:173–182.

24. Adkins HV (ed): Spinal Cord Injury. New York, Churchill Livingstone, 1985.

25. Bromley I: Tetraplegia and Paraplegia: a Guide for Physiotherapists, 5th edn. Edinburgh, New York, Churchill Livingstone, 1998.

26. Somers MF: Spinal Cord Injury: Functional Rehabilitation, 2nd edn. Upper Saddle River, NJ, Prentice Hall, 2001.

27. Crowe J, MacKay-Lyons M, Morris H: A multi-centre, randomized controlled trial of the effectiveness of positioning on quadriplegic shoulder pain. Physiother Can 2000; 52:266–273.

28. Svensson M, Siosteen A, Wetterqvist H et al: Influence of physiotherapy on leg blood flow in patients with complete spinal cord injury lesions. Physiother Theory Pract 1995; 11:97–107.

29. Schmitz TJ: Traumatic spinal cord injury. In O'Sullivan SB, Schmitz TJ (eds): Physical Rehabilitation: Assessment and Treatment. Philadelphia, FA Davis, 2000.

30. Harvey LA, McQuade L, Hawthorne S et al: Quantifying the magnitude of torque physiotherapists apply when stretching the hamstring muscles of people with spinal cord injury. Arch Phys Med Rehabil 2003; 84:1072–1075.

31. Herbert RD: The prevention and treatment of stiff joints. In Crosbie J, McConnell J (eds): Key Issues in Musculoskeletal Physiotherapy. Oxford, Butterworth Heinemann, 1993:114–141.

32. Tardieu C, Tabary JC, Tabary C et al: Adaptation of sarcomere numbers to the length imposed on muscle. In Guba F, Marechal G, Takacs O (eds): Mechanism of Muscle Adaptation of Functional Requirements. Elmsford, NY, Pergamon Press, 1981:99–113.

33. Herbert R: How muscles respond to stretch. In Refshauge K, Ada L, Ellis E (eds): Science-based Rehabilitation. Theories into Practice. Edinburgh, New York, Butterworth Heinemann, 2005:107–130.

34. Tabary JC, Tabary C, Tardieu C et al: Physiological and structural changes in the cat's soleus muscle due to immobilization at different lengths by plaster casts. J Physiol 1972; 224:231–244.
35. Tabary JC, Tardieu C, Tardieu G et al: Experimental rapid sarcomere loss with concomitant hypoextensibility. Muscle Nerve 1981; 4:198–203.
36. Herbert RD, Balnave RJ: The effect of position of immobilisation on resting length, resting stiffness, and weight of the soleus muscle of the rabbit. J Orthop Res 1993; 11:358–366.
37. Tardieu G, Tardieu C, Colbeau-Justin P et al: Muscle hypoextensibility in children with Cerebral Palsy: II. Therapeutic implications. Arch Phys Med Rehabil 1982; 63:103–107.
38. Williams PE, Goldspink G: Connective tissue changes in immobilised muscle. J Anat 1984; 138:343–350.
39. Woo SL, Mathews JV, Akeson WH et al: Connective tissue response to immobility. Correlative study of biomechanical and biochemical measurements of normal and immobilized rabbit knees. Arthritis Rheum 1975; 18:257–264.
40. Booth F: Physiological and biochemical effects of immobilisation on muscle. Clin Orthop Relat Res 1987; 219:15–20.
41. Williams PE, Goldspink G: The effect of immobilization on the longitudinal growth of striated muscle fibres. J Anat 1973; 116:45–55.
42. Williams PE, Catanese T, Lucey EG et al: The importance of stretch and contractile activity in the prevention of connective tissue accumulation in muscle. J Anat 1988; 158:109–114.
43. Williams PE: Effect of intermittent stretch on immobilised muscle. Ann Rheum Dis 1988; 47:1014–1016.
44. Goldspink G, Tarbary C, Tabary JC et al: Effect of denervation on the adaptation of sarcomere number and muscle extensibility to the functional length of the muscle J Physiol 1974; 236: 733–742.
45. Goldspink DF: The influence of immobilization and stretch on protein turnover of rat skeletal muscle. J Physiol 1977; 264:267–282.
46. Witzmann FA, Kim DH, Fitts RH: Hindlimb immobilization: length-tension and contractile properties of skeletal muscle. J Appl Physiol 1982; 53:335–345.
47. Tardieu G, Thuilleux G, Tardieu C et al: Long-term effects of surgical elongation of the tendo calcaneus in the normal cat. Dev Med Child Neurol 1979; 21:83–94.
48. Gossman MR, Sahrmann SA, Rose SJ: Review of length-associated changes in muscle. Experimental evidence and clinical implications. Phys Ther 1982; 62:1799–1808.
49. Akeson WH, Amiel D, Abel MF et al: Effects of immobilization on joints. Clin Orthop Relat Res 1987; 219:28–37.
50. Herbert R: Adaptations of muscle and connective tissue. In Refshauge KM, Gass EM (eds): Musculoskeletal Physiotherapy: Clinical Science and Practice. Oxford, Butterworth Heinemann, 2004:39–44.
51. Williams PE, Goldspink G: The effect of denervation and dystrophy on the adaptation of sarcomere number to the functional length of the muscle in young and adult mice. J Anat 1976; 122:455–465.
52. Goldspink DF: The influence of passive stretch on the growth and turnover of the denervated extensor digitorum longus muscle. Biochem J 1978; 174:595–602.
53. Hayat A, Tardieu C, Tabary JC et al: Effects of denervation on the reduction of sarcomere number in cat soleus muscle immobilized in shortened position during seven days. J Physiol (Paris) 1978; 74:563–567.
54. Williams PE: Use of intermittent stretch in the prevention of serial sarcomere loss in immobilised muscle. Ann Rheum Dis 1990; 49:316–317.
55. Harvey L, Herbert R, Crosbie J: Does stretching induce lasting increases in joint ROM? A systematic review. Physiother Res Int 2002; 7:1–13.
56. Radford JA, Burns J, Buchbinder R et al: Does stretching increase ankle dorsiflexion range of motion? A systematic review. Br J Sports Med 2006; 40:870–875.
57. Magnusson SP, Simonsen EB, Aagaard P et al: Viscoelastic response to repeated static stretching in the human hamstring muscle. Scand J Med Sci Sports 1995; 5:342–347.
58. Magnusson SP, Simonsen EB, Aagaard P et al: Biomechanical responses to repeated stretches in human hamstring muscle in vivo. Am J Sports Med 1996; 24:622–628.
59. Magnusson SP, Simonsen EB, Dhyre-Poulsen P et al: Viscoelastic stress relaxation during static stretch in human skeletal muscle in the absence of EMG activity. Scand J Med Sci Sports 1996; 6:323–328.
60. Toft E, Esperson GT, Kalund S et al: Passive tension of the ankle before and after stretching. Am J Sports Med 1989; 17:489–494.
61. Duong B, Low M, Moseley AM et al: Time course of stress relaxation and recovery in human ankles. Clin Biomech 2001; 16:601–607.
62. Magnusson SP, Simonsen EB, Aagaard P et al: A mechanism for altered flexibility in human skeletal muscle. J Appl Physiol 1996; 497:291–298.
63. Folpp H, Deall S, Harvey LA et al: Can apparent increases in muscle extensibility with regular stretch be explained by changes in tolerance to stretch? Aust J Physiother 2006; 52:45–50.

64. Harvey LA, Batty J, Crosbie J et al: A randomized trial assessing the effects of 4 weeks of daily stretching on ankle mobility in patients with spinal cord injuries. Arch Phys Med Rehabil 2000; 81:1340–1347.

65. Harvey LA, Byak AJ, Ostrovskaya M et al: Randomised trial of the effects of four weeks of daily stretch on extensibility of hamstring muscles in people with spinal cord injuries. Aust J Physiother 2003; 49:176–181.

66. Ben M, Harvey L, Denis S et al: Does 12 weeks of regular standing prevent loss of ankle mobility and bone mineral density in people with recent spinal cord injuries? Aust J Physiother 2005; 51:251–256.

67. Harvey LA, de Jong I, Geohl G et al: Twelve weeks of nightly stretch does not reduce thumb web-space contractures in people with a neurological condition: a randomised controlled trial. Aust J Physiother 2006; 52:251–258.

68. Lannin NA, Horsley SA, Herbert R et al: Splinting the hand in the functional position after brain impairment: a randomized, controlled trial. Arch Phys Med Rehabil 2003; 84:297–302.

69. Ada L, Goddard E, McCully J et al: Thirty minutes of positioning reduces the development of shoulder external rotation contractures after stroke: a randomized controlled trial. Arch Phys Med Rehabil 2005; 86:230–234.

70. Autti-Ramo I, Suoranta J, Anttila H et al: Effectiveness of upper and lower limb casting and orthoses in children with cerebral palsy: an overview of review articles. Am J Phys Med Rehabil 2006; 85:89–103.

71. Dean CM, Mackey FH, Katrak P: Examination of shoulder positioning after stroke: A randomised controlled pilot trial. Aust J Physiother 2000; 46:35–40.

72. Turton AJ, Britton E: A pilot randomized controlled trial of a daily muscle stretch regime to prevent contractures in the arm after stroke. Clin Rehabil 2005; 19:600–612.

73. Refshauge KM, Raymond J, Nicholson G et al: Night splinting does not increase ankle range of motion in people with Charcot-Marie-Tooth disease: A randomised cross-over trial. Aust J Physiother 2006; 52:193–199.

74. Seeger MW, Furst DE: Effects of splinting in the treatment of hand contractures in progressive systemic sclerosis. Am J Occup Ther 1987; 41:118–121.

75. Bohannon RW, Larkin PA: Passive ankle dorsiflexion increases in patients after a regimen of tilt table-wedge board standing. Phys Ther 1985; 65:1676–1678.

76. Mortenson P, Eng JJ: The use of casts in the management of joint mobility and hypertonia following brain injury in adults: a systematic review. Phys Ther 2003; 83:648–658.

77. Ter Woerds W, De Groot PC, van Kuppevelt DH et al: Passive leg movements and passive cycling do not alter arterial leg blood flow in subjects with spinal cord injury. Phys Ther 2006; 86:636–645.

78. Ada L, Canning A: Anticipating and avoiding muscle shortening. In Ada L, Canning A (eds): Key Issues in Neurological Physiotherapy. Oxford, Butterworth Heinemann, 1990:219–236.

79. Harvey LA, Herbert RD: Muscle stretching for treatment and prevention of contracture in people with spinal cord injury. Spinal Cord 2002; 40:1–9.

80. Hokken W, Kalkman S, Blanken WC et al: A dynamic pronation orthosis for the C6 tetraplegic arm. Arch Phys Med Rehabil 1993; 74:104–105.

81. Harvey L, Crosbie J: Effect of elbow flexion contractures on the ability of people with C5 and C6 tetraplegia to lift. Physiother Res Int 2001; 62:78–82.

82. O'Dwyer NJ, Ada L, Neilson PD: Spasticity and muscle contracture following stroke. Brain 1996; 119:1737–1749.

83. Siegler S, Carr E: A method for discriminating between spasticity and contracture at the ankle joint during locomotion in neurologically impaired persons. Study Institute and Conference: Biomechanics of Human Movement. Formia, Italy, 1986.

84. Pierson SH: Physical and occupational approaches. In Gelber DA, Jeffery DR (eds): Clinical Evaluation and Management of Spasticity. Totowa, Humana Press, 2002:47–66.

85. Pandyan AD, Gregoric M, Barnes MP et al: Spasticity: Clinical perceptions, neurological realities and meaningful measurement. Disabil Rehabil 2005; 27:2–6.

86. Harvey L: Principles of conservative management for a non-orthotic tenodesis grip in tetraplegics. J Hand Ther 1996; 9:238–242.

87. Curtin M: An analysis of tetraplegic hand grips. Br J Occup Ther 1999; 62:444–450.

88. Doll U, Maurer-Burkhard B, Spahn B et al: Functional hand development in tetraplegia. Spinal Cord 1998; 36:818–821.

89. Harvey L, Batty J, Jones R et al: Hand function in C6 and C7 quadriplegics 1–16 years following injury. Spinal Cord 2001; 39:37–43.

90. DiPasquale-Lehnerz P: Orthotic intervention for development of hand function with C-6 quadriplegia. Am J Occup Ther 1994; 48:138–144.

91. Harvey L, Simpson D, Pironello D et al: Does three months of nightly splinting reduce the extensibility of the flexor pollicis longus muscle in people with tetraplegia? Physiother Res Int 2006; 12:5–13.

Contents

Assessment 194
Neuropathic pain 195
Nociceptive pain 196
Role of psychosocial
factors in chronic pain 200

Pain management

Pain is a common complication of spinal cord injury which not only limits ability to perform motor tasks, but also has important implications for quality of life, well-being and general feelings of happiness.[1–6] Physiotherapy is one component of a comprehensive pain management programme which typically involves pharmacological, surgical, psychological and behavioural interventions.

There are many different types of pain which occur in association with spinal cord injury, and the characteristics, patterns of presentation, intensity and location are highly variable. Some types of pain present at the time of spinal cord injury while other types of pain have a more insidious onset and can present years later and involve many different areas of the body. In some circumstances pain resolves quickly with minimal intervention but at other times it appears unresponsive to any intervention, and evolves into a chronic problem adversely affecting all aspects of patients' lives.

Pain associated with spinal cord injury can be categorized as either nociceptive or neuropathic (see Table 10.1).[7,8] Neuropathic pain arises from primary lesions of the nervous system and the associated neural dysfunction, while nociceptive pain originates from musculoskeletal or visceral structures. Our understanding of the underlying causes of neuropathic and nociceptive pain in patients with spinal cord injury is limited. There is some evidence to suggest that changes within the central nervous system following spinal cord injury lead to a heightened sensitivity (or neuronal excitability) and this contributes to the development of pain. Pain may have its origins at the receptor level or may be due to abnormal firing of neurons in the central nervous system either as a result of increased excitability through receptor changes or disruption of normal local and descending pain inhibitory pathways.[6] However, most studies looking at prevalence and causative factors use cross-sectional rather than longitudinal designs, making even the identification of key prognostic factors problematic.[6] The few more recent longitudinal studies have primarily looked at predictors of pain during the first 1–2 years after injury.[4]

TABLE 10.1 Classification of pain associated with spinal cord injury proposed by the Spinal Cord Injury Pain Task Force of the International Association of the Study of Pain[8]

Broad type	Broad system	Specific structures/pathology
Nociceptive	Musculoskeletal	Bone, joint, muscle trauma or inflammation Mechanical instability Muscle spasm Secondary overuse syndromes
	Visceral	Renal calculus, bowel, sphincter dysfunction, etc. Dysreflexic headache
Neuropathic	Above-level	Compressive mononeuropathies Complex regional pain syndromes
	At-level	Nerve compression (including cauda equina) Syringomyelia Spinal cord trauma/ischaemia (transitional zone, etc.) Dual level cord and root trauma (double lesion syndrome)
	Below-level	Spinal cord trauma/ischaemia

Reproduced from Siddall P, Yezierski RP, Loeser JD: Pain following spinal cord injury: clinical features, prevalence, and taxonomy. Technical Corner Newsletter of the International Association for the Study of Pain 2000; 3:3–7, with permission of The International Association for the Study of Pain.

Assessment

The first and most important purpose of a pain assessment is to ensure that there is no reason for serious concern (e.g. fractures, infections, tumours, syringomyelia[9]). If in any doubt, patients should be assessed by a medical specialist. Symptoms which may indicate the need for further medical investigation include deterioration in motor, sensory, bladder or bowel function, recent loss of weight, deterioration in 'balance', raised temperature and night sweats. Aspects of the history which may suggest a more sinister underlying cause of pain include history of acute trauma, use of corticosteroids and history of cancer.[10] It is also important to remember that patients with spinal cord injury are typically osteoporotic, and even minor physical injuries can cause fractures (see p. 21).

The assessment of pain relies on patient self-report about the characteristics of their pain, associated symptoms, activity limitations and participation restrictions (see Table 10.2).

The common measures used to quantify pain intensity are the visual analogue scale[11] and the numerical rating scale.[12] Pain drawings can be used to identify the distribution of pain,[13] and the McGill Pain Questionnaire[14] can be used to assess the quality of the pain. There are also various questionnaire-based assessments for neuropathic pain.[15] Other symptoms, such as reduced joint mobility, can be assessed using standard assessments of impairments (as outlined in previous chapters).

A pain assessment also needs to determine the implications of pain on activity limitations and participation restrictions. This is not only important for understanding the implications of pain on different aspects of patients' lives, but also for establishing a baseline measure upon which change can be monitored. This is particularly important in patients with chronic pain. Often interventions do not change the characteristics of

TABLE 10.2 The assessment of pain includes patient's self-report of the characteristics of their pain and associated symptoms

• presenting complaint	• history of pain	• quality of symptoms
• related medical history	• intensity of pain	• other symptoms (i.e. numbness,
• previous and current interventions	• frequency of pain	limited range, joint instability,
(including medication use)	• distribution of pain	paraesthesia, allodynia and
• mechanism of onset	• duration of pain	hyperalgesia)
• implications for participation	• quality of pain	• location of symptoms
• aggravating and easing factors		• behaviour of symptoms
• social factors (work, family support,		
recreation)		

pain but rather change pain-related behaviours and coping mechanisms.[16] These changes can be captured in measures of activity limitations and participation restrictions such as the Functional Independence Measure, Quadriplegic Index of Function, Spinal Cord Independence Measure or Barthell (see Chapter 2). An assessment specific to shoulder pain in patients with spinal cord injury is The Wheelchair User's Shoulder Pain Index.[17] This quantifies implications of shoulder pain on different aspects of patients' mobility and life.

It is often also helpful for physiotherapists to consider the biopsychosocial dimension of pain, including the contribution of psychological, social and behavioural factors.[18,19] Examples of measures which capture some of these dimensions of pain include the Pain Self-Efficacy Questionnaire,[20] the Fear-avoidance Beliefs Questionnaire,[21] the SF-36[22] and the Multidimensional Pain Inventory.[15,23]

Neuropathic pain

Neuropathic pain is a term used to encompass many different syndromes of pain, and includes pain due to compressive mononeuropathies, nerve root compression and syringomyelia, as well as spinal cord trauma. The pain can be above, at, or below the level of the lesion. Typically, neuropathic pain is described as burning, electric or stabbing pain, difficult to alleviate by activity or change of position. It is commonly associated with increased sensitivity to touch or any other type of physical contact. Sometimes this type of pain occurs in two to four dermatomes between areas of no sensation and areas of normal sensation (at-level neuropathic pain). In this case, the neuropathic pain commonly presents soon after injury, and is bilateral and circumferential. Alternatively, the pain can be felt more diffusely in areas without sensation below the level of the lesion (below-level neuropathic pain). Other terms used to describe this latter type of pain are central dysaesthesias syndrome, dysaesthetic pain, central pain or phantom pain.

Neuropathic pain is difficult to treat, and is largely managed pharmacologically, although the small number of clinical trials in this area have generated conflicting results.[6,24] There is some limited evidence to suggest that physiotherapy-type interventions designed to desensitize the affected dermatomes may be useful. TENS is also widely advocated, but currently without good evidence. Perhaps the largest role for physiotherapy, in patients with this type of pain, is encouraging graded exercise and activity to minimize secondary impairments and activity limitations. It is particularly important to ensure patients do not develop secondary contractures from holding limbs in protected positions (see Chapter 9).

Nociceptive pain

Nociceptive pain can be due to trauma, disease or inflammation of musculoskeletal or visceral structures. Physiotherapy interventions used to manage nociceptive pain include exercise, massage, stretch, re-education and guided return to activity.[25] A recent Swedish study indicated that 63% of patients with spinal cord injury-related pain tried one or other of these types of pain-relieving interventions.[25] Below is a summary of some of the more common musculoskeletal problems seen in patients with spinal cord injury (readers interested in pain from visceral origins are directed to Ref. 26).

Back or neck pain associated with initial injury

Back and neck pain are common immediately after injury, and particularly in patients with extensive disruption to bony and ligamentous structures of the spine. This type of pain can be due to mechanical instability or the direct effects of extensive soft tissue trauma. It is typically managed with immobilization, pain-relieving medication and/or surgery. Medical staff determine when patients can mobilize after injury, but within these guidelines physiotherapists need to encourage activity to prevent secondary disablement. The use of hot packs with or without gentle superficial massage once patients have mobilized may provide some temporary pain relief and will often provide general comfort. However, therapists need to obtain medical clearance if there is any risk that their interventions will cause movement at the injury site and hot packs should not be applied to areas with impaired sensation.

Chronic back or neck pain

If back or neck pain persists for more than 3 months without any apparent underlying cause and develops into chronic pain, then it may be appropriate to use the existing clinical guidelines on the management of chronic neck and back pain advocated for the able-bodied population but modified in an appropriate way.[27-31] These guidelines are based on high quality evidence and recommend minimal use of passive interventions, such as massage, electrotherapeutic agents or manual therapies, but rather appropriate, graded and supported return to active exercise and 'normal' activity, combined with reassurance about good prognosis. These guidelines do not recommend continued, ongoing and detailed physiotherapy-type assessments, unless there is reason to be concerned. They also highlight the futility of trying to make a precise diagnosis on the source of musculoskeletal pain and emphasize the importance of early efforts at minimizing fear, providing reassurance and encouraging graded return to activity.[32] While these guidelines have not been systematically evaluated in patients with spinal cord injury, they would seem a reasonable starting point in the absence of more specific and relevant research. At least one clinical trial indicates the benefits of encouraging activity and exercise for relieving chronic pain in patients with spinal cord injury.[33]

Shoulder pain in patients with high levels of tetraplegia

Shoulder pain is common in patients with C5 and above tetraplegia. It is more common and intense in the first year after injury, with some estimating the incidence as high as 85%.[34] In patients with established tetraplegia the incidence is between 45 and 60%.[35-37]

Possible causes

Shoulder pain in patients with high-level tetraplegia has many features in common with the shoulder pain experienced by patients with stroke. Both groups of patients have extensive paralysis around the shoulder, with or without loss of sensation. Therefore it is arguably pertinent to examine not only what is known about shoulder pain of patients with spinal cord injury, but also what is known about shoulder pain of those following stroke.

There are many different theories about the possible causes of shoulder pain in patients with tetraplegia (and stroke) including subluxation, poor physical handling by carers, prolonged sitting and lying, and limited change of shoulder position. Typically, small studies look at the relationship between shoulder pain and some of these factors.[34,38,39] However, a theoretical argument about the importance of each factor can be mounted and, without large-scale prognostic studies, it is not known which of these factors is most important and where therapeutic attention is best directed.

Subluxation

Shoulder pain may be due to overstretching of the delicate soft tissues around the glenohumeral joint secondary to inferior subluxation. Any tendency for subluxation may be increased by downward and medial rotation of the bottom tip of the scapula. In turn, medial rotation of the scapula may be precipitated by paralysis of the serratus anterior muscles and loss of extensibility in the rhomboid muscles. Dropping of the inferior lip of the glenoid fossa diminishes the scapula's ability to support and protect the head of the humerus against distracting forces. The tendency for inferior subluxation may be further aggravated through poor physical handling from therapists and carers. These and other theories about the relationship between shoulder subluxation and pain have been widely discussed since 1957,[40] but they are still speculative and contentious.[41-43]

Recent attention has been directed at determining the most effective way to treat and prevent shoulder subluxation, although most of the clinical trials in this area have been with patients following stroke, not spinal cord injury.[42,44] Some studies indicate that shoulder support reduces subluxation[45] but does not decrease pain, while others show a treatment effect on pain but not subluxation.[42] A recent Cochrane systematic review concluded that, in patients with stroke, there is insufficient evidence to indicate whether supportive devices prevent subluxation, although they may delay the onset of shoulder pain.[46] Regardless, therapists are well advised to ensure that the arm troughs of wheelchairs are appropriately adjusted to provide shoulder support. Shoulder support can also be provided with pillows, strapping, lap boards, slings or shoulder harnesses (see Figure 10.1).[42,45,47]

Regular electrical stimulation of the deltoid and supraspinatus muscles may also help prevent subluxation and pain. However, this has only been demonstrated in patients following stroke.[44,48-50] In stroke patients the electrical stimulation may be acting as a training stimulus, helping patients regain control and strength around the shoulder. Patients with tetraplegia have a poorer prognosis for motor recovery and therefore may not respond as well to the intervention. The very time-consuming nature of administering electrical stimulation may also restrict its usefulness.

Patients with some remaining voluntary motor power in the deltoid and supraspinatus muscles may benefit from strengthening exercises (see Chapter 8). Improvements in strength, however, will be limited by the extent of paralysis. The

Figure 10.1   The arms of patients with no or limited upper limb function need to be supported to help prevent shoulder pain. Arm troughs appropriately fitted and adjusted to the wheelchair can be used for this purpose.

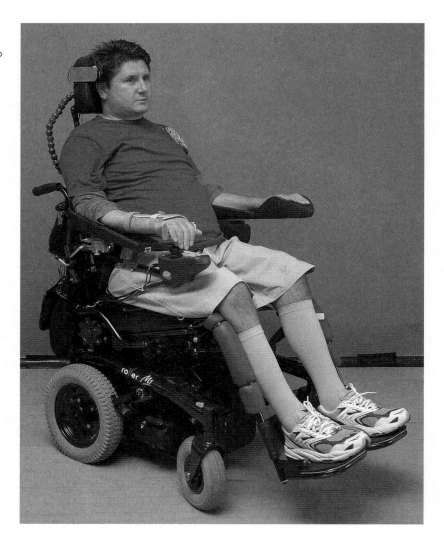

effectiveness of subtle increases in the strength of very weak patients (e.g. grade 1/5 or 2/5 motor power) for alleviating shoulder subluxation and pain is not known.

Repeated soft tissue trauma with physical handling

Shoulder pain may be due to physical handling of the paralysed arm by carers and therapists.[43] Paralysis around the shoulder prevents patients from protecting their shoulders when they are moved by others. Paralysis also prevents the normal scapulo-humeral movement which may be important for preventing impingement of the supraspinatus tendon between the humeral head and acromion. Consequently, repeated movement and/or pulling of the shoulders by others may cause impingement or other forms of soft tissue trauma.[43]

Susceptibility to impingement or trauma may be increased with secondary losses of joint range of motion, or if the scapula is not free to passively move. For example, if carers dress a lying patient by raising the arm above the head without enabling the scapula to move passively, they may damage the capsule of the glenohumeral joint or cause impingement of the supraspinatus tendon. Patients with loss of passive scapula rotation and glenohumeral flexion may be particularly vulnerable. Similarly, if carers pull on the upper limbs during a transfer, or when moving a patient from lying to sitting, they may apply a large distracting force which the patient is unable to oppose. This may cause soft tissue trauma.

The most appropriate intervention is education for patients, carers, therapists and families. In particular, patients need to be aware of the care others need to take with their shoulders. In this way, patients can reinforce the education programmes of staff and carers. The use of electrical hoists for transfers would anecdotally appear to have reduced the incidence of shoulder pain. In addition, effective prevention of contractures around the shoulder may be important.[51] This involves regular change of shoulder position and sustained stretch (see Chapter 9).

Upper and lower limb musculoskeletal pain associated with overuse

There are two common types of musculoskeletal limb pain. One is the pain seen in recently injured patients due to repeated and unaccustomed exercise. For example, patients with recently acquired C6 tetraplegia can experience wrist pain following extensive wheelchair or transfer mobility training, or during weight bearing in sitting (see Chapter 3, Figure 3.11).[52] This particular activity places large torques and compression forces on a fully extended wrist.[52] Wrist pain from such activities appears to be especially common in patients with coexisting loss of passive wrist extension. The key to management of this type of musculoskeletal pain is rest and if necessary immobilization with splints. Once the acute pain has subsided, patients need to be gradually accustomed to exercise. For example, they can practise bearing less weight through a less extended wrist (achieved by placing a sandbag under the heel of the hand).

The second type of musculoskeletal limb pain seen in patients with spinal cord injury is from years of chronic overuse. This type of pain is particularly common in shoulders, elbows, wrists, hips and knees, and is associated with the excessive loads and stresses these joints bear over many years. Shoulder[6,35,38,53–58] and wrist joints[37,59] are vulnerable to the ongoing stresses of transferring, propelling a wheelchair[17,59–62] or using walking aids. Some studies have suggested that shoulder pain is as high as 30–50% in patients with established paraplegia[35,57,63,64] and perhaps even higher in patients with tetraplegia.[35,36,54,65] Similar problems are seen around the elbow, especially in wheelchair-dependent patients with paralysis of the triceps muscles. The lower limb joints are also vulnerable to overuse type injuries in ambulating patients with limited lower limb strength.

The underlying pathology of overuse syndromes is widely debated. In the shoulder it is often attributed to impingement of soft tissues within the subacromial space with movement.[36,53,54,58,66–70] Impingement may be precipitated by a reduced subacromial space associated with anatomical abnormalities or certain movements. Some types of repetitive movement which expose soft tissues to continual friction within the subacromial space may also be problematic.

Theories about the underlying causes of shoulder and overuse syndromes have led to work examining the biomechanics and ergonomics of different functional activities such as pushing a wheelchair,[62] relieving pressure, transferring,[53] and some simple, everyday tasks such as combing the hair.[56] Others have looked at the possible benefits of different supportive devices, including wrist splints for wheelchair propulsion.[59]

Recently, attention has been directed at the possible importance of preventative exercises and stretches, especially strengthening exercises for the shoulder external rotator muscles, to restore the 'balance' between the strength of agonists and antagonists in patients with tetraplegia and partial paralysis of the shoulder muscles.[35,69,71] Stretches for the internal rotator cuff muscles of the shoulder are also widely prescribed. There are many different interventions advocated for pain associated with overuse. These are primarily based on theories about the causes of pain rather than the results of clinical trials and their effectiveness remains unclear. However, it is reasonably unambiguous that ultrasound is not useful for most musculoskeletal problems.[72–75]

The most appropriate management of musculoskeletal pain associated with overuse is, as the name implies, avoiding overuse, and decreasing repetitive and strenuous activities.[76] In addition, patients need to avoid shoulder movements which may aggravate impingement of the supraspinatus tendon (i.e. activities which involve the hand being lifted above the head). Patients need to be provided with sensible lifestyle advice about ways of minimizing stress on joints and soft-tissue structures.[76] This might include advice about limiting the number of transfers performed within a day, optimizing the way a wheelchair is propelled, minimizing the complexity of transfers, rearranging the home or work environment or reducing the amount of walking or wheelchair propulsion.[61,76] Some of these changes will require new equipment or alterations to home and work environments. For example, an ambulating patient might require a manual wheelchair or more extensive lower limb bracing and a patient with thoracic paraplegia might require a power wheelchair for some occasions. Not unreasonably, patients will be unwilling to make lifestyle changes which compromise independence in order to prevent a potential complication which *may* occur tomorrow. It is also important that advice about strategies to minimize likelihood of shoulder pain does not inadvertently discourage physical activity, as physical activity is important for general well-being (see Chapter 12).

Complex regional pain syndromes

Complex regional pain syndromes are usually categorized as a form of neuropathic pain but are a common cause of shoulder and arm pain worthy of mention. The terms complex regional pain syndromes I and II replace the old terms reflex sympathetic dystrophy and causalgia.[77] Complex regional pain syndromes are characterized by pain with associated autonomic symptoms in the affected limb such as changes in temperature, colour and sweating. Treatment is often difficult and although some patients respond to sympathetic blockade, most do not and treatment often relies on analgesia, sometimes in combination with antidepressants and anticonvulsants. Graded return to activity and desensitization programmes are also an important aspect of overall management.[78]

Role of psychosocial factors in chronic pain

Psychological, social and environmental factors play a key role in either magnifying or diminishing perceptions of pain.[6] This relationship has been well explored in chronic back and neck pain in the able-bodied population. In patients with spinal cord injury, psychosocial factors can predict more than 50% of the variance in chronic pain following spinal cord injury, and often psychosocial factors are better predictors of the severity of chronic pain than physical factors alone.[79,80] In particular, psychological stress (e.g. depression, anxiety, anger) has been associated with an increased risk of pain.[4] No association has been reported between pain and race, education or perceptions of the cause of spinal cord injury.[4] The importance of psychosocial factors highlights the importance of psychologists' involvement in the management of complex pain problems. Physiotherapists need to ensure that their interventions, assessments and approach are complementary to an integrated behavioural and psychological-based pain management programme.

References

1. Turner JA, Cardenas DD, Warms CA et al: Chronic pain associated with spinal cord injuries: a community survey. Arch Phys Med Rehabil 2001; 82:501–508.
2. Anke AGW, Stenehjem AE, Stanghell JK: Pain and life quality within 2 years of spinal cord injury. Paraplegia 1995; 33:555–559.
3. Kennedy P, Frankel HL, Gardner BP et al: Factors associated with acute and chronic pain following traumatic spinal cord injuries. Spinal Cord 1997; 35:814–817.
4. Putzke JD, Richards JS, Hicken BL et al: Interference due to pain following spinal cord injury: important predictors and impact on quality of life. Pain 2002; 100:231–242.
5. Kennedy P, Lude P, Taylor N: Quality of life, social participation, appraisals and coping post spinal cord injury: a review of four community samples. Spinal Cord 2006; 44:95–105.
6. Siddall PJ, Loeser JD: Pain following spinal cord injury. Spinal Cord 2001; 39:63–73.
7. Siddall P, Yezierski RP, Loeser JD: Pain following spinal cord injury: clinical features, prevalence, and taxonomy. Technical Corner Newsletter of the International Association for the Study of Pain 2000; 3:3–7.
8. Siddall PJ, Middleton JW: A proposed algorithm for the management of pain following spinal cord injury. Spinal Cord 2006; 44:67–77.
9. Schurch B, Wichmann W, Rossier AB: Post-traumatic syringomyelia (cystic myelopathy): a prospective study of 449 patients with spinal cord injury. J Neurol Neurosurg Psychiatry 1996; 60:61–67.
10. Bogduk N: Evidence-based clinical guidelines for the management of acute low back pain. http://www.emia.com.au/MedicalProviders/EvidenceBasedMedicine/afmm/. The Australasian Faculty of Musculoskeletal Medicine, 1999.
11. Huskisson EC: Measurement of pain. Lancet 1974; 9:127–131.
12. Downie WW, Leatham PA, Rhind VA: Studies with pain rating scales. Ann Rheum Dis 1978; 37:378–381.
13. Margolis RB, Tait RC, Krause SJ: A rating system for use with patient pain drawings. Pain 1986; 24:57–65.
14. Melzack R: The McGill Pain Questionnaire: major properties and scoring methods. Pain 1975; 1:277–299.
15. Bryce TN, Dijkers MPJM: Assessment of pain after SCI in clinical trials. Top Spinal Cord Inj Rehabil 2005; 11:50–68.
16. Butler DS, Moseley GL: Explain Pain. Adelaide, Australia, Noigroup Publications, 2003.
17. Curtis KA, Roach KE, Applegate EB et al: Reliability and validity of the Wheelchair User's Shoulder Pain Index (WUSPI). Paraplegia 1995; 33:595–601.
18. Haythornthwaite JA: Assessment of pain beliefs, coping and function. In McMahon SB, Kaltzenburg M (eds): Wall and Melzack's Textbook of Pain. Philadelphia, Elsevier Churchill Livingstone, 2006:317–328.
19. Strong J, Sturgess J, Unruh AM et al: Pain assessment and measurement. In Strong J, Unruh AM, Wright A et al (eds): Pain: A Textbook for Therapists. Edinburgh, Churchill Livingstone, 2002:123–147.
20. Asghari A, Nicholas MK: Pain self-efficacy beliefs and pain behaviour. A prospective study. Pain 2001; 94:85–100.
21. Waddell G, Newton M, Henderson I et al: A Fear-Avoidance Beliefs Questionnaire (FABQ) and the role of fear-avoidance beliefs in chronic low back pain and disability. Pain 1993; 52:157–168.
22. Ware JE: SF-36 health survey update. Spine 2000; 25:3130–3139.
23. Widerström-Noga EG, Cruz-Almeida Y, Martinez-Arizala A et al: Internal consistency, stability, and validity of the spinal cord injury version of the multidimensional pain inventory. Arch Phys Med Rehabil 2006; 87:516–523.
24. Finnerup NB, Johannesen IL, Sindrup SH et al: Pharmacological treatment of spinal cord injury pain. In Burchiel KJ, Yezierski RP (eds): Spinal Cord Injury Pain: Assessment, Mechanisms, Management. Progress in Pain Research and Management. Seattle, IASP Press, 2002:341–351.
25. Budh CN, Lundeberg T: Non-pharmacological pain-relieving therapies in individuals with spinal cord injury: a patient perspective. Complement Ther Med 2004; 12:189–197.
26. Bielefeldt K, Gebhart GF: Visceral pain: basic mechanisms. In McMahon SB, Koltzenburg M (eds): Wall and Melzack's Textbook of Pain. Philadelphia, Elsevier Churchill Livingstone, 2006.

27. Bekkering GE, Hendriks HJM, Koes BW et al: Dutch physiotherapy guidelines for low back pain. Physiotherapy 2003; 89:82–96.

28. Institute for Clinical Systems Improvement (ICSI): Assessment and Management of Chronic Pain. Bloomington, MN, Institute for Clinical Systems Improvement (ICSI), 2005.

29. Harris GR, Susman JL: Managing musculoskeletal complaints with rehabilitation therapy: summary of the Philadelphia Panel evidence-based clinical practice guidelines on musculoskeletal rehabilitation interventions. J Fam Pract 2002; 51:1042–1046.

30. Gross AR, Kay TM, Kennedy C et al: Clinical practice guideline on the use of manipulation or mobilization in the treatment of adults with mechanical neck disorders. Manual Therapy 2002; 7:193–205.

31. Koes BW, van Tulder MW, Ostelo R et al: Clinical guidelines for the management of low back pain in primary care: an international comparison. Spine 2001; 26:2504–2513.

32. Koes BW, van Tulder MW, Thomas S: Diagnosis and treatment of low back pain. BMJ 2006; 332:1430–1434.

33. Martin Ginis KA, Latimer AE, McKechnie K et al: Using exercise to enhance subjective well-being among people with spinal cord injury: the mediating influences of stress and pain. Rehabil Psychol 2003; 48:157–164.

34. Salisbury SK, Choy NL, Nitz J: Shoulder pain, range of motion, and functional motor skills after acute tetraplegia. Arch Phys Med Rehabil 2003; 84:1480–1485.

35. Curtis KA, Drysdale GA, Lanza RD et al: Shoulder pain in wheelchair users with tetraplegia and paraplegia. Arch Phys Med Rehabil 1999; 80:453–457.

36. Sie IH, Waters RL, Adkins RH et al: Upper extremity pain in the postrehabilitation spinal cord injured patient. Arch Phys Med Rehabil 1992; 73:44–48.

37. Subbarao JV, Klopfstein J, Turpin R: Prevalence and impact of wrist and shoulder pain in patients with spinal cord injury. J Spinal Cord Med 1995; 18:9–13.

38. Campbell CC, Koris MJ: Etiologies of shoulder pain in cervical spinal cord injury. Clin Orthop Relat Res 1996; 322:140–145.

39. MacKay-Lyons M: Shoulder pain in patients with acute quadriplegia. Physiother Can 1994; 46:255–258.

40. Tobin JS: Posthemiplegic shoulder pain. N Y State J Med 1957; 57:1377–1380.

41. Cailliet R: The shoulder in the hemiplegic patient. In Shoulder Pain, 3rd edn. Philadelphia, FA Davis Company, 1991:193–226.

42. Paci M, Nannetti L, Rinaldi LA: Glenohumeral subluxation in hemiplegia: An overview. J Rehabil Res Dev 2005; 42:557–568.

43. Turner-Stokes L, Jackson D: Shoulder pain after stroke: a review of the evidence base to inform the development of an integrated care pathway. Clin Rehabil 2002; 16:276–298.

44. Ada L, Foongchomcheay A: Efficacy of electrical stimulation in preventing or reducing subluxation of the shoulder after stroke: a meta-analysis. Aust J Physiother 2002; 48:257–267.

45. Dieruf K, Poole JL, Gregory C et al: Comparative effectiveness of the GivMohr sling in subjects with flaccid upper limbs on subluxation through radiologic analysis. Arch Phys Med Rehabil 2005; 86:2324–2329.

46. Ada L, Foongchomcheay A, Canning C: Supportive devices for preventing and treating subluxation of the shoulder after stroke. The Cochrane Database of Systematic Reviews 2005: Issue 1. Art. No.: CD003863. DOI: 10.1002/14651858.CD003863.pub2.

47. Hanger HC, Whitewood P, Brown G et al: A randomised controlled trial of strapping to prevent post-stroke shoulder pain. Clin Biomech 2000; 14:370–380.

48. Van Peppen RPS, Kwakkel G, Wood-Dauphinnee S et al: The impact of physical therapy on functional outcomes after stroke: What's the evidence? Clin Rehabil 2004; 18:833–862.

49. Price CIM, Pandyan AD: Electrical stimulation for preventing and treating post-stroke shoulder pain. The Cochrane Database of Systematic Reviews 2000: Issue 4. Art. No.: CD001698. DOI: 10.1002/14651858.CD001698.

50. Chae J, Yu DT, Walker ME et al: Intramuscular electrical stimulation for hemiplegic shoulder pain: a 12-month follow-up of a multiple-center, randomized clinical trial. Am J Phys Med Rehabil 2005; 84:832–842.

51. Crowe J, MacKay-Lyons M, Morris H: A multi-centre, randomized controlled trial of the effectiveness of positioning on quadriplegic shoulder pain. Physiother Can 2000; 52:266–273.

52. Hara Y: Dorsal wrist joint pain in tetraplegic patients during and after rehabilitation. J Rehabil Med 2003; 35:57–61.

53. Nawoczenski DA, Clobes SM, Gore SL et al: Three-dimensional shoulder kinematics during a pressure relief technique and wheelchair transfer. Arch Phys Med Rehabil 2003; 84:1293–1300.

54. Powers CM, Newsam CJ, Gronley JK et al: Isometric shoulder torque in subjects with spinal cord injury. Arch Phys Med Rehabil 1994; 75:761–765.

55. Gellman H, Sie I, Waters RL: Late complications of the weight-bearing upper extremity in the paraplegic patient. Clin Orthop Relat Res 1988; 233:132–135.

56. Gronley JK, Newsam CJ, Mulroy SJ et al: Electromyographic and kinematic analysis of the shoulder during four activities of daily living in men with C6 tetraplegia. J Rehabil Res Dev 2000; 37:423–432.

57. Nickols PJ, Norman P, Ennis JR: Wheelchair user's shoulder? Shoulder pain in patients with spinal cord lesions. Scand J Rehabil Med 1979; 11:29–32.
58. Silfverskiold J, Waters RL: Shoulder pain and functional disability in spinal cord injury patients. Clin Orthop Relat Res 1991; 272:141–145.
59. Malone LA, Gervais PL, Burnham RS et al: An assessment of wrist splint and glove use on wheeling kinematics. Clin Biomech 1998; 13:234–236.
60. Cooper RA, Boninger ML, Shimada SD et al: Glenohumeral joint kinematics and kinetics for three coordinate system representations during wheelchair propulsion. Am J Phys Med Rehabil 1999; 78:435–446.
61. Fitzgerald SG, Arva J, Cooper RA et al: A pilot study on community usage of a pushrim-activated, power-assisted wheelchair. Assist Technol 2003; 15:113–119.
62. Koontz AM, Cooper R, Boninbger ML et al: Shoulder kinematics and kinetics during two speeds of wheelchair propulsion. J Rehabil Res Dev 2002; 39:635–650.
63. Bayley JC, Cochran TP, Sledge CB: The weight-bearing shoulder. The impingement syndrome in paraplegics. J Bone Joint Surg (Am) 1987; 69:676–678.
64. Daylan M, Cardenas DD, Gerard B: Upper extremity pain after spinal cord injury. Spinal Cord 1999; 37:191–195.
65. Subbarao JV, Nemchausky BA, Niekelski JJ et al: Spinal cord dysfunction in older patients — rehabilitation outcomes. J Am Paraplegia Soc 1987; 10:30–35.
66. Neer CS: Anterior acromioplasty for the chronic impingement syndrome in the shoulder: a preliminary report. J Bone Joint Surg (Am) 1972; 54:41–50.
67. Matsen FA, Arntz CT: Subacromial impingement. In Rockwood CA, Matsen FA (eds): The Shoulder. Philadelphia, WB Saunders, 1990:623–636.
68. May LA, Burnham RS, Steadward RD: Assessment of isokinetic and hand-held dynamometer measures of shoulder rotator strength among individuals with spinal cord injury. Arch Phys Med Rehabil 1997; 78:251–255.
69. Burnham RS, May L, Nelson E et al: Shoulder pain in wheelchair athletes. Am J Sports Med 1993; 21:328–342.
70. Burnham M, Curtis K, Reid DB: Shoulder problems in the wheelchair athlete. In Pettrone FA (ed): Athletic Injuries of the Shoulder. New York, McGraw-Hill, 1995:375–381.
71. Curtis KA, Tyner TM, Zachary L et al: Effect of a standard exercise protocol on shoulder pain in long-term wheelchair users. Spinal Cord 1999; 37:421–429.
72. Gam AN, Johannsen F: Ultrasound therapy in musculoskeletal disorders: a meta-analysis. Pain 1995; 63:85–91.
73. Brosseau L, Tugwell P, Wells GA et al: Philadelphia Panel evidence-based clinical practice guidelines on selected rehabilitation interventions for shoulder pain. Phys Ther 2001; 81:1719–1730.
74. van der Heijden GJ, van der Windt DA, de Winter AF: Physiotherapy for patients with soft tissue shoulder disorders: a systematic review of randomised clinical trials. BMJ 1997; 315:25–30.
75. New Zealand Guidelines Group: The Diagnosis and Management of Soft Tissue Shoulder Injuries and Related Disorders. Best Practice Evidence Based Guidelines. Wellington, ACC, 2004.
76. Consortium for Spinal Cord Medicine: Preservation of upper limb function following spinal cord injury: a clinical practice guideline for health-care professionals. Washington, DC, Paralyzed Veterans of America, 2005.
77. Sutbeyaz ST, Koseoglu BF, Yeiltepe E: Case Report. Simultaneous upper and lower extremity complex regional pain syndrome type I in tetraplegia. Spinal Cord 2005; 43:568–572.
78. Harden RN, Swan M, King A et al: Treatment of complex regional pain syndrome: functional restoration. Clin J Pain 2006; 22:420–424.
79. Rintala D, Loubser PG, Castro J et al: Chronic pain in a community-based sample of men with spinal cord injury: prevalence, severity, and relationship with impairment, disability, handicap, and subjective well-being. Arch Phys Med Rehabil 1999; 79:601–614.
80. Widerstrom-Noga EG, Felip-Cuervo E, Broton JG et al: Perceived difficulty in dealing with consequences of spinal cord injury. Arch Phys Med Rehabil 1999; 80:580–586.

Contents

The direct and indirect
effects of respiratory
muscle weakness 206

Respiratory
complications in the
period immediately
after injury 210

Assessment of
respiratory function 212

Treatment options 213

Ventilation for patients
with C1–C3 tetraplegia 219

Respiratory management

Respiratory complications are a common cause of morbidity and mortality in patients with spinal cord injury.[1–21] They occur throughout patients' lives and are a leading cause of hospitalization. Patients are particularly susceptible to respiratory complications in the first few weeks after spinal cord injury. At this time, respiratory complications are the second leading cause of death.[2,21] The common respiratory complications are hypoventilation, atelectasis, secretion retention and pneumonia.[2,22,23] Each leads to a mismatch between ventilation and perfusion, resulting in hypoxaemia and, if untreated, respiratory failure.[10,15,24] Not surprisingly, patients with tetraplegia are particularly vulnerable.[1,2,21]

The respiratory function of patients with spinal cord injury is primarily determined by neurological status (see Table 11.1 for level of innervations of the key respiratory muscles)[25] and can be summarized as follows:

C1 and C2 tetraplegia. Patients with lesions at C1 and C2 have total paralysis of the diaphragm, intercostals and abdominal muscles and are therefore ventilatory-dependent. They, however, retain some voluntary control of accessory respiratory muscles such as the sternocleidomastoid muscles. These muscles receive innervation from cranial nerves and contribute to respiration in a small way, although they have little functional importance in patients with such high levels of tetraplegia requiring mechanical ventilation.[26]

C3 tetraplegia. Patients with lesions at C3 have marked but not total paralysis of the diaphragm. They have some voluntary control of the scalene muscles which assist respiration. Most, however, require long-term mechanical ventilation.[27]

C4 tetraplegia. Patients with lesions at C4 have partial paralysis of the diaphragm and total paralysis of the intercostal and abdominal muscles. Most can breathe independently, typically after short periods of invasive mechanical ventilation following injury. They have little ability to cough and a vital capacity less than one third of predicted.[23,28] They have minimal expiratory reserve.

C5–C8 tetraplegia. Patients with lesions at C5–C8 have full voluntary control of the diaphragm, partial voluntary control of the scalene and pectoralis muscles and full paralysis of the intercostal and abdominal muscles. They have a poor cough and a vital capacity of between one third and one half of predicted.[23,28] The pectoralis muscles are significant because they contribute to expiration.[29–31]

TABLE 11.1 Levels of innervation for the sternocleidomastoid, diaphragm, scalene, pectoralis, intercostal and abdominal muscles

Cranial nerve XI	Sternocleidomastoid
C3–C5	Diaphragm
C3–C8	Scalene
C5–T1	Pectoralis
T1–T11	Intercostals
T6–T12	Abdominals

See Appendix 1 for more details.[25]

Thoracic paraplegia. Patients with thoracic paraplegia have full voluntary control of the diaphragm, scalene and pectoralis muscles but varying amounts of paralysis of the intercostal and abdominal muscles. Some have a normal vital capacity[23,28] but a weak cough. It is not until the lesion is below T12 that respiratory function can be deemed normal.[32]

The direct and indirect effects of respiratory muscle weakness

Patients with spinal cord injury have a restrictive pattern of breathing with marked reductions in all lung volumes and capacities (except residual volume; see Table 11.2 and Figure 11.1).[11,12,15,18,19,26,28,33–46] Expiratory flow and peak cough flow rates are also adversely affected. All these changes are due to the direct and indirect effects of respiratory muscle weakness. They explain patients' heightened susceptibility to hypoventilation, atelectasis, secretion retention and pneumonia.

The majority of this chapter focuses on patients with C4–C8 tetraplegia capable of breathing independently. Patients with thoracic paraplegia have similar respiratory problems although less pronounced. The respiratory management of patients with C1–C3 tetraplegia is briefly covered at the end of the chapter.

Tidal volume, vital capacity and total lung capacity

In the laboratory, respiratory muscle strength is quantified by measuring mouth or pleural pressures during maximal static inspiratory and expiratory efforts, respectively.[9,47,48] Not surprisingly, there is a marked reduction in maximal inspiratory and expiratory pressures of patients with tetraplegia reflecting respiratory muscle weakness.[9,33,35,47–51] Poor inspiratory and expiratory muscle strength directly limits vital capacity, total lung capacity and their determinants.[9,10,16] Tidal volume is also reduced but this is compensated for by an increase in respiratory rate.

The decreases in lung parameters are greater than expected from muscle weakness alone.[10,33,48] For example, it has been calculated that the direct effects of inspiratory muscle weakness explain some, but not all, of the observed loss in total lung capacity.[47] This disparity is due to the indirect effects of respiratory muscle weakness and, in particular, the effects of respiratory muscle weakness on pulmonary and rib cage compliance.[9,10,33,47,49]

TABLE 11.2 Definition of lung volumes, capacities and flows

Parameter	Definition
Tidal volume	The volume of air inspired (or expired) in a quiet breath[40,46]
Vital capacity	The volume of air expired after a maximal inspiration[41–43]
Inspiratory capacity	The volume of air inspired after a normal expiration[42,43]
Inspiratory reserve	The maximum volume of air inspired after a tidal volume inhalation[46]
Expiratory reserve	The maximum volume of air expired after a tidal volume exhalation[46]
Total lung capacity	The total volume of air contained in the lungs at maximal inspiration[41–43]
Residual volume	The volume of air remaining in the lungs after a maximal expiration[41–43]
Closing capacity	The volume of air trapped by the closure of airways on expiration after a maximal inspiration[41,43]
Functional residual capacity	The volume of air remaining in the lungs after a normal expiration[41–43]
Peak expiratory flow rate	The maximal flow rate generated on expiration after a maximal inspiration[42]
Peak cough flow rate	The maximal flow rate generated during a cough after a maximal inspiration[45,77] Under normal circumstances, peak cough flow rates are higher than peak expiratory flow rates[44,45]
Forced expiratory volume in 1 second (FEV$_1$)	The volume of air expelled in the first second of a maximal forced expiration after a maximal inspiration[40,46]

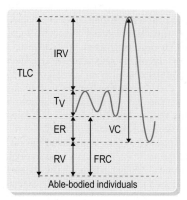
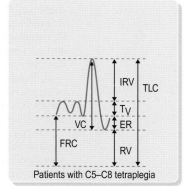

Figure 11.1 A schematic representation of the effects of respiratory muscle weakness on lung volumes and capacities in patients with C5–C8 tetraplegia. Patients with C4 tetraplegia have similar reductions in lung volumes and capacities but minimal expiratory reserve. (Abbreviations: TLC — total lung capacity; IRV — inspiratory reserve volume; T$_v$ — tidal volume; ER — expiratory reserve; RV — residual volume; VC — vital capacity; FRC — functional residual capacity.) Copyright 1985 from The Thorax by Roussos C, Macklem P (eds). Reproduced by permission of Routledge/Taylor & Francis Group, LLC.

Figure 11.2 The direct and indirect effects of respiratory muscle weakness. (Abbreviations: VC — vital capacity; FRC — functional residual capacity; CV — closing volume; TLC — total lung capacity.)

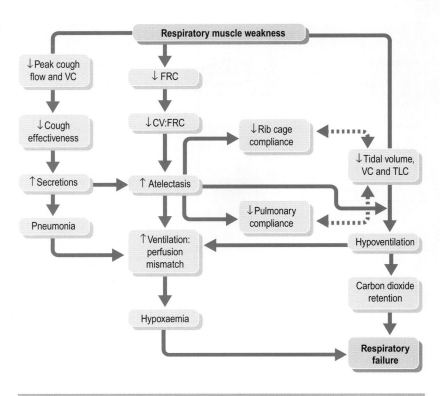

Pulmonary compliance reflects lung stiffness. It is reduced by approximately 30% in people with tetraplegia.[20,33,52,53] Decreases in pulmonary compliance are undesirable because as pulmonary compliance decreases it becomes more difficult to inflate the lungs. This is a problem for patients already having difficulty inflating the lungs due to inspiratory muscle weakness. Decreases in pulmonary compliance are typically attributed to chronic atelectasis.[54,55] Chronic atelectasis directly increases the surface tension of alveoli. It also leads to a reduction in surfactant. Both factors adversely affect the distensibility of alveoli.[56,57] However, decreases in pulmonary compliance may also be due to changes in the elasticity of lung tissue.[58] Not surprisingly, while pulmonary compliance is always reduced in patients with tetraplegia, it is further reduced during periods of acute respiratory illness characterized by secretion retention and atelectasis.[9,10,47,48,59]

Rib cage compliance reflects the stiffness of the rib cage and its resistance to movement during respiration.[20,35,49] It is decreased in people with tetraplegia, exacerbating losses in lung volumes.[10,35,49] The decrease in rib cage compliance occurs over time secondary to poor rib cage expansion. Rib cage expansion is limited because of respiratory muscle paralysis and because patients are physically inactive.[35,49] Without regular expansion and movement of the rib cage, the thoracovertebral and costosternal joints become stiff.[10,29,35,49] Rib cage expansion may also be limited by spasticity although the link between spasticity and rib cage compliance is disputed.[10,33,35,49,58,60]

The direct and indirect effects of respiratory muscle weakness on tidal volume, vital capacity, total lung capacity, and pulmonary and rib cage compliance are undesirable for many reasons (see Figure 11.2). If severe, they lead to hypoventilation characterized by carbon dioxide retention and hypoxaemia.[32,61] In addition, they lead to poorly ventilated areas of the lung which are highly susceptible to atelectasis.

Atelectasis decreases pulmonary compliance, creating a snowball effect where the effects of atelectasis on pulmonary compliance causes further atelectasis. Atelectasis is also due to other factors such as decreases in functional residual capacity and secretion retention (see below). Atelectasis is common and can cause bacterial overgrowth leading to pneumonia,[2] pleural effusion and empyema (infection within a pleural effusion).[22,23]

Functional residual capacity

Functional residual capacity is also reduced in patients with tetraplegia, especially during periods of acute respiratory illness.[9,12,20,33–36,47–49,62] Functional residual capacity is the volume of air in the lungs after a normal relaxed expiration and is determined by the balance between the tendency of the lungs to recoil inwards and the chest wall to pull outwards.[10,33,47,48,60,63] Decreases in functional residual capacity are primarily due to decreases in the outward pull of the chest wall. Changes in chest wall recoil occur over time in people with tetraplegia and are due to patients' inability to regularly expand the chest wall to large lung volumes (see discussion above).[9,33,47–49,60] During periods of acute respiratory illness reductions in functional residual capacity are common and due to underlying lung pathology.

Reductions in functional residual capacity predispose patients to atelectasis. If closing capacity is higher than functional residual capacity, the alveoli in dependent regions of the lung collapse on expiration. This occurs during normal tidal breathing, trapping air and precipitating atelectasis.[41]

Expiratory flow rates

Respiratory muscle weakness directly affects the ability to forcibly expire and generate high expiratory flow rates. This is reflected by marked reductions in forced expiratory volume in 1 second, maximal expiratory flow rate and peak cough flow.[4,10,13] These reductions are primarily due to the direct effects of abdominal and intercostal muscle weakness.

A forced expiration is dependent on generating high intrathoracic positive pressures.[64] In able-bodied individuals, these are generated when the abdominal muscles contract and pull the abdominal contents inwards and upwards, thereby increasing intrathoracic positive pressures and decreasing lung volumes.[65] The intrathoracic positive pressures are further increased by the action of the intercostal muscles on the rib cage. Without intercostal and abdominal muscle activity, large positive intrathoracic pressures cannot be generated and, consequently, expiration is largely passive and dependent on the elastic recoil of the lungs. Forced expiration is further restricted by poor inspiration. Without large volumes of air in the lungs at the commencement of expiration, the ability to generate high expiratory flow rates is further reduced.[5,8,10,13,15,17,26,29,30,36,44,64,66–70]

The inability to forcibly expire prevents an effective cough. High flow rates are required to generate turbulent air flow through the trachea and large bronchi.[64,69,71–74] This in turn creates shear forces on the walls of the airways which entrain secretions and move them up to the pharynx.[71,75] Typically, in able-bodied individuals, flow rates of between 6 and 20 $l.sec^{-1}$ are generated during coughing,[44,64] although peak flow rates as low as 2.7 $l.sec^{-1}$ can help move secretions within the airways.[44,68,73,76] As a general rule patients unable to generate maximal expiratory flow rates of at least 4.5 $l.sec^{-1}$ and with vital capacity less than 1.5 l during health will be unable to generate the critical flow rates required during periods of acute respiratory illness.[44,73,77]

Without an effective cough, patients are highly susceptible to secretion retention. The accumulation of secretions and in particular secretion plugging causes atelectasis.[5,17,30,44,66] Secretions also contribute to decreases in pulmonary compliance. Secretions act as a direct physical barrier to the ventilation of distal regions of the lungs and increase the risk of pneumonia.[5,10,17,30,44,66,72,74] Secretions are a noted problem during acute respiratory illnesses when secretion production is increased.[69,78] The loss of sympathetic supraspinal control and the resultant unchecked parasympathetic activity also increases the production of secretions.[2] Patients with C5 and below tetraplegia are less vulnerable to problems associated with sputum retention than patients with C4 tetraplegia because they retain voluntary control of the clavicular portion of the pectoralis muscles.[30,79] In the absence of intercostals and abdominal muscles, the pectoralis muscles play an important role in assisting cough and forced expiration.[29–31]

Residual volume

Residual volume is the only lung volume that is not decreased with respiratory muscle weakness. Residual volume is the amount of air left in the lungs at the end of a maximal expiration and is typically increased due to the inability to forcibly expire and remove air from the lungs.[10,34,47,80] However, residual volume can be unchanged despite expiratory muscle weakness.[33,48] This occurs if there is a corresponding decrease in the tendency for the chest wall to recoil out to functional residual capacity. Residual volume is determined by competing factors: the strength of the expiratory muscles and the inwards pull of the lungs tending to decrease residual volume, and the outward pull of the chest wall tending to increase residual volume.[10,20,47,60] Increases in residual volume are not associated with increases in total lung capacity.

Rib cage distortion

There are several patterns of rib cage distortion seen during breathing in patients with tetraplegia.[58,81] The precise pattern is determined by factors such as the level of the lesion, strength of accessory respiratory muscles, rib cage compliance and extent of spasticity. Some patients demonstrate paradoxical breathing where the negative intrathoracic pressures associated with inspiration 'suck' the upper ribs inwards. This phenomenon is *paradoxical* because in able-bodied individuals the upper ribs move up and outwards during inspiration in response to intercostal muscle activity. Patients with lesions at and below C5 have less pronounced upper rib cage indrawing because of preserved function in the scalene and other respiratory accessory muscles.[58] Rib cage indrawing is less pronounced in the lower ribs because they are 'pulled' outwards by the direct action of the diaphragm.

Respiratory complications in the period immediately after injury

While patients with tetraplegia are always susceptible to respiratory complications, they are far more susceptible in the period immediately after injury.[5,8,10,12] The reasons for this are outlined below.

Prolonged bedrest

Prolonged bedrest is often required for the management of vertebral instability but it has a dampening effect on respiratory function.[82–84] In particular, it decreases functional residual capacity[16] and vital capacity, promotes atelectasis and increases susceptibility to pneumonia. While the period of bedrest can often be reduced if vertebral instability is managed surgically, this approach exposes patients to the respiratory risks associated with anaesthesia.[82,84–88] Often, medical staff weigh up the relative respiratory risk of conservative versus surgical management after taking into account all aspects of patients' care.

Pain and sedation

Pain and sedation decreases patients' ability and willingness to take deep breaths, cough and cooperate with therapy.[15]

Aspiration

Patients with recent tetraplegia are at increased risk of aspiration and subsequent pneumonia, particularly if they are elderly and have recently undergone anterior cervical spine surgery.[23] Aspiration is also common in those susceptible to vomiting, especially if they are nursed in the supine position and unable to turn the head.

Paralytic ileus

The respiratory function of patients with recently-acquired tetraplegia is further compromised by the associated paralytic ileus. Paralytic ileus is a condition in which the gastrointestinal system temporarily ceases to function (see Chapter 1).[82,84] The condition develops within the first 48 hours after injury and can usually last for a few days.[82,84] The development of a paralytic ileus increases the risk of pulmonary complications because it distends the abdomen.[4] Abdominal distension is undesirable because it impedes the movement of the diaphragm, increases the work of breathing and heightens susceptibility to basal atelectasis.[4,22] In addition, a paralytic ileus predisposes patients to vomiting which can cause aspiration.[4]

Respiratory muscle fatigue

Immediately after injury the remaining non-paralysed respiratory muscles must compensate for the loss of other important respiratory muscles. This is a sudden change in function and the remaining non-paralysed respiratory muscles are not sufficiently adapted to perform the additional work of breathing.[16,22,31,50,89] With time, non-paralysed respiratory muscles adapt and are better able to compensate for the loss of other respiratory muscles.[90] That is, there is an improvement in respiratory muscle strength and endurance.[90,91] The respiratory training effect which occurs in the early days and weeks after injury is accompanied by a gradual increase in vital capacity. For example, vital capacity can almost double in patients with C4–C6 tetraplegia over the first 3 months.[15] Improvements in vital capacity are also due to other factors, including neurological recovery.[2]

Associated respiratory injuries

Injuries severe enough to cause vertebral damage often also cause other injuries. The common injuries seen with spinal cord injuries which have respiratory implications are fractured ribs (with or without haemo/pneumothoraces), head injuries and abdominal injuries.[23] Patients who sustain injuries during water-related activities often also develop aspiration pneumonias secondary to inhaling water at the time of injury.[4] Pulmonary emboli and pleural effusions are also common complications which may or may not be a direct consequence of associated chest injuries.

Some of the other key factors which increase a patient's risk of respiratory complications are increased age, excessive weight, history of substance abuse, history of smoking and past history of respiratory problems.[22] Patients deemed at high risk of respiratory complications need to be carefully monitored for both respiratory and neurological deterioration, particularly in the early days after injury and particularly in those with C6 and above tetraplegia.

Assessment of respiratory function

The respiratory assessment of patients with tetraplegia is not dissimilar to the respiratory assessments of other types of patients and includes an assessment of factors such as:

- level of distress and/or anxiety
- ease of breathing
- shortness of breath
- alertness
- pattern of breathing
- effectiveness of cough
- respiratory rate
- breath sounds
- body temperature
- pulse rate
- need for additional oxygen
- volume and tenacity of secretions
- vital capacity
- forced expiratory volume in 1 second
- arterial blood gases
- oxygen saturation
- end-tidal CO_2[22]
- X-ray changes

It is also important to ascertain the extent of respiratory muscle weakness. This can be gauged from patients' overall neurological status. For example, upper and lower limb paralysis consistent with complete C5 tetraplegia (and no zones of partial preservation) suggests profound respiratory muscle paralysis. In contrast, incomplete C5 motor paralysis with extensive lower limb movement suggests preservation of intercostal and abdominal muscles. A more direct assessment of respiratory muscle weakness can be attained by measuring (forced) vital capacity. This is a key parameter to measure because it strongly correlates with other lung volumes and reflects patients' ability to ventilate and cough.[23,92] It also provides a sensitive and easy way to detect early and subtle changes in respiratory function. Vital capacity should be tested at least every 8 hours in patients deemed at high respiratory risk, and hourly in patients who are on the verge of requiring mechanical ventilation.[22] A vital capacity of less than 1 l is of concern and in some patients indicative of the need for mechanical ventilation.[1,22]

In the early days after injury it is not unusual for the level of the lesion to temporarily ascend one or two segments with the effects of spinal cord oedema.[1,22] This can increase the extent of respiratory muscle paralysis with notable effects on respiratory function. Often only a slight deterioration in respiratory function is required to tip the balance between managing with and without invasive mechanical ventilation. The tip can occur rapidly and if undetected leads to respiratory failure.

Treatment options

The treatment and prevention of respiratory complications in patients with tetraplegia is of paramount importance, and few would dispute the potential life-saving effects of physiotherapy. However, the efficacy of different respiratory techniques has not been well researched and there are few clinical trials to guide the decision-making process.[22,23,93–95] The lack of research in this area is partly due to the ethical problems of performing trials involving respiratory treatments which have long become accepted standard practice. However, it is also due to the inherent difficulties of performing respiratory trials in patients with tetraplegia (see Chapter 14).[93]

In the absence of clinical trials, decisions about respiratory management need to be based, wherever possible, on the results of studies from other patient populations and preferably on the results of clinical trials including patients with neuromuscular weakness (i.e. muscle dystrophy or multiple sclerosis). However, even in these patient populations there is a paucity of good quality evidence and uncertainty about the broad applicability of these results to patients with tetraplegia. Below is an overview of current practice and the evidence which underpins it. Most of the treatment options are for patients with the ability to breathe spontaneously and not for patients requiring invasive mechanical ventilation.

Physiotherapy is primarily aimed at assisting the removal of secretions and improving ventilation. The techniques commonly used to assist the removal of secretions include assisted cough, percussion, vibrations, shaking, suctioning and gravity assisted drainage. The techniques commonly used to increase ventilation include positioning for ventilation, breathing exercises, inspiratory muscle training and non-invasive positive airway pressure support. A brief description of each is provided below.

Assisted cough

An assisted cough is the main technique used by physiotherapists to help clear secretions in patients with respiratory muscle weakness.[2,94] An assisted cough can increase peak expiratory flow rates by up to seven-fold.[72,75,96] The technique requires therapists to use the palms of their hands to apply a sudden and forceful overpressure to the chest or abdominal wall as the patient attempts to voluntarily cough.[61,65,97,98] Chest wall overpressure can be applied anteriorly or at the costophrenic angles. One or two therapists can be used to perform an assisted cough (see Figure 11.3). The external pressure substitutes for the paralysed intercostal and abdominal muscles. Patients may benefit from nebulized saline to help moisten secretions prior to coughing. Bronchodilators may also be helpful. These counteract the bronchoconstricting effects of unchecked parasympathetic activity.

An assisted cough is difficult to administer effectively in obese patients[71,72,74,96] and care needs to be taken when treating children or patients with stiff or distorted chest walls. In addition, direct pressure should not be applied over the abdomen in

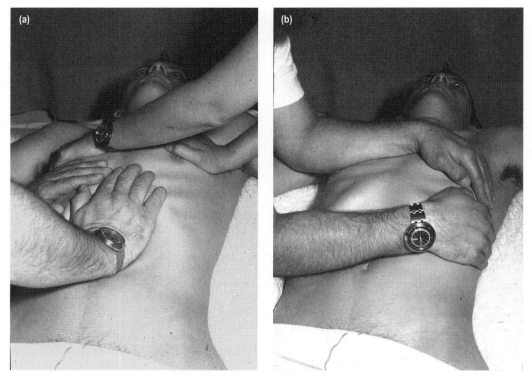

Figure 11.3 Four different ways of applying an assisted cough. Some techniques require one physiotherapist and others two.

patients who have just eaten[61] or who may have internal injuries. Importantly, vigorous assisted coughs need to be used cautiously in patients with unstable and recent tetraplegia. In these patients, advice should be sought from the treating medical officer. The neck of patients with recent cervical injuries should be stabilized during assisted coughs. This can be done either manually by a suitably qualified person or with appropriate bracing.

The effectiveness of an assisted cough can be enhanced by mechanically inflating the lungs prior to each cough (see section below on non-invasive positive airway pressure support). With a large initial lung volume it is possible to generate higher expiratory flow rates during the subsequent cough.[4,61,71,94] The cough can also be augmented by mechanical in-exsufflators (see Figure 11.4).[44,69,71,73,74,99] These devices apply a gradually increasing positive pressure to the airways during inspiration (up to 40 cm H_2O).[61,100] The pressure then suddenly changes to a large negative pressure which stimulates and augments coughing. Mechanical in-exsufflators can increase peak cough flow rates by approximately three times.[68,72] While there has been a recent resurgence in mechanical in-exsufflators, similar devices were widely used during the 1940 poliomyelitis epidemic.[74,101]

The effectiveness of an assisted cough can also be improved with electrical stimulation of the intercostal and abdominal muscles[65,75,102–104] or magnetic stimulation of the thoracic nerve roots innervating these muscles.[104,105] These augment stimulated and non-stimulated cough. Patients may also attain long-term benefit from

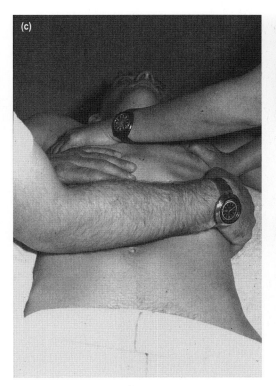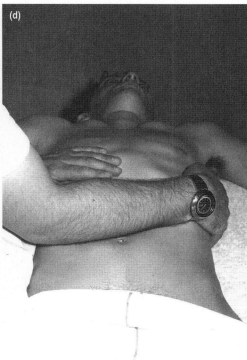

Figure 11.3 Continued

strengthening the clavicular portion of the pectoralis muscles using the principles of progressive resistance training (see Chapter 8).[31] These muscles, while not usually considered important respiratory muscles, take on a key role during expiration and cough in patients with paralysis of the intercostals and abdominal muscles.[30,79] Coughing is unlikely to be enhanced by the use of abdominal binders.[106]

Percussion, vibration and shaking

Percussion, vibration and shaking of the chest wall are used to improve secretion clearance. All these interventions can potentially move the spine. For this reason they should be used cautiously in acutely-injured patients and only with medical approval. The evidence base supporting the use of percussion, vibration and shaking in people with tetraplegia is poor.[40,74,94] The best support for these interventions comes from recent clinical trials involving children with cystic fibrosis[94,107] and patients with bronchiectasis.[108] These trials indicate modest short-term effects. The applicability of these trials to patients with tetraplegia is unknown.

Suctioning

Suctioning is used to move secretions from the trachea. However, this is an unpleasant and invasive technique which should only be used when other interventions fail. In non-intubated patients access to the upper airways is gained by either the

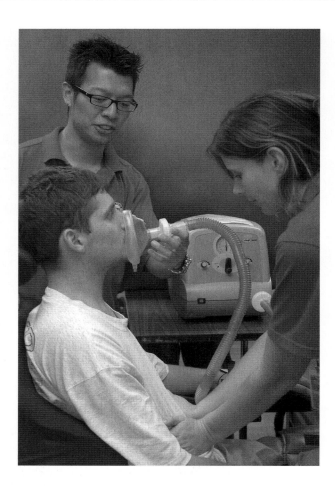

Figure 11.4 Mechanical in-exsufflator.

oropharanx or nasopharanx. If repeated suctioning is required, then minitra-cheostomies can be used.[109] These provide direct tracheal access and are a more comfortable and effective way of suctioning secretions. Minitracheostomies cannot, however, be used for other purposes (e.g. to provide invasive ventilation).

Suctioning can elicit a vagal reflex response which can cause a cardiac arrest.[4] This is due to loss of supraspinal control of the sympathetic nervous system and is precipitated by hypoxia. It is an unusual complication of suctioning which is best avoided with pre-oxygenation.[110] Atropine should be readily available as an additional safety precaution (this is administered intravenously).

Positioning

The effect of body position on respiratory function is complex because it influences both ventilation and perfusion.[111] The effects of position on ventilation also depend on the underlying pathology. However, it is generally desirable to regularly change the position of patients if medically possible and some positions can improve ventilation to specific areas of the lung. Gravity can also be used to help move secretions up the airways although the classic postural drainage positions, once the 'bread and butter' of respiratory physiotherapists, are less commonly used in patients with tetraplegia.[94,112] Clearly, acutely-injured patients should never be moved without prior medical clearance.

In other patient populations, respiratory function is usually improved by sitting patients out of bed as soon as feasible. However, moving patients *with* tetraplegia from the supine to sitting position will not always assist ventilation, although it may help ventilate specific parts of the lung. This is because of the deleterious effects of gravity on vital capacity in patients with respiratory muscle weakness.[28,34] Normally, the diaphragm maintains its high arched position in sitting. This is due to the intrinsic activity of the abdominal muscles which maintain abdominal pressure, pushing the abdominal contents up and under the diaphragm. However, in patients with tetraplegia and paralysis of the abdominal muscles there is no corresponding way of maintaining abdominal pressure. Not only do these patients have no ability to contract their abdominal muscles, but the paralysed abdominal muscles lengthen and become very compliant with time (hence they develop the typical 'quad pop belly').[64] Without abdominal pressure under the diaphragm it drops into a flattened position with the effects of gravity. The flattened position of the diaphragm places it in a less mechanically advantageous position, adversely affecting its length–tension relationship and its ability to expand the lower ribs.[34] Consequently, residual volume is increased and vital capacity is decreased. Total lung capacity is also increased despite concurrent increases in residual volume.

Abdominal binders help maintain vital capacity when patients move from lying to sitting.[113,114] They act like tight elastic corsets substituting for paralysis of the abdominal muscles and maintaining abdominal pressure.[114,115] Abdominal binders also help prevent venous pooling, thereby improving venous return and possibly assisting lung perfusion.

Inspiratory muscle training

Inspiratory muscle training is used to increase the strength and/or endurance of remaining non-paralysed (or partially paralysed) inspiratory muscles.[16,89–91,116–126] Hand-held devices which incorporate one-way valves are typically used. The valves allow unimpeded expiration but provide resistance to inspiration via small diameter tubes or mesh. Some valves control inspiratory flow while others control inspiratory pressure. Less commonly, inspiratory muscle training is done by placing weights on the abdomen.[91,126]

Like any strength and endurance training programme, the key parameter is overload (see Chapter 8).[90] A typical inspiratory training protocol requires patients to generate additional inspiratory pressures for 15–30 minutes, two to three times a day.[90,122,125,127] The optimal inspiratory pressures are not known, although excessive pressures may cause respiratory muscle fatigue and hypercapnia.[95] The response to strength and endurance training is reversible, implying that the effects of training will cease once training stops unless normal breathing and activities can be expected to maintain the gains.[90] While the rationale for inspiratory muscle training is strong, the results from the small number of clinical trials in the area are inconclusive.[89,91,116,120,123,127]

Non-invasive positive airway pressure support

Non-invasive positive airway pressure support is used to provide positive airway pressure during inspiration and/or expiration. As the name implies it is administered *non-invasively* (i.e. not through intubation tubes associated with invasive mechanical ventilation). There are different types of non-invasive positive airway pressure support but the three most widely used types are continuous positive airway pressure, bi-level positive airway pressure and intermittent positive pressure breathing. Typically, the pressure is delivered through tight-fitting nasal or oronasal masks. Alternatively, it is delivered through a mouthpiece or through soft rubber or silicone pledgets sitting in the nostrils. Most types of non-invasive positive airway pressure support are used in patients capable of breathing spontaneously. However, occasionally, non-invasive positive airway pressure support is used to ventilate patients with paralysis of the diaphragm who are unable (or barely able) to ventilate. Non-invasive positive airway pressure support can cause aspiration if delivered through tight-fitting masks in patients unable to remove them and at risk of vomiting.

Continuous positive airway pressure

Continuous positive airway pressure (CPAP) is used to administer low levels of pressure throughout the respiratory cycle. Typically, pressures of between 5 and 10 cm H_2O are used (higher pressures are occasionally used in patients with complex underlying respiratory disease[74]). The pressures are maintained through devices which provide a constant stream of compressed air. The expiratory pressures are particularly beneficial. They are transmitted throughout the airways helping to splint the airways open during expiration. In this way the expiratory pressures maintain functional residual capacity above closing capacity, preventing airway collapse.[128] They also facilitate collateral ventilation, increasing gas pressure behind secretions.[129] The low levels of inspiratory pressure assist tidal volume.

Continuous positive airway pressure is primarily used to treat acute episodes of atelectasis, respiratory distress and secretion retention, and to wean patients from invasive mechanical ventilation.[74,94,130] However, continuous positive airway pressure is also widely used to manage sleep apnoea. Sleep apnoea is a common problem in patients with tetraplegia, especially if they are elderly and overweight.[22,131,132] The expiratory pressures help splint the upper airways open during sleep preventing obstruction.

Bi-level positive airway pressure support

Bi-level positive airway pressure support is used to provide different levels of positive inspiratory and expiratory pressure support during the respiratory cycle.[133] The expiratory pressures are typically low and used to splint the airways open during expiration (as above). The inspiratory pressures can be varied and are used to augment tidal volume. However, it is the difference between the inspiratory and expiratory pressures which determines the precise effect of bi-level positive airway pressure support on tidal volume. Bi-level positive airway pressure support is used for the same reasons as continuous positive airway pressure but with the added benefit of providing extra assistance for inspiration if needed.

Bi-level positive airway pressure support is administered through pressure-limited intensive care-type ventilators or 'bi-level' devices (e.g. BiPAP® machines). Inspiratory airflow continues until a pre-set pressure is reached. Inspiratory flow is typically triggered by patients' spontaneous attempts at inspiration while expiration is passive and commences once the inspiratory airflow finishes. Pressure during expiration is maintained with a constant airflow during expiration.

The settings of most ventilators and 'bi-level' devices can be adjusted to determine variables such as:

- how quickly peak pressures (or volumes) are reached;
- whether additional breaths are delivered if patients fail to make a minimum number of spontaneous breaths; and
- how quickly inspiratory pressures (or volumes) drop off at the end of each breath.

'Bi-level' devices, rather than pressure-limited intensive care-type ventilators, are increasingly used in patients with tetraplegia because they are relatively cheap, light, portable and easy to use.[61] However, they do not always enable the administration of additional oxygen or very high inspiratory pressures, and they have limited adjustability.[61] In addition, most do not have alarm systems essential for very disabled patients reliant on them for ventilation.

Intermittent positive pressure breathing

Intermittent positive pressure breathing is used to provide large breaths to patients who are breathing spontaneously.[2,134] Large inspiratory pressures are administered, typically with an intensive care-type ventilator through a mouth piece. The delivery of airflow is triggered by patients' inspiration. Intermittent positive pressure breathing was widely used 20 years ago as a treatment modality by physiotherapists but is less commonly used today.[135]

The regular expansion of the lungs with intermittent positive pressure breathing may have lasting beneficial effects on pulmonary and chest wall compliance and may help to treat and prevent atelectasis, hypoventilation and secretion retention (see Figure 11.2). However, no clinical trials have been done in this area and its lasting effectiveness is unclear.[134,136,137] Presumably, however, any beneficial effects on pulmonary and chest wall compliance are reliant on its regular application over a sustained period of time.[61] Intermittent positive pressure breathing is also used to augment coughing in much the same way as in-exsufflators but without the added benefit of large negative pressures during expiration. Intermittent positive pressure breathing is applied on a breath-by-breath basis with each attempt at coughing (see discussion above). Interestingly, intermittent positive pressure breathing is not an effective way of administering aerosols but can be used to provide humidification.[49,61] An equivalent but less precise way of providing patients with deep breaths is by inflating the lungs manually with a resuscitation bag and mouthpiece (or face mask).

Non-invasive ventilation

Non-invasive positive airway pressure support can be used to ventilate patients. If used in this way, it is called *non-invasive* ventilation. High inspiratory pressures (up to 40 cm H_2O) with or without expiratory pressures are administered through intensive care-type ventilators or 'bi-level' devices. Non-invasive ventilation is used in patients with profound respiratory muscle weakness and/or fatigue unable to maintain adequate ventilation.[61,137] It is commonly used as an interim measure to get patients through acute episodes of respiratory distress and avoid the need for mechanical invasive ventilation. In these patients it is used either intermittently or continuously throughout the day. It is also used by some patients on an ongoing basis to provide sustained periods of respiratory rest each day and to prevent respiratory complications.[138–140] In these patients it is typically used at night while sleeping.

Ventilation for patients with C1–C3 tetraplegia

Invasive mechanical ventilation

Most patients with lesions at C1–C3 are managed with invasive mechanical ventilation via tracheostomy. The life expectancy of these, and other patients requiring long-term invasive mechanical ventilation, is reduced with 25% of patients surviving the first year and 17% surviving 15 years.[141] Not surprisingly, respiratory complications are the leading cause of their death.[141] This is due to increased susceptibility to pneumonia, atelectasis and secretion retention.[141]

Patients with high levels of tetraplegia requiring long-term ventilation have many nursing, social, vocational and psychological needs. They require portable ventilators and suction units which can be attached to their wheelchairs. They also require warning systems and secondary back-up equipment in case the primary ventilator fails. These patients cannot be left unattended and personnel responsible for their care require extensive training on all aspects of respiratory management.

A less obvious implication of invasive mechanical ventilation is its deleterious effects on speech. Speech is possible by deflating the cuff of the tracheal tube and increasing tidal volume.[142] However, patients lose the ability to control and time expiration. Both these factors are important precursors to the natural speech pattern. For this reason speech becomes dependent on the fixed and passive phases of expiration. In addition, they have little ability to change the quality or volume of their speech, and invariably patients run out of breath before they have finished a sentence or phrase. The typical speech pattern of a ventilated patient with tetraplegia is soft and inappropriately disrupted with each inspiration. This adversely affects the spontaneity of their speech and verbal communication with others.

Diaphragmatic pacing

The ventilation of some patients with C1 or C2 tetraplegia can be managed with diaphragmatic pacing, where ventilation is controlled by cyclic electrical stimulation of the phrenic nerve. In these patients the electrodes are surgically implanted but controlled by an external device.[65,103,143–146] Most patients using phrenic nerve stimulation continue to require a tracheostomy for the removal of secretions and use mechanical ventilation at night. The success of diaphragmatic pacing depends on an intact phrenic nerve which is responsive to electrical stimulation. Consequently, most patients with C3 tetraplegia and damage to the anterior horn cells of the diaphragm are unsuitable for diaphragmatic pacing.

Non-invasive negative ventilation

Artificial ventilation can also be provided by generating negative pressures around the thorax with body ventilators such as the iron lung.[147,148] The iron lung is a shell which encompasses the trunk and expands the lungs during inspiration by generating an external negative pressure over the thorax. These devices were primarily used to manage the poliomyelitis epidemic which left thousands with chronic respiratory muscle paralysis. Today, negative ventilatory support systems are rarely used. This is for several reasons, including their tendency to cause upper airway collapse.[148]

Glossopharyngeal breathing

Glossopharyngeal breathing, also called 'frog breathing', is a technique used by patients with severe respiratory muscle paralysis.[40] The tongue and pharyngeal muscles are used to generate a repeated wave-like action of the tongue which moves it up and down against the palate. Each cyclic movement of the tongue forces up to 150 ml of air into the trachea. The glottis closes each time the tongue is lowered to prevent escape of air. If this action is quickly repeated many times over without escape of air, an inspiratory breath of approximately 500 ml can be achieved. Expiration is then passive.[61,149]

Glossopharyngeal breathing is used by some ventilated patients to enable them to be removed from the ventilator for short periods of time. This can be useful when patients are being moved about (e.g. when being transferred from the bed to the wheelchair). It is also used by some non-ventilated patients to augment coughing. Glossopharyngeal breathing is, however, a difficult technique to master and for therapists to teach. It cannot be used for sustained periods of time.

References

1. Ragnarsson KT, Hall KM, Wilmot CB et al: Management of pulmonary, cardiovascular and metabolic conditions after spinal cord injury. In Stover S, DeLisa JA, Whiteneck GG (eds): Spinal Cord Injury: Clinical Outcomes from the Model Systems. Gaithersburg, Aspen Publishers, 1995:79–99.
2. McCrory DC, Samsa GP, Hamilton BB et al: Treatment of pulmonary disease following cervical spinal cord injury. Evidence report/technology assessment. Agency for Healthcare Research and Quality. US Department of Health and Human Services, Duke Evidence-based Practice Center, Center for Clinical Health Policy Research, 2001:1–60.
3. Bellamy R, Pitts FW, Stauffer ES: Respiratory complications in traumatic quadriplegia. Analysis of 20 years' experience. J Neurosurg 1973; 39:596–600.
4. Brownlee S, Williams SJ: Physiotherapy in the respiratory care of patients with high spinal injury. Physiotherapy 1987; 73:148–152.
5. Carter RE: Respiratory aspects of spinal cord injury management. Paraplegia 1987; 25:262–266.
6. Chen CF, Lien IN: Spinal cord injuries in Taipei, Taiwan, 1978–1981. Paraplegia 1985; 23:364–370.
7. Cheshire DJ: Respiratory management in acute traumatic tetraplegia. Paraplegia 1964; 1: 252–261.
8. Clough P, Lindenauer D, Hayes M et al: Guidelines for routine respiratory care of patients with spinal cord injury. A clinical report. Phys Ther 1986; 66:1395–1402.
9. De Troyer A, Deisser P: The effects of intermittent positive pressure breathing on patients with respiratory muscle weakness. Am Rev Respir Dis 1981; 124:132–137.
10. De Troyer A, Pride NB: The respiratory system in neuromuscular disorders. In Roussos C, Macklem P (eds): The Thorax. New York, Dekker, 1985:1089–1121.
11. Forner JV, Llombart RL, Valledor MC: The flow-volume loop in tetraplegics. Paraplegia 1977; 15:245–251.
12. Forner JV: Lung volumes and mechanics of breathing in tetraplegics. Paraplegia 1980; 18:258–266.
13. Fishburn MJ, Marino RJ, Ditunno JF: Atelectasis and pneumonia in acute spinal cord injury. Arch Phys Med Rehabil 1990; 71:197–200.
14. Hackler RH: A 25-year prospective mortality study in the spinal cord injured patient: comparison with the long-term living paraplegic. J Urol 1977; 117:486–488.
15. Ledsome JR, Sharp JM: Pulmonary function in acute cervical cord injury. Am Rev Respir Dis 1981; 124:41–44.
16. Hornstein S, Ledsome JR: Ventilatory muscle training in acute quadriplegia. Physiother Can 1986; 38:145–149.
17. Mansel JK, Norman JR: Respiratory complications and management of spinal cord injuries. Chest 1990; 99:1446–1452.
18. McMichan JC, Michel L, Westbrook PR: Pulmonary dysfunction following traumatic quadriplegia. Recognition, prevention, and treatment. JAMA 1980; 243:528–531.
19. Ohry A, Molho M, Rozin R: Alterations of pulmonary function in spinal cord injured patients. Paraplegia 1975; 13:101–108.
20. Scanlon PD, Loring SH, Pichurko BM et al: Respiratory mechanics in acute quadriplegia. Lung and chest wall compliance and dimensional changes during respiratory maneuvers. Am Rev Respir Dis 1989; 139:615–20.
21. De Vivo MJ, Krause JS, Lammertse DP: Recent trends in mortality and causes of death among persons with spinal cord injury. Arch Phys Med Rehabil 1999; 80:1411–1419.
22. Consortium for Spinal Cord Medicine: Respiratory management following spinal cord injury: a clinical practice guideline for health-care professionals. Washington, DC, Paralyzed Veterans of America, 2005.
23. Peterson WP, Kirshblum S: Pulmonary management of spinal cord injury. In Kirshblum S, Campagnolo DI, DeLisa JA (eds): Spinal Cord Medicine. Philadelphia, Lippincott Williams & Wilkins, 2002:108–122.

24. Schmidt-Nowara WW, Altman AR: Atelectasis and neuromuscular respiratory failure. Chest 1984; 85:792–795.
25. Williams PL, Bannister LH, Berry MM et al: Gray's Anatomy, 38th edn. New York, Churchill Livingstone, 1995.
26. De Troyer A, Estenne M, Heilporn A: Mechanism of active expiration in tetraplegic subjects. N Engl J Med 1986; 314:740–744.
27. Wicks AB, Menter RR: Long-term outlook in quadriplegic patients with initial ventilator dependency. Chest 1986; 90:406–410.
28. Linn WS, Adkins RH, Gong H et al: Pulmonary function in chronic spinal cord injury: a cross-sectional survey of 222 southern California adult outpatients. Arch Phys Med Rehabil 2000; 81:757–763.
29. Estenne M, Yernault JC, De Troyer A: Rib cage and diaphragm–abdomen compliance in humans: effects of age and posture. J Appl Physiol 1985; 59:1842–1848.
30. Estenne M, De Troyer A: Cough in tetraplegic subjects: an active process. Ann Intern Med 1990; 112:22–28.
31. Estenne M, Knopp C, Vanvaerenbergh J et al: The effect of pectoralis muscle training in tetraplegic subjects. Am Rev Respir Dis 1989; 139:1218–1222.
32. Padman R, Alexander M, Thorogood C et al: Respiratory management of pediatric patients with spinal cord injuries: Retrospective review of the duPont experience. Neurorehabil Neural Repair 2003; 17:32–36.
33. De Troyer A, Heilporn A: Respiratory mechanics in quadriplegia. The respiratory function of the intercostal muscles. Am Rev Respir Dis 1980; 122:591–600.
34. Estenne M, De Troyer A: Mechanism of the postural dependence of vital capacity in tetraplegic subjects. Am Rev Respir Dis 1987; 135:367–371.
35. Estenne M, De Troyer A: The effects of tetraplegia on chest wall statics. Am Rev Respir Dis 1986; 134:121–124.
36. Fugl-Meyer AR, Grimby G: Ventilatory function in tetraplegic patients. Scand J Rehabil Med 1971; 3:151–160.
37. Loveridge BM, Dubo HI: Breathing pattern in chronic quadriplegia. Arch Phys Med Rehabil 1990; 71:495–499.
38. Maloney FP: Pulmonary function in quadriplegia: effects of a corset. Arch Phys Med Rehabil 1979; 60:261–5.
39. McCool FD, Brown R, Mayewski RJ et al: Effects of posture on stimulated ventilation in quadriplegia. Am Rev Respir Dis 1988; 138:101–105.
40. Jones M, Moffatt F: Cardiopulmonary Physiotherapy. Oxford, BIOS Scientific Publishers, 2002.
41. West JB: Respiratory Physiology: The Essentials, 7th edn. Philadelphia, Lippincott Williams & Wilkins, 2005.
42. Ellis E, Alison J: Key Issues in Cardiorespiratory Physiotherapy. Oxford, Butterworth Heinemann, 1992.
43. Frownfelter DL, Dean EW: Principles and Practice of Cardiopulmonary Physical Therapy, 3rd edn. St Louis, Mosby-Year Book, 1996.
44. Anderson JL, Hasney KM, Beaumont NE: Systematic review of techniques to enhance peak cough flow and maintain vital capacity in neuromuscular disease: the case for mechanical insufflation-exsufflation. Phy Ther Reviews 2005; 10:25–33.
45. Suarez AA, Pessolano FA, Monteiro SG et al: Peak flow and peak cough flow in the evaluation of expiratory muscle weakness and bulbar impairment in patients with neuromuscular disease. Am J Phys Med Rehabil 2002; 81:506–511.
46. des Jardins TR: Cardiopulmonary Anatomy & Physiology: Essentials for Respiratory Care. Albany, Australia, Delmar/Thomson Learning, 2002.
47. De Troyer A, Borenstein S, Cordier R: Analysis of lung volume restriction in patients with respiratory muscle weakness. Thorax 1980; 35:603–610.
48. Gibson GJ, Pride NB, Davis JN et al: Pulmonary mechanics in patients with respiratory muscle weakness. Am Rev Respir Dis 1977; 115:389–395.
49. Estenne M, Heilporn A, Delhez L et al: Chest wall stiffness in patients with chronic respiratory muscle weakness. Am Rev Respir Dis 1983; 128:1002–1007.
50. Gross D, Ladd HW, Riley EJ et al: The effect of training on strength and endurance of the diaphragm in quadriplegia. Am J Med 1980; 68:27–35.
51. Leith DE, Bradley M: Ventilatory muscle strength and endurance training. J Appl Physiol 1976; 41:508–516.
52. Bergofsky EH: Mechanism for respiratory insufficiency after cervical cord injury; a source of alveolar hypoventilation. Ann Intern Med 1964; 61:435–447.
53. Stone DJ, Keltz H: The effect of respiratory muscle dysfunction on pulmonary function. Studies in patients with spinal cord injuries. Am Rev Respir Dis 1963; 88:621–629.
54. Sybrecht GW, Garrett L, Anthonisen NR: Effect of chest strapping on regional lung function. J Appl Physiol 1975; 39:707–713.
55. Stubbs SE, Hyatt RE: Effect of increased lung recoil pressure on maximal expiratory flow in normal subjects. J Appl Physiol 1972; 32:325–331.

56. De Troyer A, Borenstein S, Bastenier-Geens J: Acute changes in respiratory mechanics after pyridostigmine injection in patients with myasthenia gravis. Effects of neuromuscular blockade on respiratory mechanics in conscious man. Am Rev Respir Dis 1980; 121:629–638.

57. Young SL, Tierney DF, Clements JA: Mechanism of compliance change in excised rat lungs at low transpulmonary pressure. J Appl Physiol 1970; 29:780–785.

58. Estenne M, De Troyer A: Relationship between respiratory muscle electromyogram and rib cage motion in tetraplegia. Am Rev Respir Dis 1985; 132:53–59.

59. Blossom R, Affeldt J: Chronic poliomyelitic respirator deaths. Am J Med 1956; 20:77–87.

60. De Troyer A, Bastenier-Geens J: Effects of neuromuscular blockade on respiratory mechanics in conscious man. J Appl Physiol 1979; 47:1162–1168.

61. Mehta S, Hill NS: Noninvasive ventilation. Am J Respir Crit Care Med 2001; 163:540–577.

62. Fugl-Meyer AR, Grimby G: Rib-cage and abdominal volume ventilation partitioning in tetraplegic patients. Scand J Rehabil Med 1971; 3:161–167.

63. Altose MD: The physiological basis of pulmonary function testing. Clin Symp 1979; 31:1–39.

64. McCool FD: Global physiology and pathophysiology of cough: ACCP evidence-based clinical practice guidelines. Chest 2006; 129:48S–53S.

65. Zupan A, Savrin R, Erjavec T et al: Effects of respiratory muscle training and electrical stimulation of abdominal muscles on respiratory capabilities in tetraplegic patients. Spinal Cord 1997; 35:540–545.

66. De Troyer A, Estenne M: The expiratory muscles in tetraplegia. Paraplegia 1991; 29:359–363.

67. Wang AY, Jaeger RJ, Yarkony GM et al: Cough in spinal cord injured patients: the relationship between motor level and peak expiratory flow. Spinal Cord 1997; 35:299–302.

68. Bach JR: Mechanical insufflation–exsufflation. Comparison of peak expiratory flows with manually assisted and unassisted coughing techniques. Chest 1993; 104:1553–1562.

69. Miske LJ, Hickey EM, Kolb SM et al: Use of the mechanical in-exsufflator in pediatric patients with neuromuscular disease and impaired cough. Chest 2004; 125:1406–1412.

70. Kang SW, Shin JC, Park CI et al: Relationship between inspiratory muscle strength and cough capacity in cervical spinal cord injured patients. Spinal Cord 2005; 44:242–248.

71. Sivasothy P, Brown L, Smith IE et al: Effect of manually assisted cough and mechanical insufflation on cough flow of normal subjects, patients with chronic obstructive pulmonary disease (COPD), and patients with respiratory muscle weakness. Thorax 2001; 56:438–444.

72. Bach JR, Smith WH, Michaels J et al: Airway secretion clearance by mechanical exsufflation for post-poliomyelitis ventilator-assisted individuals. Arch Phys Med Rehabil 1993; 74:170–177.

73. Tzeng AC, Bach JR: Prevention of pulmonary morbidity for patients with neuromuscular disease. Chest 2000; 118:1390–1396.

74. Hardy KA, Anderson BD: Noninvasive clearance of airway secretions. Respir Care Clin N Am 1996; 2:323–345.

75. Jaeger RJ, Turba RM, Yarkony GM et al: Cough in spinal cord injured patients: comparison of three methods to produce cough. Arch Phys Med Rehabil 1993; 74:1358–1361.

76. Bach JR, Ishikawa Y, Kim H: Prevention of pulmonary morbidity for patients with Duchenne muscular dystrophy. Chest 1997; 112:1024–1028.

77. Sancho J, Servera E, Díaz J et al: Comparison of peak cough flows measured by pneumotachograph and a portable peak flow meter. Am J Phys Med Rehabil 2004; 83:608–612.

78. Mier-Jedrzejowicz A, Brophy C, Green M: Respiratory muscle weakness during upper respiratory tract infections. Am Rev Respir Dis 1988; 138:5–7.

79. Estenne M, Van Muylem A, Gorini M et al: Evidence of dynamic airway compression during cough in tetraplegic patients. Am J Respir Crit Care Med 1994; 150:1081–1085.

80. Leith DE, Mead J: Mechanisms determining residual volume of the lungs in normal subjects. J Appl Physiol 1967; 23:221–227.

81. De Troyer A, Estenne M, Vincken W: Rib cage motion and muscle use in high tetraplegics. Am Rev Respir Dis 1986; 133:1115–1119.

82. Buchanan LE, Nawoczenski DA: Spinal Cord Injury: Concepts and Management Approaches. Baltimore, Williams & Wilkins, 1987.

83. Cloward RB: Acute cervical spine injuries. Clin Symp 1980; 32:1–32.

84. Zejdlick CP: Management of Spinal Cord Injury. Monterey, CA, Wardsworth Health Sciences Division, 1983.

85. Don HF, Wahba M, Cuadrado L et al: The effects of anesthesia and 100 per cent oxygen on the functional residual capacity of the lungs. Anesthesiology 1970; 32:521–529.

86. Don HF, Wahba WM, Craig DB: Airway closure, gas trapping, and the functional residual capacity during anesthesia. Anesthesiology 1972; 36:533–539.

87. Gilmour I, Burnham M, Craig DB: Closing capacity measurement during general anesthesia. Anesthesiology 1976; 45:477–482.

88. Hedenstierna G, McCarthy G, Bergstrom M: Airway closure during mechanical ventilation. Anesthesiology 1976; 44:114–123.

89. Loveridge B, Badour M, Dubo H: Ventilatory muscle endurance training in quadriplegia: effects on breathing pattern. Paraplegia 1989; 27:329–339.

90. Reid WD, Loveridge BM: Physiotherapy management of patients with chronic obstructive airways disease. Physiother Can 1983; 35:183–195.

91. Derrickson J, Clesia N, Simpson N et al: A comparison of two breathing exercise programs for patients with quadriplegia. Phys Ther 1992; 72:763–769.

92. Roth EJ, Nussbaum SB, Berkowitz M et al: Pulmonary function testing in spinal cord injury: correlation with vital capacity. Paraplegia 1995; 33:454–457.

93. Samsa GP, Govert J, Matchar DB et al: Use of data from nonrandomized trial designs in evidence reports: An application to treatment of pulmonary disease following spinal cord injury. J Rehabil Res Dev 2002; 39:41–52.

94. McCool FD, Rosen MJ: Nonpharmacologic airway clearance therapies: ACCP evidence-based clinical practice guidelines. Chest 2006; 129:S250–S259.

95. Sheel AW, Reid WD, Townson AF et al: Respiratory management following spinal cord injury. In Eng JJ, Teasell RW, Miller WC et al (eds): Spinal Cord Injury Rehabilitation Evidence. Vancouver, SCIRE, 2006:8.1–8.30.

96. Braun SR, Giovannoni R, O'Connor M: Improving the cough in patients with spinal cord injury. Am J Phys Med 1984; 63:1–10.

97. Pryor JA, Webber BA: Physiotherapy for Respiratory and Cardiac Problems, 2nd edn. Edinburgh, Sydney, Churchill Livingstone, 1998.

98. Ward TA: Spinal injuries. In Pryor JA, Webber BA (eds): Physiotherapy for Respiratory and Cardiac Problems. Edinburgh, Churchill Livingstone, 1998:429–438.

99. Chatwin M, Ross E, Hart N et al: Cough augmentation with mechanical insufflation/exsufflation in patients with neuromuscular weakness. Eur Respir J 2003; 21:502–508.

100. Whitney J, Harden B, Keilty S: Assisted cough. A new technique. Physiotherapy 2002; 88:201–207.

101. Barach AL, Beck GJ: Exsufflation with negative pressure; physiologic and clinical studies in poliomyelitis, bronchial asthma, pulmonary emphysema, and bronchiectasis. AMA Arch Intern Med 1954; 93:825–841.

102. Cheng PT, Chen CL, Wang CM et al: Effect of neuromuscular electrical stimulation on cough capacity and pulmonary function in patients with acute cervical cord injury. J Rehabil Med 2006; 38:32–36.

103. Linder SH: Functional electrical stimulation to enhance cough in quadriplegia. Chest 1993; 103:166–169.

104. Estenne M, Pinet C, De Troyer A: Abdominal muscle strength in patients with tetraplegia. Am J Respir Crit Care Med 2000; 161:707–712.

105. Lin VW, Singh H, Chitkara RK et al: Functional magnetic stimulation for restoring cough in patients with tetraplegia. Arch Phys Med Rehabil 1998; 79:517–522.

106. Estenne M, Van Muylem A, Gorini M et al: Effects of abdominal strapping on forced expiration in tetraplegic patients. Am J Respir Crit Care Med 1998; 157:95–98.

107. Thomas J, Cook DJ, Brooks D: Chest physical therapy management of patients with cystic fibrosis. A meta-analysis. Am J Respir Crit Care Med 1995; 151:846–850.

108. Irwin RS, Boulet LP, Cloutier MM et al: Managing cough as a defense mechanism and as a symptom: a consensus panel report of the American College of Chest Physicians. Chest 1998; 114:133S–181S.

109. Gupta A, McClelland MR, Evans A et al: Minitracheotomy in the early respiratory management of patients with spinal injuries. Paraplegia 1989; 27:269–277.

110. Phillips WT, Kiratli BJ, Sarkarati M et al: Effect of spinal cord injury on the heart and cardiovascular fitness. Curr Probl Cardiol 1998; 23:649–716.

111. Dean E: Body positioning. In Frownfelter D, Dean E (eds): Cardiovascular and Pulmonary Physical Therapy. St Louis, Mosby Elsevier, 2006:307–324.

112. Jones AP, Rowe BH: Bronchopulmonary hygiene physical therapy for chronic obstructive pulmonary disease and bronchiectasis. The Cochrane Database of Systematic Reviews 1998: Issue 4. Art. No.: CD000045. DOI: 10.1002/14651858.CD000045.

113. Boaventura CD, Gastaldi AC, Silveira JM et al: Effect of an abdominal binder on the efficacy of respiratory muscles in seated and supine tetraplegic patients. Physiotherapy 2003; 89:290–295.

114. Hart N, Laffont I, de la Sota AP et al: Respiratory effects of combined truncal and abdominal support in patients with spinal cord injury. Arch Phys Med Rehabil 2005; 86:1447–1451.

115. McCool FD, Pichurko BM, Slutsky AS et al: Changes in lung volume and rib cage configuration with abdominal binding in quadriplegia. J Appl Physiol 1986; 60:1198–1202.

116. Brooks D, O'Brien K, Geddes EL et al: Is inspiratory muscle training effective for individuals with cervical spinal cord injury? A qualitative systematic review. Clin Rehabil 2005; 19:237–246.

117. Gutierrex CJ, Harrow J, Haines F: Using an evidence-based protocol to guide rehabilitation and weaning of ventilator-dependent cervical spinal cord injury patients. J Rehabil Res Dev 2003; 40:99–110.

118. Fanta CH, Leith DE, Brown R: Maximal shortening of inspiratory muscles: effect of training. J Appl Physiol 1983; 54:1618–1623.

119. Biering-Sorensen F, Lehmann Knudsen J, Schmidt A et al: Effect of respiratory training with a mouth-nose-mask in tetraplegics. Paraplegia 1991; 29:113–119.

120. Gounden P: Progressive resistive loading on accessory expiratory muscles in tetraplegia. S Afr J Physiother 1990; 46:4–12.

121. Gallego J, Perez de al Sota A, Vardon G et al: Learned activation of thoracic inspiratory muscles in tetraplegics. Am J Phys Med Rehabil 1993; 72:312–317.

122. Rutchik A, Weissman AR, Almenoff PL et al: Resistive inspiratory muscle training in subjects with chronic cervical spinal cord injury. Arch Phys Med Rehabil 1998; 79:293–297.

123. Stiller K, Huff N: Respiratory muscle training for tetraplegic patients: a literature review. Aust J Physiother 1999; 45:291–299.

124. Huldtgren AC, Fugl-Meyer AR, Jonasson E et al: Ventilatory dysfunction and respiratory rehabilitation in post-traumatic quadriplegia. Eur J Respir Dis 1980; 61:347–356.

125. Wang TG, Wang YH, Tang FT et al: Resistive inspiratory muscle training in sleep-disordered breathing of traumatic tetraplegia. Arch Phys Med Rehabil 2002; 83:491–496.

126. Ciesla N: Physical therapy associated with respiratory failure. In DeTurk WE, Cahalin LP (eds): Cardiovascular and Pulmonary Physical Therapy: An Evidence-based Approach. New York, McGraw-Hill, 2004:541–588.

127. Liaw MY, Lin MC, Cheng PT et al: Resistive inspiratory muscle training: its effectiveness in patients with acute complete cervical cord injury. Arch Phys Med Rehabil 2000; 81:752–756.

128. Harvey LA, Ellis ER: The effect of continuous positive airway pressures on lung volumes in tetraplegic patients. Paraplegia 1996; 34:54–58.

129. Groth S, Stafanger G, Dirksen H et al: Positive expiratory pressure (PEP-mask) physiotherapy improves ventilation and reduces volume of trapped gas in cystic fibrosis. Clin Resp Phys 1985; 21:339–343.

130. Ehrlich M, Manns PJ, Poulin C: Respiratory training for a person with C3–C4 tetraplegia. Aust J Physiother 1999; 45:301–307.

131. Burns S, Little J, Hussey J et al: Sleep apnea syndrome in chronic spinal cord injury: associated factors and treatment. Arch Phys Med Rehabil 2000; 81:1334–1339.

132. Fanfulla F, Delmastro M, Berardinelli A et al: Effects of different ventilator settings on sleep and inspiratory effort in patients with neuromuscular disease. Am J Respir Crit Care Med 2005; 172:619–624.

133. Tromans AM, Mecci M, Barrett FH et al: The use of the BiPAP biphasic positive airway pressure system in acute spinal cord injury. Spinal Cord 1998; 36:481–484.

134. Sorenson HM, Shelledy DC, AARC: AARC clinical practice guideline. Intermittent positive pressure breathing — 2003 revision & update. Respir Care 2003; 48:540–546.

135. Frownfelter D, Baskin MW: Respiratory care practice review. In Frownfelter D, Dean E (eds): Cardiovascular and Pulmonary Physical Therapy. St Louis, Mosby Elsevier, 2006:759–771.

136. Thomas JA, McIntosh JM: Are incentive spirometry, intermittent positive pressure breathing, and deep breathing exercises effective in the prevention of postoperative pulmonary complications after upper abdominal surgery? A systematic overview and meta-analysis. Phys Ther 1994; 74:10–16.

137. Anonymous: Clinical indications for noninvasive positive pressure ventilation in chronic respiratory failure due to restrictive lung disease, COPD, and nocturnal hypoventilation — a consensus conference report. Chest 1999; 116:521–534.

138. Bach JR, Alba AS: Management of chronic alveolar hypoventilation by nasal ventilation. Chest 1990; 97:52–57.

139. Ellis ER, Bye PT, Bruderer JW et al: Treatment of respiratory failure during sleep in patients with neuromuscular disease: positive-pressure ventilation through a nose mask. Am Rev Respir Dis 1987; 135:148–152.

140. Bach JR, Alba AS, Saporito LR: Intermittent positive pressure ventilation via the mouth as an alternative to tracheostomy for 257 ventilator users. Chest 1993; 103:174–182.

141. De Vivo MJ, Ivie CS: Life expectancy of ventilator-dependent persons with spinal cord injuries. Chest 1995; 108:226–232.

142. Frownfelter D, Sigg Mendelson L: Care of the patient with an artificial airway. In Frownfelter D, Dean E (eds): Cardiovascular and Pulmonary Physical Therapy. St Louis, Mosby Elsevier, 2006: 773–784.

143. DiMarco AF, Takaoka Y, Kowalski KE: Combined intercostal and diaphragm pacing to provide artificial ventilation in patients with tetraplegia. Arch Phys Med Rehabil 2005; 86:1200–1207.

144. Creasey G, Elefteriades J, DiMarco AF et al: Electrical stimulation to restore respiration. J Rehabil Res Dev 1996; 33:123–132.

145. Carter RE: Experience with ventilator dependent patients. Paraplegia 1993; 31:150–153.

146. Weese-Mayer DE, Silvestri JM, Kenny AS et al: Diaphragm pacing with a quadripolar phrenic nerve electrode: an international study. Pacing Clin Electrophysiol 1996; 19:1311–1319.

147. Drinker P, Shaw LA: An apparatus for the prolonged administration of artificial respiration: I. Design for adults and children. JCI 1929; 7:229–247.

148. Smith IE, King MA, Shneerson JM: Choosing a negative pressure ventilation pump: are there are important differences? Eur Respir J 1995; 8:1792–1795.

149. Warren V: Glossopharyngeal and neck accessory muscle breathing in a young adult with C2 complete tetraplegia resulting in ventilator dependency. Phys Ther 2002; 82:590–600.

Contents

Assessment of
cardiovascular fitness 228

The response of
people with spinal
cord injury to exercise 231

Exercise prescription 234

Exercise in the
community 237

Cardiovascular fitness training

Poor cardiovascular fitness is an impairment which commonly prevents patients with spinal cord injury from performing motor tasks.[1-4] The performance of motor tasks with paralysis is often an inefficient way of moving[5] and is physically demanding.[6,7] For example, ambulating with partial paralysis of the lower limbs is associated with a greater oxygen cost than walking as an able-bodied individual.[8] Similarly, pushing a wheelchair up a slope is physically strenuous. The added physical stress of moving with paralysis is particularly pronounced in the early days after injury when patients have not yet mastered efficient ways of moving.[1] At this time, patients may also be deconditioned from extended periods of bedrest[9] and may still be recovering from the effects of associated chest or lung injuries.

The importance of cardiovascular fitness is sometimes only apparent when patients participate in real life activities. For example, patients may be able to walk or propel their wheelchairs quite easily in the physiotherapy gymnasium but may experience difficulties going to a park with family and friends. Mobilizing outdoors generally requires more cardiovascular fitness than mobilizing about a physiotherapy gymnasium.

Cardiovascular fitness is also important for good long-term health and quality of life.[2,10-12] Poor cardiovascular fitness predisposes patients to cardiovascular disease, a leading cause of death in patients with spinal cord injury.[13-16] Seventeen per cent of patients with established spinal cord injury develop ischaemic heart disease (compared to 7% in the general community)[13] and 50% die of cardiovascular-related diseases.[17] The high rate of cardiovascular-related disease is due to sedentary lifestyles[18] and the high incidence of obesity,[19,20] glucose intolerance,[21] diabetes[22] and smoking.[10,23-26] It is also due to deleterious changes in lipid profiles including decreases in the concentration of high density lipoprotein-cholesterol (this is the type of cholesterol which helps prevent cardiovascular disease).[19,22,27] Regular and ongoing exercise decreases the incidence of cardiovascular-related disease in the able-bodied population and is believed to be equally important for patients with spinal cord injury.[5,23] Patients are probably most likely to regularly exercise in the community if fitness-training programmes are an integral part of the rehabilitation process and if patients have access to appropriate opportunities and facilities.

Fitness-training programmes need to be based on appropriate exercise testing and prescription. Both pose unique problems in people with spinal cord injury, especially those with high thoracic and cervical lesions. These patients have marked or complete loss of supraspinal sympathetic control (see Chapter 1). The sympathetic nerves innervate the smooth muscles of arteries, veins and airways, as well as the heart and adrenal medullae.[4] They are important for cardiac, respiratory, thermoregulatory and metabolic responses to exercise.[20] Circulating catecholamines can mimic sympathetic activity but their effects are delayed and often less pronounced.[4,28]

There are still many unanswered questions about different aspects of cardiovascular fitness training and testing for patients with spinal cord injury[24,39] and few randomized controlled trials to provide definitive answers.[12,29–32] Most of what is known comes from quasi-experimental trials,[33,34] cross-sectional studies,[35–37] knowledge about the short-term effects of exercise in patients with spinal cord injury, and the generic benefits of exercise for other patient and able-bodied populations.[6,11,35–39] The important trial examining the effectiveness of cardiovascular fitness training for preventing cardiovascular-related disease in patients with spinal cord injury is yet to be done. With these limitations in mind, the purpose of this chapter is to outline the effects of spinal cord injury on patients' responses to exercise and to provide guidelines for exercise testing and prescription. This chapter focuses on patients who are wheelchair-dependent with sufficient upper limb strength to actively exercise (i.e. patients with lesions between C5 and T12). However, regular exercise is also important for ambulating patients and the underlying principles of exercise testing and training are the same.

Assessment of cardiovascular fitness

The assessment of cardiovascular fitness is important for setting exercise programmes and monitoring response to training. Strenuous exercise can precipitate adverse cardiovascular events and for this reason usual care and precautions need to be followed. A medical specialist should assess elderly patients and those at high risk of cardiovascular disease before they engage in strenuous physical activity.

Assessments of cardiovascular fitness need to be done under reproducible test situations. Factors such as the wheelchair, cushion, trunk constraint and the position of the patient all need to be standardized. It is particularly important that the wheelchair is standardized for tests involving wheelchair propulsion. Different wheelchairs are associated with different mechanical efficiencies.

There are three main ways to assess cardiovascular fitness.[40] Each is summarized below.

Peak oxygen consumption tests

The most accurate way to assess cardiovascular fitness is with a peak oxygen consumption ($\dot{V}O_{2peak}$) test.[8,20,41] The $\dot{V}O_{2peak}$ test measures the maximal capacity of the body to deliver oxygen from the lungs to the mitochondria of exercising muscles.[42] The test can be performed with any type of exercise, although ideally with exercise incorporating as much available muscle mass as possible. It is typically performed with patients rotating arm ergometers, or propelling wheelchairs on treadmills or ergometers.[20,40,43,44] Expired gases are collected during the test through a mouthpiece connected to a gas analysis system.[45,46] Results are expressed as either the greatest absolute ($l.min^{-1}$) or relative ($ml.kg^{-1}.min^{-1}$) rate of oxygen consumption.[46]

The $\dot{V}O_{2peak}$ test requires patients to exercise at gradually increasing intensities until exhaustion. Short rests of between 20 and 30 seconds are sometimes provided between each increment.[11,47,48] For example, an arm ergometer test in a patient with paraplegia might start at 30 watts (W) and then increase by 10–15 W every 2 minutes.[11,49,50] The maximal power output these patients are likely to achieve is between 50 W and 100 W. The equivalent test for a patient with tetraplegia might start at 5 W or less, and increase by between 2.5 W and 10 W, depending on the level of fitness and spinal cord injury. The maximal power output a patient with tetraplegia is likely to attain ranges from 10 W to 50 W.[45] The power output of an arm ergometer can be adjusted by changing the externally applied resistance and cranking velocity. Cranking velocities between 30 and 90 rpm are commonly used.

The $\dot{V}O_{2peak}$ test is equivalent to the $\dot{V}O_{2max}$ test in able-bodied people. The different terminology is used to reflect the lower maximal rate of oxygen consumption with arm versus leg exercise.[11] Arm exercise is associated with a lower maximal rate of oxygen consumption because of the lower demand for oxygen from the smaller exercising upper limb muscles and the circulatory implications of arm exercise (see pp. 231–234 for details).

The $\dot{V}O_{2peak}$ test is the most accurate way of measuring cardiovascular fitness in patients with spinal cord injury but is not commonly used in spinal cord injury units because it is unnecessarily complex for the needs of clinicians. It has been included here because it is the 'gold standard' and the basis for understanding the exercise response of patients with spinal cord injury.

Submaximal exercise tests

Cardiovascular fitness is most commonly assessed in wheelchair-dependent patients with submaximal arm tests. Expired gases can be collected with portable and easy-to-use expired gas analysis systems although it is more common in spinal cord injury units to just measure heart rate.[41] Submaximal arm tests are performed in a similar way to maximal arm tests but are terminated before exhaustion. Different testing protocols are used. A commonly used protocol includes three 7-minute bouts of exercise at 40%, 60% and 80% of predicted maximal exercise capacity. For example, a patient with paraplegia and a high level of fitness might exercise at 40 W, 60 W and 80 W. Patients with lower levels of cardiovascular fitness and patients with tetraplegia would exercise at three lower power outputs (e.g. 20 W, 30 W and 40 W).

In able-bodied individuals, submaximal tests with expired gas analysis are used to estimate $\dot{V}O_{2max}$. Estimations are based on the assumption that there is a linear relationship between oxygen consumption and heart rate.[46,55,56] Oxygen consumption data are extrapolated to the point which corresponds with predicted maximal heart rate. The same process can be used to predict maximal power output because there is also a linear relationship between oxygen consumption and power output.[45] It is, however, more difficulty to estimate $\dot{V}O_{2peak}$ from submaximal arms tests, especially in patients with spinal cord injury and loss of supraspinal sympathetic control.[55] Formulae for predicting $\dot{V}O_{2peak}$ from the results of submaximal tests have been proposed but are yet to be validated.[11,43,57,58]

The results of submaximal tests which solely rely on heart rate are primarily used to monitor the response of patients to training.[51] For example, improvements in cardiovascular fitness are indicated by a decrease in heart rate at the same power output with training. It is also possible to gauge improvements in fitness by patients' perceptions of exertion. The Borg exertion scale is widely used for this purpose (see Table 12.1).[41,52–54] Improvements in fitness are indicated by lower levels of perceived exertion with exercise at the same power output.

TABLE 12.1 **Borg scale of exertion**			
6	no exertion at all	14	
7	extremely light	15	hard (heavy)
8		16	
9	very light	17	very hard
10		18	
11	light	19	extremely hard
12		20	maximal exertion
13	somewhat hard		

After References 52 and 53 with permission of Borg Products USA, Inc.

TABLE 12.2 **Guidelines to estimating fitness from distance pushed in a manual wheelchair over 12 minutes**		
Fitness level	Distance (km)	$\dot{V}O_{2peak}$ (ml.kg^{-1}.min^{-1})
Poor	<1	<7.7
Below average	1–1.39	7.7–4.5
Fair	1.4–2.1	14.6–29.1
Good	2.2–2.5	29.2–36.2
Excellent	>2.5	>36.3

Reprinted from Archives of Physical Medicine and Rehabilitation, Vol 71, Franklin BA, Swaantek KI, Grais SL et al, Field test estimation of maximal oxygen consumption in wheelchair users, pp 574–578. Copyright 1990, with permission from the American Congress of Rehabilitation Medicine and the American Academy of Physical Medicine and Rehabilitation.

Field exercise tests

Cardiovascular fitness can also be assessed by measuring the distance walked, pushed, cycled or swam over a set time period.[51] Alternatively, instead of measuring the distance covered in a set time, the distance can be standardized and the time taken to cover the distance measured. The more standardized tests include the 6- and 12-minute wheelchair propulsion tests.[3,59,60] In these tests, patients are required to push their wheelchairs as far and as fast as possible in 6 or 12 minutes over flat ground. Variations can be used where the speed of pushing and/or incline are gradually increased.[61] $\dot{V}O_{2peak}$ can be estimated from the 12-minute wheelchair propulsion test (see Table 12.2).[59,60]

TABLE 12.3 Key determinants of heart rate, stroke volume and a-$\bar{v}O_2$ difference

Heart rate	Stroke volume	a-$\bar{v}O_2$ difference
Sympathetic nervous system	Venous return	Size of exercising muscle mass
Parasympathetic nervous system	After-load	Ability of muscles to extract oxygen:
Circulating noradrenalin	Contractility	– capillarization
Intrinsic heart rhythm	Blood volume	– number of mitochondria
		– blood flow through exercising muscles
		– oxidative enzyme activity

The response of people with spinal cord injury to exercise

The response of patients with spinal cord injury to exercise is influenced by the extent and level of neurological involvement. Patients with the ability to ambulate respond to exercise in a similar way as their able-bodied counterparts. In contrast, the response to exercise of wheelchair-dependent patients with complete upper thoracic paraplegia or tetraplegia is quite different. Their exercise response is adversely affected by three main factors, namely, reliance on arm exercise, lower limb paralysis and loss of supraspinal sympathetic nervous control.[4,20] Each of these three factors adversely effect cardiac output and arterio-venous oxygen difference (a-$\bar{v}O_2$ difference): the two determinants of $\dot{V}O_{2peak}$ (see Table 12.3).

The relationship between cardiac output, arterio-venous oxygen difference and $\dot{V}O_{2peak}$ can be summarized by Fick's principle:

$$\dot{V}O_{2peak} = \text{cardiac output} \times (\text{a-}\bar{v}O_2 \text{ difference})$$

where: cardiac output = heart rate $\times$ stroke volume.

Cardiac output is the 'central' determinant of $\dot{V}O_{2peak}$ and the a-$\bar{v}O_2$ difference is the 'peripheral' determinant. The next section outlines the implications of spinal cord injury and arm exercise on cardiac output and a-$\bar{v}O_2$ difference.

Cardiac output

Maximal cardiac output is reduced in patients with spinal cord injury. This is predominantly due to a decrease in maximal stroke volume but also due to a decrease in maximal heart rate.[14,48]

Fitness training typically increases maximal cardiac output in able-bodied individuals and patients with lower levels of spinal cord injury capable of exercising with larger muscle masses. However, in wheelchair-dependent patients with spinal cord injury, and especially in those with tetraplegia, arm exercise does not commonly place a sufficient demand on the heart to prompt a central training effect on cardiac output unless patients are very deconditioned.[48] The exercising muscles are too small and the body's demand for oxygen too low to stress and hence train the heart.[4,5,62,63]

Heart rate

The balance between sympathetic and parasympathetic activity determines heart rate. Sympathetic control to the heart is via T1–T4 nerve roots, while parasympathetic control is via the vagal nerve.[20,48] Sympathetic activity increases and parasympathetic activity decreases heart rate.[4,20,48] Without input from either source, the heart will beat at approximately 70–80 beats.min^{-1}. This is due to the intrinsic firing rate of the sinoatrial node in the heart.

Patients with lesions above T1 have complete loss of supraspinal sympathetic control to the heart. Consequently, heart rate is primarily increased by the withdrawal of excitatory input from the vagal nerve.[4,20,64] Circulating humoral factors such as catecholamines can further increase heart rate[65,66] but there is a time lag between their release and effect. The maximal heart rate of patients with lesions above T1 can be as low as 110–130 beats.min^{-1}.[4,49] In contrast, the maximal heart rate of able-bodied individuals is approximately 200 beats.min^{-1} depending on age.

Unlike able-bodied individuals, fitness training may increase maximal heart rate in patients with spinal cord injury.[41] The mechanisms underlying this possible training effect are not well understood, but may be due to changes in the body's ability to release and respond to circulating humoral factors. Alternatively, it may be due to the local effects of training on the arm muscles. Training delays the onset of muscle fatigue during maximal exercise testing. Consequently, trained patients can exert themselves more than untrained patients placing a greater demand on the body for oxygen. This demand is met by an increase in heart rate.[41]

Stroke volume

Patients with spinal cord injury have a lower maximal stroke volume.[48,67] The decrease in stroke volume is primarily due to the loss of supraspinal sympathetic control and the implications of arm exercise. Both have deleterious effects on the two primary determinants of stroke volume, namely venous return (also called pre-load) and contractility.

Venous return

Normally, 65–70% of the body's total blood volume sits within the venous system. In able-bodied individuals, at least half of this blood volume is redistributed from inactive tissues to working muscles during exercise.[48,68] However, in patients with spinal cord injury this blood volume stays largely pooled within the venous system.[34,69,70] Venous pooling is due to the loss of the lower limb and intra-thoracic muscle pumps secondary to abdominal and lower limb muscle paralysis. It is also due to loss of supraspinal sympathetic control.

Venous return is important because it determines end-diastolic filling. That is, the amount of blood which returns to the ventricles for subsequent redistribution. In turn, end-diastolic filling dictates stroke volume by the Frank-Starling mechanism.[69] A poor venous return limits stroke volume which in turn limits cardiac output and $\dot{V}O_{2peak}$.

Venous return and stroke volume can be improved with lower limb elevation[56,69] and electrical stimulation.[50,71] Leg stockings and binders do not make a notable difference to venous return during exercise.[69]

Contractility

Contractility refers to the heart's ability to contract the cardiac muscles and forcibly expel blood. In able-bodied individuals, sympathetic activity is the most important and direct determinant of contractility. Without sympathetic activity, contractility and hence stroke volume is reduced.

After-load and blood volume

After-load and blood volume also determine stroke volume (see Table 12.3).[46] The effects of spinal cord injury on these two factors are not well understood, although exercising blood pressure is lower than normal in patients with tetraplegia[4] and blood volume may be reduced.[72]

Arterio-venous oxygen difference

The a-$\bar{v}O_2$ difference is the peripheral determinant of $\dot{V}O_{2peak}$. It reflects the ability to extract and utilize oxygen and is expressed as the difference in the oxygen content of blood entering and leaving the pulmonary arteries (a-$\bar{v}O_2$ difference). There are two key factors determining the a-$\bar{v}O_2$ difference. They are the size of the exercising muscle mass and the ability of muscles to extract oxygen. Both are adversely affected by spinal cord injury but not to the same extent as cardiac output.

Fitness training improves the a-$\bar{v}O_2$ difference in people with spinal cord injury, delaying the onset of muscle fatigue. This is particularly important for patients with tetraplegia and little active muscle mass. Their ability to maximally exercise is primarily limited by muscle fatigue. If muscle fatigue can be delayed, $\dot{V}O_{2peak}$ can be increased.[5]

Size of the exercising muscle mass

The most important determinant of the a-$\bar{v}O_2$ difference is the size of the exercising muscle mass. Patients with tetraplegia and partial paralysis of the upper limbs have a smaller active muscle mass than their paraplegic counterparts. Their ability to actively utilize their upper limbs during exercise is capped by neurological involvement.[4,20,49] Exercise in small muscles is associated with a lower a-$\bar{v}O_2$ difference than exercise in large muscles because there is less opportunity, need and ability to extract and utilize oxygen.[4,20] It is partly for this reason that, even in able-bodied individuals, $\dot{V}O_{2peak}$ with arm exercise is approximately 70% of $\dot{V}O_{2max}$ with leg exercise.[8,45,47]

Fitness training in patients with spinal cord injury induces muscle hypertrophy, thereby increasing muscle mass and the a-$\bar{v}O_2$ difference.

Ability of muscles to extract oxygen

The ability of muscles to extract oxygen is also an important determinant of the a-$\bar{v}O_2$ difference and hence $\dot{V}O_{2peak}$. Oxygen extraction is determined by factors including the size and type of muscle fibres, the density of capillaries, the regulation of blood flow, the size and number of mitochondria and the type of metabolism.[8] These factors are relatively unaffected by the implications of spinal cord injury, although the loss of supraspinal sympathetic control adversely affects the ability to redirect blood from non-essential organs to exercising muscles.[48] Sympathetic activity with exercise in able-bodied individuals causes vasoconstriction in non-essential organs. This increases blood flow to exercising muscles. Without sympathetic activity, the blood flow to exercising muscles is restricted. This is partially counteracted in patients with spinal cord injury by the local vasodilating effects within muscles by factors such as changes in pH, metabolites, temperature and interstitial fluid. However, local vaso-dilation without compensatory vasoconstriction elsewhere can be problematic causing exercise-induced hypotension.[4]

Fitness training increases the ability of muscles to extract oxygen in all patients, including those with higher levels of spinal cord injury. This training effect is one of the key factors increasing $\dot{V}O_{2peak}$ in patients with spinal cord injury. A better ability to extract oxygen delays the onset of local muscle fatigue and increases maximal exercise capacity. This training response is due to an increase in the concentration of mitochondria and myoglobia, better utilization of free fatty acids (rather than carbohydrates), increased capillary density, better glycogen storage and increased capacity for glycogen synthesis.[4] Associated with these changes is a decreased accumulation of lactic acid, especially at the commencement of exercise when there is an interim, but high, reliance on the anaerobic system. This is particularly relevant because build-up of lactic acid and its associated local feelings of muscle soreness and fatigue are important limiting factors when exercising with small muscle masses.[4,5,45,73]

Exercise prescription

The key parameters for exercise prescription are frequency, intensity and duration.[43,74] The generic guidelines, set down by the American College of Sports Medicine for people with disabilities, recommend at least 20 minutes of exercise three to five times a week at an intensity which corresponds with 50–80% of maximal exercise capacity (i.e. $\dot{V}O_{2peak}$).[43,74,75] This is equivalent to working at 70–85% of maximal heart rate.[47] These guidelines are similar to exercise protocols recommended specifically for patients with spinal cord injury,[18,43,49,76,77] although the reliance on heart rate for exercise prescription is clearly problematic for patients with loss of supraspinal sympathetic control.[56] Importantly, as patients improve, exercise intensity needs to increase so patients continue to work at 50–80% of their maximal exercise capacity.

Setting the intensity

The results of submaximal tests can be used to estimate a power output which corresponds with 50–80% of maximal exercise capacity. However, this is only helpful if training is done on ergometers which measure power output. Alternatively, portable heart rate monitors can be used to get an indication of exercise intensity, although with less certainty in patients with loss of supraspinal sympathetic control.[58]

Arguably, the most appropriate way to determine exercise intensity in the clinical situation is to rely on patients' perceptions of exertion. Patients are encouraged to exercise at an intensity which corresponds with 12–16 on the 20-point Borg scale of perceived exertion. Portable heart rate monitors can then be used to determine the relationship between heart rate and Borg levels of exertion. In this way, both can be used interchangeably to indicate exercise intensity.

Selecting the type of exercise

The appropriate type of exercise will depend on many factors and in particular whether power output needs to be monitored. However, training effects are quite specific to the way patients exercise.[47] So training on arm ergometers will improve patients' exercise capacity when performing this type of exercise but the benefits will not be fully transferable to other forms of exercise (see Figure 12.1). For this reason exercise involving wheelchair propulsion is usually most appropriate during the initial rehabilitation phase when the aim of treatment is to improve a patient's ability to mobilize in a wheelchair. Pushing a wheelchair around a hospital, rather than as part of a structured and physically demanding programme, is not normally of sufficient intensity to attain a training effect.[1,20,24,48,78] The exception is in the early days after injury when patients are very deconditioned.

Continuous or short-interval training programmes can be used.[49,79] Some would argue that interval training and its effects on the anaerobic system better match the

Figure 12.1 Training with an arm ergometer while the legs are passively moved.

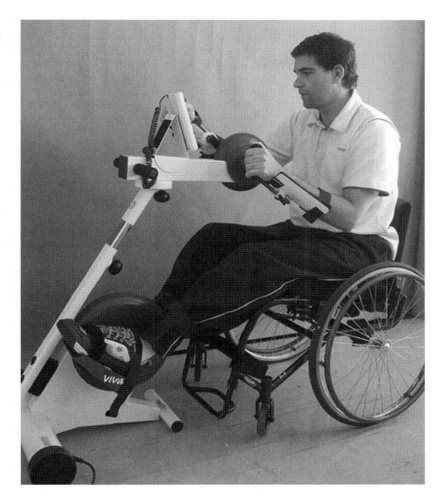

physical demands placed on patients with spinal cord injury during their normal daily routines, although a combination of the two is arguably most appropriate.

It is important to design exercise programmes which promote patient adherence. Patient adherence will be improved if exercise programmes are varied, interesting, structured and monitored. Exercises performed within group settings are most likely to maintain patients' interest and motivation. Programmes which consist of rotating arm ergometers at a fixed velocity and resistance for 20 minutes a day with minimal supervision are unlikely to be continued. Rather, programmes need to be broken up with rapid low-resistance bouts mixed with slower and more sustained high-resistance bouts. One day patients might use an arm ergometer, the next day they might push their wheelchair around a circuit. Wheelchair mobility can be varied by pushing on the flat, pushing up and down ramps, pushing forwards, pushing backwards, pushing in a standard wheelchair and pushing in a racing wheelchair. Exercise intensity can be monitored and progress recorded with the use of stopwatches, portable heart rate monitors and the Borg exertion scale.

The practice of motor tasks can also be used to train cardiovascular fitness during the early phases of rehabilitation. For instance, repeated but physically demanding practice of transfers within a set time frame can be useful for this purpose (e.g. the patient performs repeated transfers within a series of 3-minute bouts, each bout separated by a short rest). Alternatively, ambulating patients can practise aspects of their gait while training cardiovascular fitness. For example, a patient can practise sit to stand from a low chair repeatedly. The emphasis is placed on a high number of repetitions within a set time frame. Again portable heart rate monitors can be used to ensure patients work at a minimum predetermined heart rate for a sufficiently long period of time. This type of fitness training is less precise than other forms of fitness training but arguably provides patients with functional fitness appropriate for activities of daily living. Training fitness in this way is also often more acceptable to patients.

Exercise which is part of recreational and sporting pursuits is more likely to be continued throughout patients' lives. Swimming, boxing, wheelchair racing, wheelchair basketball or rugby are all increasingly popular and are a good way to enable wheelchair-dependent patients to engage in regular physical activity.[43,80] However, initially patients need information and exposure to the range of exercises and recreational activities appropriate for their level of disability and interest.[81] This type of assistance is commonly provided by recreational therapists within spinal cord injury units. The same form of assistance also needs to be provided for patients living in the community. There are numerous sporting organizations for the disabled in most countries which provide assistance in this area.

Incorporating electrical stimulation

Electrical stimulation can be used to help patients with spinal cord injury exercise. A hybrid cycle ergometer can be used where the arms and legs cycle together but the paralysed legs are driven by electrical stimulation. The primary advantage of electrically stimulating the legs is that it enables exercise with a large muscle mass.[4,20] This, combined with improved venous return from the cyclic contraction and movement of the paralysed legs,[50,71] leads to a greater stroke volume,[50,71] $\dot{V}O_{2max}$[50,82] and a better central training effect than arm exercise alone.[20,82,83] Electrical stimulation also has additional neural, metabolic, vascular and endocrine effects, and increases the stimulated 'strength' of paralysed muscles.[84–89] There is also initial evidence to indicate that it prevents bone loss.[90,91]

Despite initial evidence supporting the benefits of hybrid exercise, it is not yet part of most patients' routine and ongoing care. Instead it is primarily used for research purposes. This is partly because hybrid exercise requires expensive equipment[92] and is time-consuming to set up. Often patients need to travel to specialized clinics to participate in hybrid-exercise programmes. Hybrid exercise is unlikely to be more widely used or advocated until high quality clinical trials provide convincing evidence that the long-term benefits justify the associated cost, time and commitment.

Considering the needs of the frail and elderly

Initially patients may be unable to exercise at an optimal training intensity for 20 minutes at a time. This may be because of the effects of local muscle fatigue, age, musculoskeletal pain, general deconditioning or merely limited tolerance to the discomfort and effort associated with exercise. In these patients, the intensity and frequency of exercise may need to be gradually built up over many weeks, if not months.[51] These patients may also better tolerate programmes consisting largely of interval rather than continuous training. Overzealous prescription of exercise in the early days after injury may be counter-productive and only serve to discourage patients from good long-term exercise habits.

Maintaining thermoregulation

Patients with spinal cord injury have a limited ability to dissipate heat with exercise.[93,94] This is primarily due to disruption of the sympathetic nervous system and the resultant limited ability to sweat and redirect blood flow to the skin.[95,96] Patients will not necessarily sense an increase in temperature with strenuous exercise but any elevation in core body temperature needs to be avoided. This is best achieved by not exercising in hot conditions and ensuring adequate hydration and appropriate clothing.[97]

Exercise in the community

Ongoing regular exercise is not only important for cardiovascular health[43,81,98] but also for general well-being. Regular exercise promotes social integration and satisfaction with life.[20,32,98–100] It reduces anxiety,[101] pain and depression,[29,102,103] and increases self-esteem and efficacy.[104] It may also reduce the incidence of urinary tract infections, and helps prevent pressure ulcers, osteoporosis, respiratory infections and spasticity.[2,3,37,105] Some of these and other generic benefits of regular exercise have been well established in other patient groups[106] and in the able-bodied community.[101]

Just as it is difficult to encourage regular exercise in the able-bodied population, it is also difficult to encourage regular exercise in patients with spinal cord injury.[107] The long-term exercise habits of patients with spinal cord injury are closely related to their pre-injury exercise habits[98,108] and innate motivation.[107] In addition, there are real and perceived barriers preventing patients exercising in the community. These include cost, time and difficulties accessing transport, appropriate facilities and assistance.[1,12,102,107,109,110]

The challenge for health care providers is to remove barriers and promote healthy lifestyles. This firstly requires widespread education which not only addresses the importance of exercise but also encourages good diet and the cessation of smoking.[111] Secondly, resources and support need to be directed at enabling patients to easily and cheaply access community-based exercise programmes. A variety of different programmes need to be provided to cater for patients' different lifestyles and exercise choices. Exercise opportunities should, where possible, be provided in patients' local communities, preferably within the context of an enjoyable sport or recreational activity which is likely to be continued. Alternatively, patients can exercise at home. Importantly, exercise programmes need to be realistic, appreciating that patients with spinal cord injury have many demands on their time. They are not only being encouraged to perform exercises to address cardiovascular fitness but are also being encouraged to stand (see Chapter 6), perform strengthening exercises (see Chapter 8), wear splints, stretch (see Chapter 9) and use electrical stimulation. It is perhaps not realistic to expect patients to devote more than a few hours a week to all these aspects of their long-term physical health. The future challenge for researchers is to determine which aspects are most important and cost-effective.

References

1. Janssen TW, van Oers CA, Rozendaal EP et al: Changes in physical strain and physical capacity in men with spinal cord injuries. Med Sci Sports Exerc 1996; 28:551–559.
2. Noreau L, Shephard RJ: Spinal cord injury, exercise and quality of life. Sports Med 1995; 20:226–250.

3. Laskin JJ, James SA, Cantwell BM: A fitness and wellness program for people with spinal cord injury. Top Spinal Cord Inj Rehabil 1997; 3:16–33.
4. Figoni SF: Exercise responses and quadriplegia. Med Sci Sports Exerc 1992; 25:433–441.
5. Chase TM: Physical fitness strategies. In Lanig IS, Chase TM, Butt LM et al (eds): A Practical Guide to Health Promotion after Spinal Cord Injury. Gaithersburg, MD, Aspen Publishers, 1996:243–291.
6. Pang MY, Eng JJ, Dawson AS et al: The use of aerobic exercise training in improving aerobic capacity in individuals with stroke: a meta-analysis. Clin Rehabil 2006; 20:97–111.
7. Meek C, Pollock A, Potter J et al: A systematic review of exercise trials post stroke. Clin Rehabil 2003; 17:6–13.
8. Waters RL, Mulroy S: The energy expenditure of normal and pathologic gait. Gait Posture 1999; 9:207–231.
9. Hjeltnes N: Control of medical rehabilitation of para- and tetraplegics by repeated evaluation of endurance capacity. Int J Sports Med 1984; 5:171–174.
10. Duran FS, Lugo L, Ramirez L et al: Effects of an exercise program on the rehabilitation of patients with spinal cord injury. Arch Phys Med Rehabil 2001; 82:1349–1354.
11. Davis G, Glaser RM: Cardiorespiratory fitness following spinal cord injury. In Ada L, Canning C (eds): Key Issues in Neurological Physiotherapy. Oxford, Butterworth Heinemann, 1990:155–196.
12. Martin Ginis KA, Hicks AL: Exercise research issues in the spinal cord injured population. Exerc Sport Sci Rev 2005; 33:49–53.
13. Yekutiel M, Brooks ME, Ohry A et al: The prevalence of hypertension, ischaemic heart disease and diabetes in traumatic spinal cord injured patients and amputees. Paraplegia 1989; 27:58–62.
14. Figoni S: Perspectives on cardiovascular fitness and SCI. J Am Paraplegia Soc 1990; 13:63–71.
15. Whiteneck GG, Charlifue SW, Frankel HL et al: Mortality, morbidity, and psychosocial outcomes of persons spinal cord injured more than 20 years ago. Paraplegia 1992; 30:617–630.
16. De Vivo MJ, Krause JS, Lammertse DP: Recent trends in mortality and causes of death among persons with spinal cord injury. Arch Phys Med Rehabil 1999; 80:1411–1419.
17. Cardus D, Ribas-Cardu F, McTaggart WG: Coronary risk in spinal cord injury: assessment following a multivariate approach. Arch Phys Med Rehabil 1992; 73:930–933.
18. Warburton DER, Sproule S, Krassioukov A et al: Cardiovascular health and exercise following spinal cord injury. In Eng JJ, Teasell RW, Miller WC et al (eds): Spinal Cord Injury Rehabilitation Evidence. Vancouver, SCIRE, 2006:7.1–7.28.
19. Maki KC, Briones ER, Langbein WE et al: Associations between serum lipids and indicators of adiposity in men with spinal cord injury. Paraplegia 1995; 33:102–109.
20. Ragnarsson KT: The cardiovascular system. In Whiteneck GG, Charlifue SW, Gerhart KA (eds): Aging with Spinal Cord Injury. New York, Demos Publications, 1993.
21. Bauman WA, Spungen AM: Disorders of carbohydrate and lipid-metabolism in veterans with paraplegia or quadriplegia: a model of premature aging. Metabolism 1994; 43:749–756.
22. Manns PJ, McCubbin JA, Williams DP: Fitness, inflammation, and the metabolic syndrome in men with paraplegia. Arch Phys Med Rehabil 2005; 86:1176–1181.
23. Dearwater SR, LaPorte RE, Robertson RJ et al: Activity in the spinal cord-injured patient: an epidemiologic analysis of metabolic parameters. Med Sci Sports Exerc 1986; 18:541–544.
24. Janssen TW, van Oers CA, van der Woude LH et al: Physical strain in daily life of wheelchair users with spinal cord injuries. Med Sci Sports Exerc 1994; 26:661–670.
25. Nuhlicek DN, Spurr GB, Barboriak JJ et al: Body composition of patients with spinal cord injury. Eur J Clin Nutr 1988; 42:765–773.
26. Spungen AM, Lesser M, Almenoff PL et al: Prevalence of cigarette smoking in a group of male veterans with chronic spinal cord injury. Mil Med 1995; 160:308–311.
27. Zlotolow SP, Levy E, Baurnan WA: The serum lipoprotein profile in veterans with paraplegia: the relationship to nutritional factors and body mass index. J Am Paraplegia Soc 1992; 15:158–162.
28. Gass G, Gass EM, Climstein M et al: Effect of exercise and water immersion (39°C) on core temperature, sweat rate and catecholamines in tetraplegics. Med Sci Sports Exerc 1991; 23:S102.
29. Hicks AL, Martin KA, Ditor DS et al: Long-term exercise training in persons with spinal cord injury: effects on strength, arm ergometry performance and psychological well-being. Spinal Cord 2003; 41:34–43.
30. Martin Ginis KA, Latimer AE, McKechnie K et al: Using exercise to enhance subjective well-being among people with spinal cord injury: the mediating influences of stress and pain. Rehabil Psychol 2003; 48:157–164.
31. Baldi JC, Jackson RD, Moraille R et al: Muscle atrophy is prevented in patients with acute spinal cord injury using functional electrical stimulation. Spinal Cord 1998; 36:463–469.
32. Rimmer JH, Braddock D, Pitetti KH: Research on physical activity and disability: an emerging national priority. Med Sci Sports Exerc 1996; 28:1366–1372.
33. DiCarlo SE, Supp MD, Taylor HC: Effect of arm ergometry training on physical work capacity of individuals with spinal cord injuries. Phys Ther 1983; 63:1104–1107.

34. Gass G, Watson J, Camp EM et al: The effects of physical training on high level spinal lesion patients. Scand J Rehabil Med 1980; 12:61–65.
35. Zwiren LD, Bar-Or O: Responses to exercise of paraplegics who differ in conditioning level. Med Sci Sports Exerc 1975; 7:94–98.
36. Noreau L, Shephard RJ, Simard C et al: Relationship of impairment and functional ability to habitual activity and fitness following spinal cord injury. Int J Rehabil Res 1993; 16:265–275.
37. Hjeltnes N, Jansen T: Physical endurance capacity, functional status and medical complications in spinal cord injured subjects with long-standing lesions. Paraplegia 1990; 28:428–432.
38. Van Peppen RPS, Kwakkel G, Wood-Dauphinnee S et al: The impact of physical therapy on functional outcomes after stroke: what's the evidence? Clin Rehabil 2004; 18:833–862.
39. Saunders DH, Greig CA, Young A et al: Physical fitness training for stroke patients. The Cochrane Database of Systematic Reviews 2004: Issue 1. Art. No.: CD003316. DOI: 10.1002/14651858.CD003316.pub2.
40. Fehr L, Langbein WE, Edwards LC et al: Diagnostic wheelchair exercise testing. Top Spinal Cord Inj Rehabil 1997; 3:34–48.
41. Stewart MW, Melton-Rogers SL, Morrison S et al: The measurement properties of fitness measures and health status for persons with spinal cord injuries. Arch Phys Med Rehabil 2000; 81:394–400.
42. Barstow TJ, Scremin AME, Mutton DL et al: Changes in gas exchange kinetics with training in patients with spinal cord injury. Med Sci Sports Exerc 1996; 28:1221–1228.
43. Jacobs PL, Nash MS: Exercise recommendations for individuals with spinal cord injury. Sports Med 2004; 34:727–751.
44. Gass EM, Harvey LA, Gass GC: Maximal physiological responses during arm cranking and treadmill wheelchair propulsion in T4–T6 paraplegic men. Paraplegia 1995; 33:267–270.
45. Jacobs PL, Beekhuizen KS: Appraisal of physiological fitness in persons with spinal cord injury. Top Spinal Cord Inj Rehabil 2005; 10:32–50.
46. Astrand P, Rodahl K: Textbook of Work Physiology: Physiological Bases of Exercise, 2nd edn. New York, McGraw-Hill, 1977.
47. Franklin BA: Exercise testing, training and arm ergometry. Sports Med 1985; 2:100–119.
48. Phillips WT, Kiratli BJ, Sarkarati M et al: Effect of spinal cord injury on the heart and cardiovascular fitness. Curr Probl Cardiol 1998; 23:649–716.
49. Bizzarini E, Saccavini M, Lipanje F et al: Exercise prescription in subjects with spinal cord injuries. Arch Phys Med Rehabil 2005; 86:1170–1175.
50. Raymond J, Davis GM, Clarke J et al: Cardiovascular responses during arm exercise and orthostatic challenge in individuals with paraplegia. Eur J Appl Physiol 2001; 85:89–95.
51. Russo P: Cardiovascular responses associated with activity and inactivity. In Ada L, Canning C (eds): Key Issues in Neurological Physiotherapy. Oxford, Butterworth Heinemann, 1990:127–154.
52. Borg G: Psychophysical basis of perceived exertion. Med Sci Sports Exerc 1982; 14:371–381.
53. Borg G: Borg's Perceived Exertion and Pain Scales. Champaign, IL, Human Kinetics, 1998.
54. Capodaglio P, Grilli C, Bazzini G: Tolerable exercise intensity in the early rehabilitation of paraplegic patients. A preliminary study. Spinal Cord 1996; 34:684–690.
55. Sawka MN: Physiology of upper body exercise. Exerc Sport Sci Rev 1986; 14:175–211.
56. McLean KP, Jones PP, Skinner JS: Exercise prescription for sitting and supine exercise in subjects with quadriplegia. Med Sci Sports Exerc 1995; 27:15–21.
57. Kofsky PR, Davis GM, Shephard RJ et al: Field testing: assessment of physical fitness of disabled adults. Eur J Appl Physiol Occup Physiol 1983; 51:109–120.
58. Rimmer JH: Spinal cord injury. In Rimmer JH (ed): Fitness and Rehabilitation Programs for Special Populations. Madison, WI, WCB Brown and Benchmark Publishers, 1994:206–246.
59. Franklin BA, Swaantek KI, Grais SL et al: Field test estimation of maximal oxygen consumption in wheelchair users. Arch Phys Med Rehabil 1990; 71:574–578.
60. Rhodes EC, McKenzie DC, Coutts KD et al: A field test for the prediction of aerobic capacity in male paraplegics and quadriplegics. Can J Appl Sport Sci 1981; 6:182–186.
61. Vinet A, Bernard PL, Poulain M et al: Validation of an incremental field test for the direct assessment of peak oxygen uptake in wheelchair-dependent athletes. Spinal Cord 1996; 34:288–293.
62. Figoni SF: Circulorespiratory effects of arm training and detraining in one C5–6 quadriplegic man. Phys Ther 1986; 66:779.
63. Hjeltnes M: Capacity for physical work and training after spinal injuries and strokes. Scand J Rehabil Med 1982; 29:245–251.
64. Birk TJ, Nieshoff R, Gray G et al: Metabolic and cardiopulmonary responses to acute progressive resistive exercise in a person with C4 spinal cord injury. Spinal Cord 2001; 39:336–339.
65. Kjaer M, Pott F, Mohr T et al: Heart rate during exercise with leg vascular occlusion in spinal cord-injured humans. J Appl Physiol 1999; 86:806–811.
66. Raymond J, Davis GM, van der Plas M: Cardiovascular responses during submaximal electrical stimulation-induced leg cycling in individuals with paraplegia. Clin Physiol Funct Imaging 2002; 22:92–98.

67. Hopman MT, Houtman S, Groothius JT et al: The effect of varied fractional inspired oxygen on arm exercise performance in spinal cord injury and able-bodied persons. Arch Phys Med Rehabil 2004; 85:319–323.

68. Rothe CF: Point: active venoconstriction is/is not important in maintaining or raising end-diastolic volume and stroke volume during exercise and orthostasis. J Appl Physiol 2006; 101:1262–1264.

69. Hopman MT, Monroe M, Dueck C et al: Blood redistribution and circulatory responses to submaximal arm exercise in person with spinal cord injury. Scand J Rehabil Med 1998; 30:167–174.

70. Teasell RW, Arnold JM, Krassioukov A et al: Cardiovascular consequences of loss of supraspinal control of the sympathetic nervous system after spinal cord injury. Arch Phys Med Rehabil 2000; 81:506–516.

71. Davis GM, Servedio FJ, Glaser RM et al: Cardiovascular responses to arm cranking and FNS-induced leg exercise in paraplegics. J Appl Physiol 1990; 69:671–677.

72. Houtman S, Oeseburg B, Hopman MT: Blood volume and hemoglobin after spinal cord injury. Am J Phys Med Rehabil 2000; 79:260–265.

73. Olive JL, Slade JM, Dudley GA et al: Blood flow and muscle fatigue in SCI individuals during electrical stimulation. J Appl Physiol 2003; 94:701–708.

74. Rimmer JH: Exercise prescription for special populations. In Rimmer JH (ed): Fitness and Rehabilitation Programs for Special Populations. Madison, WI, WCB Brown and Benchmark Publishers, 1994:1–21.

75. Figoni SF: Spinal cord injury. In Durstine JL (ed): ACSM's Exercise Management for Persons with Chronic Diseases and Disabilities/American College of Sports Medicine. Champaign, IL, Human Kinetics, 1997:175–179.

76. Hooker SP, Wells CL: Effects of low and moderate intensity training in spinal cord-injured persons. Med Sci Sports Exerc 1989; 21:18–22.

77. Crane L, Klerk K, Ruhl A et al: The effect of exercise training on pulmonary function in persons with quadriplegia. Paraplegia 1994; 32:435–441.

78. Hjeltnes N, Vokac Z: Circulatory strain in everyday life of paraplegics. Scand J Rehabil Med 1979; 11:67–73.

79. Tordi N, Dugue B, Klupzinski D et al: Interval training program on a wheelchair ergometer for paraplegic subjects. Spinal Cord 2001; 39:532–537.

80. Bar-Or O: The Wingate anaerobic test. An update on methodology, reliability and validity. Sports Med 1987; 4:381–394.

81. Chase TM, Lanig IS: Fitness awareness during acute SCI rehabilitation. Top Spinal Cord Inj Rehabil 1997; 3:49–55.

82. Raymond J, Davis GM, Climstein M et al: Cardiovascular responses to arm cranking and electrical stimulation leg cycling in people with paraplegia. Med Sci Sports Exerc 1999; 31:822–828.

83. Wheeler GD, Andrews B, Lederer R et al: Functional electrical stimulation-assisted rowing: increasing cardiovascular fitness through functional electrical stimulation rowing training in persons with spinal cord injury. Arch Phys Med Rehabil 2002; 83:1093–1099.

84. Aydin G, Tomruk S, Keles I et al: Transcutaneous electrical nerve stimulation versus baclofen in spasticity: clinical and electrophysiologic comparison. Am J Phys Med Rehabil 2005; 84:584–592.

85. Carraro U, Rossini K, Mayr W et al: Muscle fiber regeneration in human permanent lower motoneuron denervation: relevance to safety and effectiveness of FES-training, which induces muscle recovery in SCI subjects. Artif Organs 2005; 29:187–191.

86. Chao CY, Cheing GL: The effects of lower-extremity functional electric stimulation on the orthostatic responses of people with tetraplegia. Arch Phys Med Rehabil 2005; 86:1427–1433.

87. de Groot P, Crozier J, Rakobowchuk M et al: Electrical stimulation alters FMD and arterial compliance in extremely inactive legs. Med Sci Sports Exerc 2005; 37.

88. van der Salm A, Veltink PH, IJzerman MJ et al: Comparison of electric stimulation methods for reduction of triceps surae spasticity in spinal cord injury. Arch Phys Med Rehabil 2006; 87:222–228.

89. Sampson E, Burnhams R, Andrews B: Functional electrical stimulation effect on orthostatic hypotension after spinal cord injury. Arch Phys Med Rehabil 2000; 81:139–143.

90. Chen SC, Lai CH, Chan WP et al: Increases in bone mineral density after functional electrical stimulation cycling exercises in spinal cord injured patients. Disabil Rehabil 2005; 27:1337–1341.

91. Maimoun L, Fattal C, Micallef JP et al: Bone loss in spinal cord-injured patients: from physiopathology to therapy. Spinal Cord 2006; 44:203–210.

92. Ragnarsson KT: Functional electrical stimulation systems: what have we accomplished, where are we going? J Rehabil Res Dev 1996; 33:vii–iii.

93. Ellenberg M, MacRitchie M, Franklin B et al: Aerobic capacity in early paraplegia: implications for rehabilitation. Paraplegia 1989; 27:261–268.

94. Yaggie JA, Nieme TJ, Buono MJ: Adaptive sweat gland response after spinal cord injury. Arch Phys Med Rehabil 2002; 83:802–805.

95. Price MJ, Campbell IG: Thermoregulatory responses of spinal cord injured and able-bodied athletes to prolonged upper body exercise and recovery. Spinal Cord 1999; 37:772–779.

96. Price MJ, Campbell IG: Effects of spinal cord lesion level upon thermoregulation during exercise in the heat. Med Sci Sports Exerc 2003; 35:1100–1107.

97. Petrofsky JS: Thermoregulatory stress during rest and exercise in heat in patients with a spinal cord injury. Eur J Appl Physiol Occup Physiol 1992; 64:503–507.

98. Wu SK, Williams T: Factors influencing sport participation among athletes with spinal cord injury. Med Sci Sports Exerc 2001; 33:177–182.

99. Manns PJ, Chad KE: Determining the relation between quality of life, handicap, fitness, and physical activity for persons with spinal cord injury. Arch Phys Med Rehabil 1999; 80:1566–1571.

100. Hanson CS, Nabavi D, Yuen HK: The effect of sports on level of community integration as reported by persons with spinal cord injury. Am J Occup Ther 2001; 55:332–338.

101. Petruzzello SJ, Landers DM, Hatfield BD et al: A meta-analysis on the anxiety-reducing effects of acute and chronic exercise. Outcomes and mechanisms. Sports Med 1991; 11:143–182.

102. Ditor DS, Latimer AE, Martin Ginis KA et al: Maintenance of exercise participation in individuals with spinal cord injury: effects on quality of life, stress and pain. Spinal Cord 2003; 41:446–450.

103. Orenczuk S, Slivinski J, Teasell RW: Depression following spinal cord injury. In Eng JJ, Teasell RW, Miller WC et al (eds): Spinal Cord Injury Rehabilitation Evidence. Vancouver, SCIRE, 2006:10.1–10.19.

104. Shephard RJ: Benefits of sport and physical activity for the disabled: implications for the individual and for society. Scand J Rehabil Med 1991; 23:51–59.

105. Curtis KA, McClanahan S, Hall KM et al: Health, vocational, and functional status in spinal cord injured athletes and nonathletes. Arch Phys Med Rehabil 1986; 67:862–865.

106. Gowans SE, deHueck A, Voss S et al: Effect of a randomized, controlled trial of exercise on mood and physical function in individuals with fibromyalgia. Arthritis Rheum 2001; 45:519–529.

107. Scelza WM, Kalpakjian CZ, Zemper ED et al: Perceived barriers to exercise in people with spinal cord injury. Am J Phys Med Rehabil 2005; 84:576–583.

108. Godin G, Colantonio A, Davis GM et al: Prediction of leisure time exercise behavior among a group of lower-limb disabled adults. J Clin Psychol 1986; 42:272–279.

109. Rimmer JH, Rubin SS, Braddock D: Barriers to exercise in African American women with physical disabilities. Arch Phys Med Rehabil 2000; 81:182–188.

110. Rimmer JH, Riley B, Wang E et al: Physical activity participation among persons with disabilities: Barriers and facilitators. Am J Prev Med 2004; 26:419–425.

111. Rimmer JH: Health promotion for people with disabilities: the emerging paradigm shift from disability prevention to prevention of secondary conditions. Phys Ther 1999; 79:495–502.

Environmental factors

CHAPTER 13

Wheelchair seating

245

Contents

Wheelchair cushions 245
Manual wheelchairs 249
Power wheelchairs 267
Sitting in vehicles 269

Wheelchair seating

Appropriate wheelchair seating is an integral aspect of the overall management of people with spinal cord injury. It not only determines patients' mobility but also has implications for skin, posture, pain and contracture management.

Over recent years a highly commercialized industry has evolved around mobility and seating equipment for the disabled. Consequently, there are hundreds of different types of cushions, wheelchairs, backrests and accessories, making selection of appropriate equipment increasingly complex. In specialized spinal units, wheelchair seating and prescription is predominantly done by seating teams comprising engineers, technicians, physiotherapists and occupational therapists. These teams are solely devoted and specifically trained for wheelchair prescription, and have an in-depth knowledge of locally available products and pressure management. Typically, commercial products are used but then individually modified to suit patients' specific needs and to minimize the deleterious effects of pressure.

This chapter outlines some of the key features of wheelchairs and cushions which need to be considered when this equipment is selected and adjusted for patients. The first section provides an overview of wheelchair cushions with particular emphasis on the effects of upright sitting on pressure distribution. The second section summarizes different types of wheelchairs and the effects of wheelchair set-up on mobility, stability and pressure. Those who require more information are well advised to refer to the excellent books solely devoted to this topic.[1-3]

Wheelchair cushions

It is important that patients sit on appropriate cushions to prevent pressure ulcers. A poorly fitted, maintained or prescribed cushion or a cushion placed upside down or around the wrong way can cause debilitating pressure ulcers necessitating months of bedrest. The soft tissues overlying the ischial tuberosities are most vulnerable to damage from sitting and cushions are primarily designed to protect these areas (see Chapter 1 for discussion on causes and management of pressure ulcers).

Figure 13.1 Most cushions are air- (a), foam- (b) or gel-based (c).

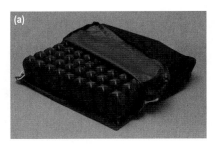

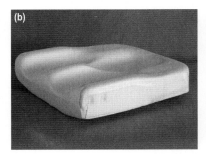

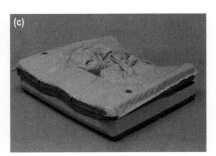

Most of the commercially-available cushions are air-, foam- or gel-based (see Figure 13.1a–c).[4] A recent Cochrane systematic review found insufficient evidence to recommend one type of cushion over another, suggesting that decisions about appropriate cushions for patients need to be based on rationale and clinical reasoning and cannot yet be based on good quality evidence.[5] Often a cushion which provides adequate pressure relief for one patient will be inappropriate for another. This is partly because the pressure-relieving features of cushions are influenced by many factors, including the wheelchair and its set-up, and patients' mobility, skin integrity, nutrition and weight. Cushions need to be prescribed on a case-by-case basis after examining their effects on pressure distribution.

The pressure-relieving qualities of cushions need to be assessed every time a new cushion is trialled. This can be done using simple or sophisticated equipment to measure skin-interface pressures.[4,6–8] These pressures are measured with patients sitting on their cushions in their wheelchairs. However, there is not one critical pressure below which patients will be safe from skin damage and above which they will not. The appropriate pressure is determined by patients' susceptibility to pressure ulcers and their ability to relieve pressure.[2] However, as a general rule, peak pressures over vulnerable sites should be kept well below 60 mm Hg.[4,7,9,10]

The pressure-relieving qualities of cushions should also be assessed by examining skin integrity immediately after patients return to bed following a period of sitting in their wheelchairs. When a new cushion is trialled, patients should only sit for between 30 minutes and 1 hour. The length of time spent sitting can be gradually increased but the skin should continue to be checked after patients return to bed and always checked at least once a day. If the skin looks red and does not blanch with localized pressure, the cushion is not providing adequate protection.[5] Either the cushion needs to be modified or changed, or the length of time spent sitting needs to be reduced. Alternatively, pressure needs to be more effectively or frequently relieved when sitting, or the set-up of the wheelchair needs to be changed.

Air-based cushions

Air-based cushions relieve pressure by distributing air from pockets of high pressure to pockets of low pressure. In this way, they mould to the shape of patients and distribute pressure over a larger surface area.[5] The ischial tuberosities should submerge into the cushion but should not press hard up against the seat of the wheelchair. The effectiveness of air-based cushions is dependent on appropriate inflation. An under-inflated cushion provides little or no protection because the ischial tuberosities bury through the cushion onto the hard seat of the wheelchair. An over-inflated cushion prevents submersion and mimics the effects of sitting on a hard seat. Therapists can use their fingers to crudely check the inflation of air-based cushions by ensuring there is enough room to slide two fingers between the ischial tuberosities and seat. Insufficient space for the fingers indicates that the cushion is under-inflated.

Some air-based cushions are power operated, cycling air between different compartments. They constantly vary pressure, avoiding long periods of high pressure in any one spot.[5] These types of cushions are primarily used for patients in power wheelchairs with ongoing pressure problems.

Gel-based cushions

Gel-based cushions work on a similar principle to air-based cushions. They dissipate pressure by allowing gel to move from areas of high pressure to areas of low pressure. Most have a contoured foam base upon which the gel sits.[4] The foam base has a specially-designed hollow or 'well' for the ischial tuberosities (see Figure 13.2). This helps ensure that most pressure is borne by the soft tissues over the lateral aspect of the thighs, leaving the ischial tuberosities free to submerge within the gel-filled well. Needless to say, if the well is too wide both the lateral thighs and ischial tuberosities fall into it with a high risk of the ischial tuberosities burying through the gel, pressing up hard against the base of the cushion or wheelchair.

Figure 13.2 The ischial tuberosities sit in a well filled with gel. The lateral thigh bears weight through the firmer outer rim of the cushion.

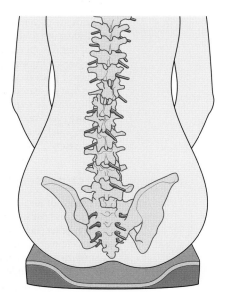

It is a common mistake to prescribe obese patients cushions with inappropriately wide wells. It is wrongly assumed that all obese patients have broad bony pelvises. These patients need to be prescribed cushions according to the width of their pelvises, not according to the width of their hips or the size of their wheelchairs. Often these patients require cushions with narrow wells individually modified to accommodate excessive adipose tissue around the hips.

Foam-based cushions

Foam-based cushions also redistribute pressure. Their effectiveness is dependent on the compressibility of the foam and the cut of the cushion. Some cushions use two or more types of foam, typically with firmer foam under the lateral aspect of the thighs and more compressible foam under the ischial tuberosities. This encourages more weight to be borne through the thighs and less weight through the vulnerable ischial tuberosities.

Foam-based cushions can be cut and contoured to meet the individual needs of patients but this is best done by trained seating specialists. Technology is also available to cut and shape foam-based cushions from plaster moulds of patients. This technology provides individualized and sophisticated seating solutions but often requires a commitment to expense without an opportunity to trial the cushion first. If the cushion is not effective, money is wasted. For this reason foam-based cushions cut and shaped from plaster moulds of patients are primarily used for particularly difficult seating and postural problems.

Other considerations

Ease of maintenance

The choice of an appropriate cushion is not only dictated by its pressure-relieving qualities but also by its ease of maintenance and its durability. For example, air-based cushions need to be regularly checked for correct inflation. Air-based cushions are also vulnerable to puncture, rendering them immediately useless until repaired. Air-based cushions are therefore not generally recommended for non-compliant patients, those with little hand function or carer support, or those in situations where punctures are a substantial risk. In contrast, gel- and foam-based cushions require little maintenance. It is, however, important that users of gel-based cushions ensure that the gel is evenly distributed prior to sitting on the cushion. Those living in cold climates also need to ensure that gel-based cushions are not stored in subzero temperatures.

All cushions require replacing. For example, foam-based cushions can require replacing every year because the foam compresses with time, decreasing its pressure-relieving qualities. Gel- and air-based cushions generally last longer, sometimes for several years.

Effect on seating stability, mobility and posture

The choice of an appropriate cushion is also determined by its effect on stability, mobility and posture.[11] Some patients feel unstable on air-based cushions and prefer the rigidity provided by foam- or gel-based cushions. More rigid cushions are also easier to transfer from because the cushion does not compress under the hands and patients do not lose height on the vertical lift of the transfer. Transferring from cushions with deep wells can be difficult if patients struggle to get their buttocks up and out of the well.

Cushions also influence seating posture.[11] For example, foam can be strategically placed on cushions to prevent legs falling into abduction or sweeping to one side. Similarly, foam can be used to lift one side of the pelvis for patients with a tendency to sit asymmetrically. However, it can be difficult to attain optimal seating posture while also ensuring sufficient pressure protection, especially in patients with deformities and complex seating and skin problems. To improve seating posture it is often necessary to increase pressure over vulnerable bony prominences. The solution is the best possible seating posture which provides adequate pressure protection. It is advisable to compromise on posture before compromising on pressure protection. Foam- and gel-based cushions generally provide greater potential to correct posture but air-based cushions provide greater skin protection.

Weight

Air- and foam-based cushions are lighter than gel-based cushions. This can be a consideration for patients doing a lot of wheelchair pushing or needing to regularly lift their cushions in and out of cars.

Cost considerations

The cost of cushions is variable but foam-based cushions are usually the cheapest. The cost can be prohibitive, particularly for those in developing countries and those with limited financial resources. In third world countries, cushions can be cheaply made with a sharp knife, an appropriate piece of foam and some initial training.[2,12,13] Alternatively, bicycle inner-tubes can be bound together to create an air-based cushion.[1] Cushions made in this way are not ideal but they provide some skin protection and are a better option than sitting directly on the hard base of a wheelchair.

Manual wheelchairs

Like cushions, there are hundreds of different types of wheelchairs. Large international companies supply wheelchairs to the majority of countries with ongoing customer support. There are also local manufacturers of wheelchairs in most countries. All wheelchairs come with an array of different features and accessories which need to be considered. Some features are critical and determine safety, comfort, pressure distribution and manoeuvrability, while others are less important and may reflect personal preference.

Wheelchair prescription not only involves finding the appropriate product but also ensuring it is appropriately fitted and set up for the patient. For example, a poorly fitted wheelchair which is too narrow for a patient can cause skin breakdown, and an excessively 'tippy' wheelchair can cause a backward fall (see Chapter 4). Most wheelchairs have substantial adjustability, although highly specialized sports wheelchairs do not.

Ideally, the set-up of a wheelchair should enable patients to sit comfortably with weight borne through the buttocks and thighs. Sitting posture should be as 'normal' as possible. The wheelchair set-up should provide sufficient upright stability to enable patients to sit without needing to grasp the wheelchair or rest the elbows on armrests to prop themselves upright. Those with upper limb function should also be able to raise their arms without toppling forwards and propel themselves up a slope without tipping the wheelchair backwards. If patients are unable to sit or move in these ways, it is usually indicative that their wheelchairs are inappropriately set up for them.

Inevitably wheelchair set-up is a compromise between providing optimal mobility, stability, skin protection and posture. Therapists and patients need to trial different set-ups until the best solution is reached. Sometimes appropriate seating *cannot* be achieved with the adjustability provided in commercial products. This is particularly common in patients with complex seating needs and spinal deformities. Often these patients require sophisticated custom-made seating systems, a service which can only be provided with appropriate technical and engineering support.

The optimal set-up of a wheelchair often changes over the first year following injury as patients' function and mobility changes. For example, with time and better wheelchair control it may be appropriate to move the back wheels forwards, increase the tilt of the seat or position the wheels higher on the frame (the effects of all these changes are discussed below). For this reason it is often advisable for patients' first wheelchairs to be highly adjustable. Alternatively, the prescription of first wheelchairs can be delayed until mobility and function have stabilized and patients have a better understanding of what they want and need. If there are no financial constraints then a first wheelchair can be prescribed or provided on loan soon after injury and a second and better suited wheelchair can be provided 6–12 months later.

Below is an overview of some of the key issues which need to be considered for fitting, setting up and choosing a manual wheelchair. Several generic issues are equally relevant to power wheelchairs and will be briefly discussed at the end of the chapter.[1–3,14,15]

Type of frame

There are two types of wheelchair frames, *rigid* (see Figure 13.3a) or *folding* (see Figure 13.3b). Rigid frames are primarily prescribed for active patients. They are generally lighter, sturdier, more adjustable and easier to push. Folding fames are better suited to ambulating patients because the footrests can be lifted when standing up. Folding frames are also used by patients who rely on car hoists to stow their wheelchairs on the roofs of cars. However, folding frames are more likely to break and do not always provide a comfortable ride. Some wheelchairs are fitted with suspension to provide a smoother ride; however, suspension is expensive and increases the weight of the wheelchair.

Seat

The seat of a wheelchair can be either flexible (sling) or rigid. Most manual wheelchairs have sling seats because they are lighter and enable the wheelchair to be readily collapsed. However, sling seats often sag with time and, depending on the rigidity of the cushion, can create skin and postural problems. This problem can be overcome by placing a rigid but removable base on a sling seat. Alternatively, the tension of some sling seats can be adjusted, with similar mechanisms used to change the tension of sling backrests (see Figure 13.7).

Seat-to-floor height

The seat-to-floor height determines the overall height of the wheelchair (see Figure 13.4). The back of the seat is usually lower than the front of the seat; consequently, the seat-to-floor height at the rear of the wheelchair is usually less than the seat-to-floor height at the front of the wheelchair. Seat-to-floor height is varied primarily to

Figure 13.3 A rigid (a) and folding (b) framed wheelchair.

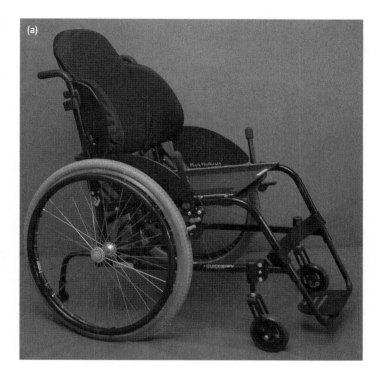

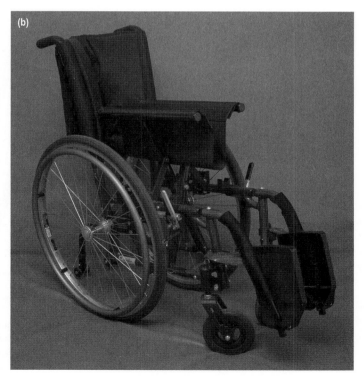

Figure 13.4 Key features of a wheelchair essential for ensuring appropriate fit.[2]

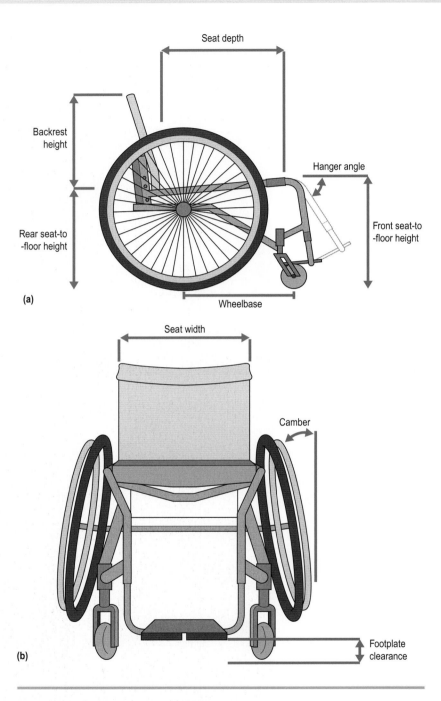

accommodate heel-to-knee length and to ensure adequate footplate clearance. Taller patients generally require higher seats. However, if the seat is *too high*, patients are unable to get their knees under tables. They may also have problems with head clearance when sitting in wheelchair-accessible vans. A high seat is also less stable than a low seat, increasing the risk of tipping. In contrast, if patients are short and the seat is *low*, they cannot comfortably rest and use their arms on the top of a table. A seat which is inappropriately low for a patient raises the knees, concentrating pressure under the pelvis. Patients propelling wheelchairs with their feet require a low seat to enable the feet to touch the ground.

The seat-to-floor distance can be changed by moving the back wheels on the wheelchair frame. To increase the seat-to-floor distance the back wheels are positioned low on the frame (see Figure 13.5a), and to decrease the seat-to-floor distance the back wheels are positioned high on the frame (see Figure 13.5b).

Different systems are used to change the vertical position of the back wheels on the frame. All systems rely on providing a range of strategically placed holes for the axle of the back wheels (see Figure 13.6a,b). However, changing the position of the back wheels changes other characteristics of the wheelchair, including the slope of its seat (i.e. rake) and slope of its backrest (i.e. recline; see Figure 13.5b). The rake of the seat and recline of the backrest can, however, be maintained when changing the position of the back wheels if the length of the front castors is appropriately adjusted. The position of the back wheels also affects the angle of the front castor forks. The front castor forks should always be vertical to ensure the castors sit squarely on the ground (see section on front castors).

The position of the back wheels on the frame of a wheelchair also determines the proportion of the wheels sitting above the seat. If the back wheels are placed high on

Figure 13.5 The back wheels can be placed low (a) or high (b) on the frame of the wheelchair. This changes the seat-to-floor distance, the rake of the seat and recline of the backrest. The vertical position of the back wheels determines how far above the seat the top of the wheels protrude. This has implications for transferring and for propulsion.

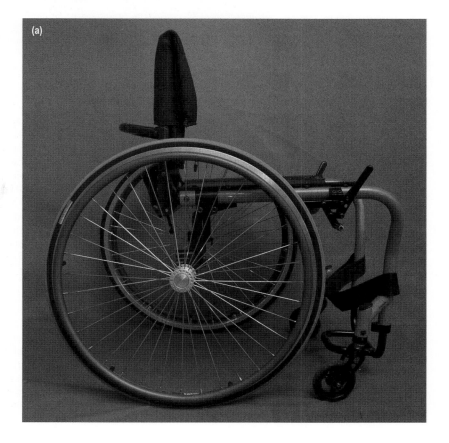

(a)

Figure 13.5   Continued

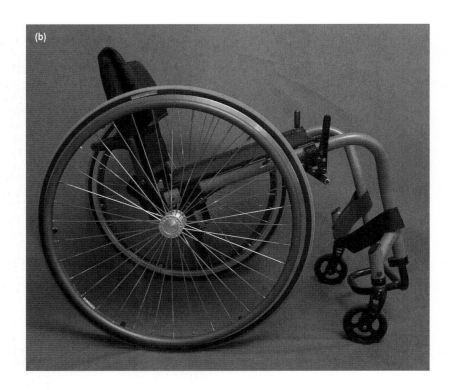

the frame, then a large proportion of each wheel sits above the seat (see Figure 13.5b). This has implications for wheelchair propulsion because it changes the distance between patients' shoulders and the top of the wheels; patients push with the shoulders more extended and the elbows more flexed. The position of the back wheels also has implications for transfers. If the wheels extend well above the seat, they can obstruct patients' attempts at moving sidewards. The opposite effect is achieved by placing the wheels low on the frame of a wheelchair. This reduces the amount of wheel sitting above the seat and increases the distance between the shoulders and wheels (see Figure 13.5a). Some of these effects of wheel position can by manipulated by changing the thickness of cushions and/or size of the back wheels. For example, a particularly tall patient can be sat on a thick cushion and be provided with extra large wheels.

Seat depth

The depth of the seat is determined by the length of the thighs (see Figure 13.4). At least 3 or 4 cm should be allowed between the end of the seat and back of the knees. If the seat is *too deep* for a patient, the front edge pushes up hard against the back of the knees. This can cause compression of the blood vessels and nerves in the popliteal fossa and encourage patients to slide forwards on the seat. If the depth of the seat is *too shallow*, there will be a large space between the front edge of the seat and the back

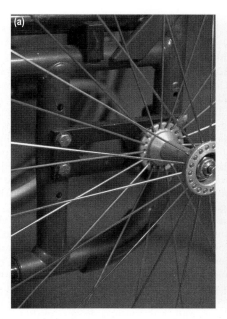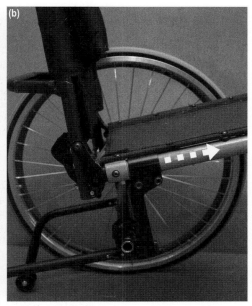

Figure 13.6   There are different systems for adjusting the position of the back wheels on the frame of a wheelchair. The wheels attach to plates (a) or brackets (b), which can be moved on the frame of the wheelchair.

of the knees. This is undesirable because it reduces the area under the thighs available for pressure distribution and encourages unwanted movement of the legs.

Seat width

The width of the seat is determined by the width of the hips (see Figure 13.4). Not surprisingly, larger patients require wider seats. If the seat is particularly wide, access through doorways and within tight spaces can be difficult. Excessive width also places the wheels further apart, necessitating more shoulder abduction when propelling the wheelchair. However, if the seat is *too narrow* for a patient, it makes it difficult for patients to get in and out of the wheelchair. In addition, the lateral aspects of the hips can rub the inside of the back wheels, causing damage to skin or clothing.

If possible, a few extra centimetres should be provided each side of the hips. This enables patients to easily position their hands onto the lateral edges of the cushion when lifting their body weight. It also protects clothing from dirt thrown up from the back wheels. Side guards attached to the outside of the seat can be used to help protect clothing, although they can be inconvenient to remove when transferring or folding the wheelchair (see Figure 13.9).

It is not advisable to prescribe a tight-fitting wheelchair if a patient's weight is fluctuating. Weight changes are particularly common in previously large patients who lose a lot of weight in the period immediately after injury. These patients often return to their original weight over time. Patients with high levels of tetraplegia also commonly gain weight. It is advisable either to prescribe a slightly wider wheelchair to accommodate potential weight gain or alternatively delay wheelchair prescription until weight has stabilized.

Seat rake

Wheelchairs typically have an inclined seat with the back of the seat sloping downwards (see Figure 13.5b). This is called 'rake' and is determined by the difference between the distance to the ground at the front and rear of the seat (see Figure 13.4).

Rake is important for posture and balance. If the seat is horizontal (see Figure 13.5a), the pelvis tends to slide forwards creating shearing forces under the ischial tuberosities as the patient slides. It also leads to a slumped sitting position with posterior pelvic rotation which can increase pressure on the sacrum. The slumped position can also cause skin problems over the ischial tuberosities, especially if patients are sitting on cushions with wells (see Figure 13.2). The rotated position of the pelvis can press the ischial tuberosities hard against the front lip of the cushion well. Patients tend to slide on horizontal seats because there is less tissue under the distal thighs than under the buttocks and consequently the thighs do not sit vertically. This tilts the pelvis posteriorly, encouraging forward slide.

Rake not only has implications for the tendency to slide but also for the rolling resistance and 'tippiness' of a wheelchair. If the rake is increased, weight is moved posteriorly off the front castors and over the back wheels. This makes it easier to get into a wheelstand position and easier to propel the wheelchair. While this may be advantageous for some, patients with limited function cannot control a 'tippy' wheelchair and may topple over backwards, especially when pushing up slopes. Therefore, the amount of rake is dictated by patients' wheelchair skills and, in particular, their ability to control a wheelstand and lean forwards when pushing up slopes. Excessive rake also makes it difficult to move forwards in the wheelchair when transferring. This is a consideration for those struggling with transfers. Some of the beneficial effects of rake can be mimicked by placing a foam wedge under the front lip of the cushion or by using an appropriately contoured cushion.

Backrest

Most wheelchairs are supplied with a soft fabric backrest. The tautness and shape of the backrest influences seating posture. The tension in some backrests can be adjusted with velcro straps (see Figure 13.7). Decreasing the tautness of the backrest enables it to wrap laterally around the patient's trunk, providing some trunk stability. Selective adjustment of tension up and down the backrest can also help control pelvic and lumbar position.

There are commercially available backrests which can be used instead of the backrests supplied with most wheelchairs (see Figure 13.8). These provide greater adjustability and are particularly useful for patients with complex seating needs. For example, some backrests wrap well around the trunk, helping to hold patients upright. Others can be angled or contoured to accommodate kyphotic or lordotic areas of the spine. These types of backrests do, however, add complexity when folding or collapsing a wheelchair, as well as extra weight and cost.

Backrest width

Most wheelchairs are supplied with backrests matching the width of the seat. This is not always appropriate. For example, patients with particularly broad shoulders but small hips require a narrow seat but a wide backrest. If provided with a backrest which matches the narrow hips, it will be too small, causing pressure and skin problems. In contrast, some patients, particularly women, have wide hips but narrow shoulders. A backrest the same width as the seat for these patients will be excessively

Figure 13.7 The tautness of some fabric backrests can be adjusted with velcro straps. A similar system can be used to adjust the tautness of sling seats.

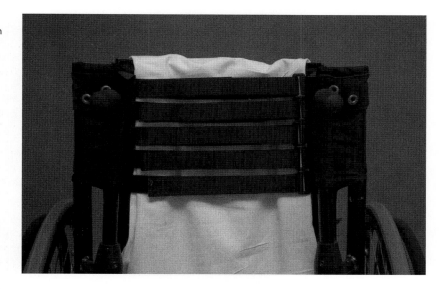

Figure 13.8 A commercially available backrest can be fitted to a wheelchair to provide lateral trunk support. The backrest is high and appropriate for most patients with tetraplegia.

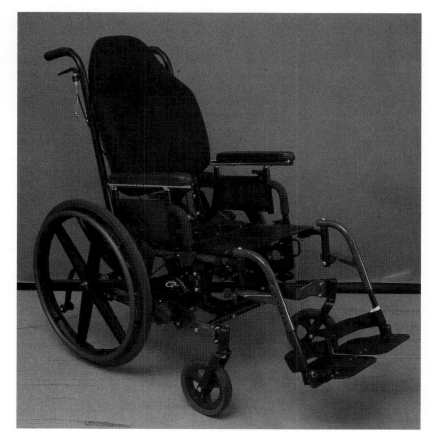

Figure 13.9 A wheelchair appropriate for a patient with thoracic paraplegia. The backrest is low and the wheels placed on the front of the frame. The wheelchair is also fitted with side guards to protect clothing from dirt thrown up from the wheels.

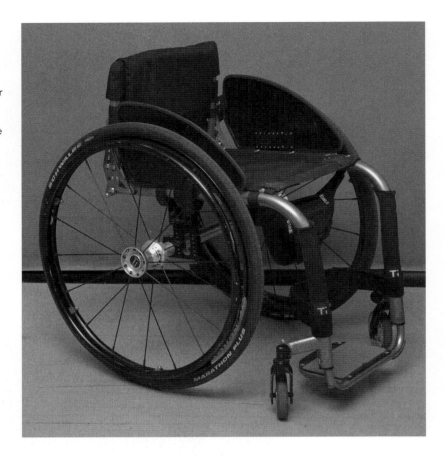

wide and fail to provide trunk support. If the backrest is too wide it also limits arm movement, making wheelchair propulsion difficult.

Backrest height

The optimal height of the backrest is not only determined by patients' height but also by the level of the spinal cord injury. Patients with tetraplegia require higher backrests than those with paraplegia (see Figures 13.8 and 13.9). High backrests are essential for ensuring patients do not fall backwards out of their wheelchairs. Falling backwards is most likely to happen when ascending steep slopes. As a general rule patients with trunk paralysis require a backrest which extends just above the inferior tip of the scapula. However, if the backrest is unnecessarily *high* it can interfere with propelling the wheelchair. High backrests prevent patients placing their hands at the back of the wheel when commencing each stroke. A high backrest can also impede the ability of patients with C6 tetraplegia to move forwards in their wheelchairs and hook their arms around the backrests for support (see Chapter 3, Table 3.8). It is advisable to experiment with backrests of different heights, observing effects on posture, function and stability. The thickness of the cushion also influences the effective height of a backrest.

Backrest inclination

Patients with extensive paralysis of the trunk *cannot* sit in a wheelchair with a vertical back, regardless of whether the seat is or is not horizontal. They do not have the ability to remain upright and therefore need the backrest to be reclined. However, a reclined backrest encourages forward sliding on the seat. This problem is overcome by introducing rake. That is, by dropping the back of the seat down and reducing the rear seat-to-floor height. The angle of the backrest can be measured with respect to the seat or with respect to the horizontal. The two measurements are only the same when the seat is horizontal. The disparity between these two measurements is often a source of confusion to the unwary.

A reclined backrest shifts pressure from under the ischial tuberosities to under the back. This can be advantageous provided the pressure is not excessive and provided the backrest is appropriate. However, it is not advisable to tilt the backrest too much because this encourages patients to flex the neck and upper trunk so as to see and use their hands in front of them.

Distance between the front castors and back wheels

The distance between the front castors and back wheels is called the 'wheelbase'. It determines a wheelchair's rolling resistance, turning circle and 'tippiness' (see Chapter 4). The distance can be adjusted by moving the back wheels forwards or backwards on the frame. These adjustments can be made using similar systems which enable the back wheels to be raised or lowered (see Figure 13.6).

By moving the back wheels forwards, the distance between the back wheels and front castors is reduced, providing a tighter turning circle (see Figure 13.9). This adjustment also moves weight from the front castors to the back wheels, decreasing overall rolling resistance and making it easier to push the wheelchair. However, it also increases the wheelchair's 'tippiness'. That is, the wheelchair will more readily rotate backwards into a wheelstand position (see Chapter 4). This may or may not be advantageous depending on whether patients can or cannot control 'tippiness'. More disabled patients generally cannot, and therefore require their back wheels positioned posteriorly for stability (see Figure 13.3). This increases the stability of the wheelchair but also increases the weight borne through the front castors, making propulsion more difficult. (Large castors provide a partial solution to this problem as discussed in the next section.)

Front castors

The front castors of wheelchairs are usually *solid* although some are *pneumatic*. They come in different sizes ranging from 5 to 19.8 cm (see Figures 13.3 and 13.9). The size of the castor has important implications for the manoeuvrability of the wheelchair and ease of pushing. Small castors have less contact area with the floor and therefore provide a tighter turning circle. However, small castors offer more resistance to rolling, increasing the effort associated with pushing a wheelchair. The effect of castor size on wheelchair propulsion is only important if large amounts of weight are borne through the front castors. If only small amounts of weight sit over the front castors, then the size will have minimal influence on the ease of propelling a wheelchair. However, if large amounts of weight are borne through the front castors then the size of the front castors will be an important consideration, particularly for very disabled patients with some but limited ability to propel a wheelchair. If using large castors it is important to ensure they do not rub the back of patients' heels when the castors rotate.

While most active patients opt for smaller castors because they provide improved manoeuvrability, there is a downside. Notably, small castors dig into soft ground and get caught in cracks. In addition, they transmit bumps up through the seat, providing a rougher ride. More skilled patients overcome most of these problems by performing small wheelstands to lift the front castors over uneven or bumpy ground. Alternatively, castors with suspension are used to provide some buffering, although the suspension increases weight.

The stem of the castor and its housing should be perpendicular to the floor (see Figure 13.10). If they are not, the castors will vibrate and wheelchair propulsion will be more difficult. Most changes to the set-up of a wheelchair tip the stem of the castor from its vertical position. This needs to be corrected.

Back wheels

The standard size of back wheels is 60 cm (or 24 in). There are two types of back wheels, *solid* or *pneumatic*. Solid wheels do not puncture and require very little

Figure 13.10   The stems of the castors (a) need to be perpendicular to the floor, otherwise they vibrate and the wheelchair is more difficult to push.

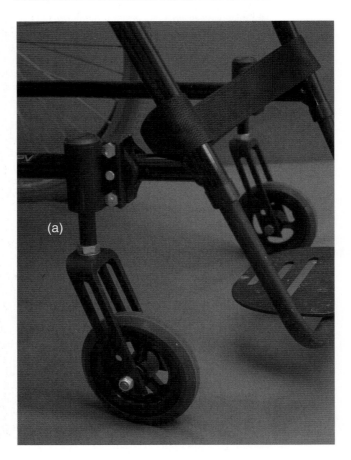

maintenance. However, they are heavy, bury into soft surfaces and transmit bumps up through the seat, providing a rougher ride. In contrast, pneumatic wheels are easier to push and manoeuvre and provide a smoother ride. However, they require higher maintenance and are vulnerable to puncture. They are not generally recommended if patients are unable to fix punctures and have limited carer support. Wheelchairs can be fitted with high tread tyres, particularly useful for patients living in rural areas.

There are different types of pushrims but the most common are *aluminium*, *plastic* or *rubber* coated (see Figures 13.11–13.13). More capable patients generally prefer aluminium pushrims because they do not burn their hands when controlling wheelchairs down steep slopes and they are more durable. However, more disabled patients without hand grasp usually opt for plastic- or rubber-coated pushrims. When used in conjunction with textured gloves, patients can better control the wheels (see Figure 13.11). Knobs (also called capstans) are sometimes placed on pushrims so patients can wedge their hands behind them to rotate the wheels, negating the need to grasp

Figure 13.11 Textured gloves used in conjunction with a rubberized pushrim help patients with limited hand function push. The tyre is solid.

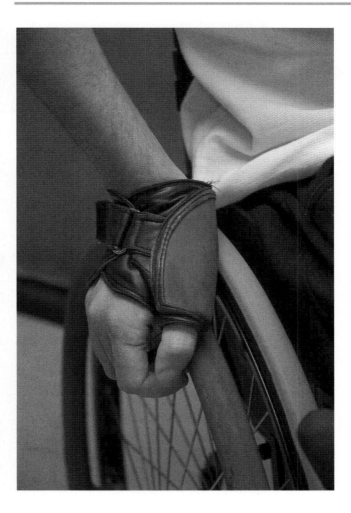

Figure 13.12 A plastic pushrim with knobs (also called capstans) appropriate for patients with C5 tetraplegia. Spoke guards are used to prevent the paralysed hand from injury. The tyre is solid.

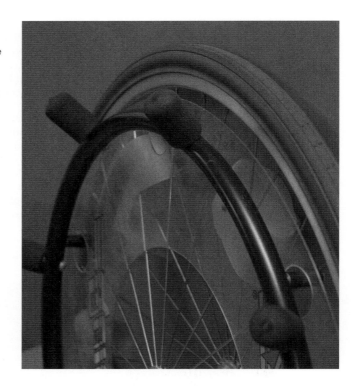

Figure 13.13 An aluminium pushrim. The tyre is solid.

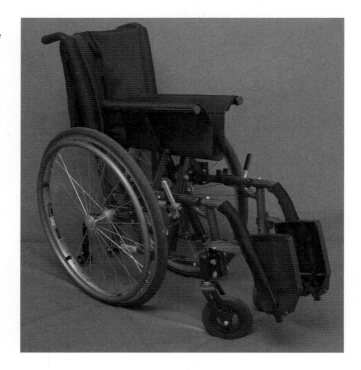

the rims (see Figure 13.12). Often patients with tetraplegia require *spoke guards*. These are plastic shields which sit over the outside of the spokes, preventing the paralysed fingers from injury (see Figure 13.12).

Wheels can be either fixed or removable. Clearly, those which can be quickly and easily removed are more convenient but they are also more expensive. There are special types of release mechanisms for patients with limited hand function.

Wheel camber

The back wheels of a wheelchair can be either vertical or cambered (see Figure 13.4). Cambered wheels are tilted with more distance between the bottoms of the two wheels than the top. The main advantages of cambered wheels are that they provide greater lateral stability and make it easier to turn. However, they also increase the width of wheelchairs, making them more difficult to manoeuvre in tight spaces and get through narrow doorways.

Brakes

Most patients require brakes to stabilize the wheelchair when transferring. However, more able patients often discard them because they get in the way of pushing. There are different types of brakes. The two most common varieties are *push/pull* and *scissor* brakes (see Figure 13.14a–c). The push/pull brakes are typically positioned within an easy arm reach, high on the frame of the wheelchair. Patients with limited arm function may, however, require extra extensions on the brakes to avoid the need to lean forwards when applying them (see Figure 13.14c). The extensions also increase the leverage arm, making the application of the brakes easier. More capable patients often prefer scissor-type brakes placed out of the way and low on the frame of wheelchairs. Brakes positioned low on the frame of wheelchairs are only appropriate if patients can reach down and independently apply them. The position of brakes needs to be adjusted every time the position of the back wheels is changed. If this is not done, the brakes will be ineffectual or impossible to apply.

Special types of brakes, called *grade-aids*, can be used to help more disabled patients push up slopes (see Figure 13.14c). When engaged, they only allow the back wheels to rotate in one direction, preventing wheelchairs rolling backwards while pushing up slopes.

Anti-tip bars

Anti-tip bars are supplied as options with most wheelchairs to help prevent them toppling over backwards (see Figure 13.15). They are small wheels located at the back of the wheelchair several centimetres above the ground. If the wheelchair tips backwards the small wheels hit the ground and prop the wheelchair up. Anti-tip bars cannot be solely relied upon to prevent wheelchairs toppling backwards. For example, they may be ineffectual when pushing up steep slopes. Occasionally severe and sudden spasticity in the hip extensor muscles tips the wheelchair backwards regardless of anti-tip bars.

Footplates and leg rests

Footplates can be either rigid, fold-up or swing-away (see Figure 13.3a,b). Some are detachable (see Figure 13.16) and others are not (see Figure 13.9). The type of

Figure 13.14 Push/pull (a and c) and scissor brakes (b). Grade-aids and brake extensions can be fitted to brakes for more disabled patients (a). The grade-aids prevent rolling backwards down a hill and the brake extensions make it easier to apply the brakes. Sometimes the brakes are fitted low on the frame of a wheelchair to prevent them interfering with propulsion (c).

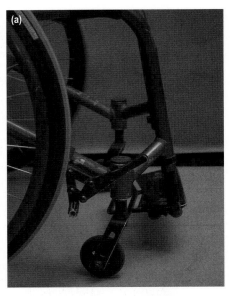

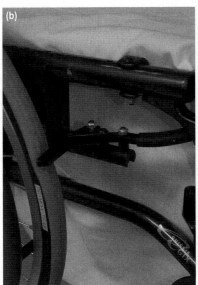

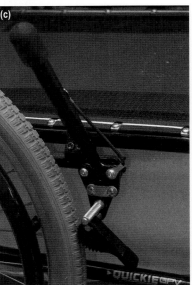

footplate is primarily determined by whether patients can or cannot stand up from the wheelchair. If patients can stand up, then they require footplates which can be lifted up or swung away. If patients cannot stand up then the choice is less important. Needless to say folding wheelchairs require folding or swing-away footplates. In addition to the footplates, there are different types of leg rests. Some can be elevated to manage postural hypotension and lower limb oedema, although these types of leg rests add weight and length to the wheelchair.

Figure 13.15 Anti-tip bars are attached to the back of wheelchairs to prevent them toppling over backwards.

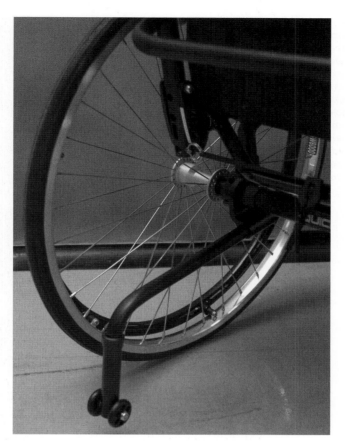

Leg rest length

The length of leg rests is determined by the length of the lower leg (i.e. distance between the knees and base of foot; see Figure 13.4). However, the length of the leg rest is also influenced by the thickness of the cushion. Patients sitting on thicker cushions require shorter leg rests than patients sitting on thinner cushions. The length needs to be appropriate to ensure a small amount of weight is borne through the feet. The feet should sit flat on the footplates with the ankles in a neutral position. This needs to be assessed when patients are wearing shoes sitting on their own cushions. In tall patients it is not always appropriate merely to adjust the length of the leg rests. This alone can cause the footplates to hit the ground. Instead, the frame of the wheelchair needs to be raised or the patient needs to sit on a thicker cushion (see section on Seat-to-floor height).

If the length of the leg rests is *too short* the feet will bear too much weight, lifting the knees and throwing excessive weight back onto the ischial tuberosities. In contrast, if the length of the leg rests is *too long*, the feet will be unsupported with no weight borne through them and the ankles will fall into plantarflexion. This is undesirable because it increases the tendency for ankle plantarflexion contractures and for the feet to come off the footplates.

Figure 13.16   A wheelchair appropriate for a patient with C4 tetraplegia. The backrest is high and moulded to provide trunk stability. The seat is tilted down at the back and the backrest is reclined. The whole frame of the wheelchair can also be tilted as one. In addition the wheelchair is fitted with arm- and headrests. The footplates and armrests are removable.

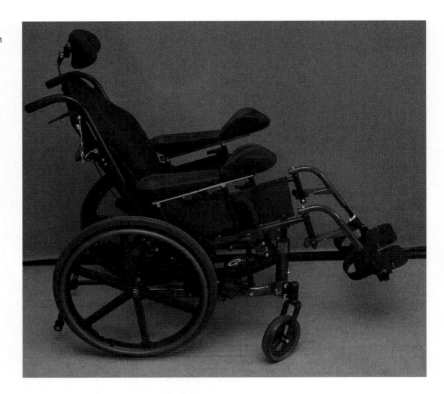

Footplate position

The *hanger angle* determines how far in front of the wheelchair the footplates sit, the overall length of a wheelchair and the angle of the knees (see Figure 13.4). There has been an increasing tendency to place the knees in more flexion with the legs tucked under the body. The main advantage of a tucked knee position is that it decreases the overall length of the wheelchair, improving its manoeuvrability. However, the tucked knee position exacerbates spasticity in some patients. Most taller patients also prefer more knee extension because it provides a way of attaining extra footplate clearance without raising the height of the seat.

Armrests

Manual wheelchairs can be supplied with armrests, although most active users find they interfere with mobility and do not have them. However, patients with high levels of tetraplegia require arm rests to support the upper limbs (see Figure 13.16). Armrests can consist of horizontal rubberized bars to support the elbows or can be extensive moulded forearm trays with inbuilt splinting for the hand. Some swing away, while others lift entirely off the wheelchair. Patients with reasonable or good arm movement may only require short armrests which primarily support the elbows. The main advantage of shorter armrests is they enable patients to position the wheelchair at a table front on. For patients with limited arm function but the potential to transfer, it is important to ensure that patients can remove the armrests independently. Special easy release options may be required.

The armrests should be positioned so the elbows are supported at 60° and shoulders are level. The position of armrests need to change if patients move onto thicker or thinner cushions. If the armrests are *too low*, the elbows fall into more extension and the shoulders drop. Alternatively, patients slide forwards on the seat to attain a more comfortable position for the arms. In contrast, if the armrests are *too high* the elbows will be excessively flexed and the shoulders elevated.

Headrest

Patients with high levels of tetraplegia require headrests especially if their wheelchairs tilt (see Figure 13.16). It is important that the headrest sits at the back of the head without thrusting the neck into flexion. Headrests are also highly recommended, and in some countries compulsory, when travelling in a wheelchair within a vehicle.

Power wheelchairs

Selecting an appropriate power wheelchair is equally, if not more, complex than selecting a manual wheelchair with just as many options and product choices. Power wheelchairs need to be fitted and appropriately set up for patients. However, most of the general principles applicable for manual wheelchair prescription, which have already been discussed, are the same for power wheelchairs. For example, considerations when determining seat and backrest width, footplate length, hanger angle, backrest height and seat depth are the same for all types of wheelchairs. In addition, tilting the backrest and seat of a power wheelchair has the same effect on seating posture and pressure management for a power wheelchair as for a manual wheelchair. Most power wheelchairs have large heavy motors positioned in front of the back wheels, which prevent the wheelchair from tipping backwards.

Some power wheelchairs are primarily designed for indoor use and are light and small, with little power and tight turning circles. They also have smaller wheels with less tread. Other power wheelchairs are designed for outdoor use and are bigger, heavier, more powerful and highly stable. They tend to have larger wheels at the back with more tread for friction. They also often incorporate more sophisticated seating systems. Power wheelchairs are either middle or rear wheel drive (see Figures 13.17 and 13.18). Mid-wheel drive wheelchairs provide good manoeuvrability and are most commonly prescribed for all-round use. Rear-wheel power wheelchairs are, however, easier to control in difficult terrains.

Like manual wheelchairs some power wheelchairs are highly adjustable with lots of moving parts and others are not. Power wheelchairs appropriate for people with high levels of tetraplegia generally have a backrest which can be tilted either manually or electronically. More sophisticated (and expensive) chairs also have 'tilt-in-space' features which rotate the whole wheelchair frame as one in space. This achieves a similar effect as dropping the seat and reclining the back together. This feature is commonly recommended as a way of relieving pressure from under the ischial tuberosities. Some wheelchairs also have leg rests which can be raised manually or electronically.

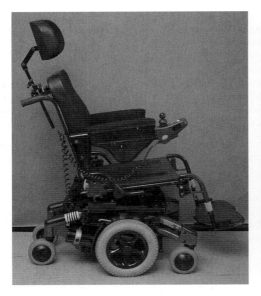

Figure 13.17　A mid-wheel drive power wheelchair.

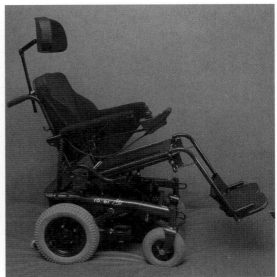

Figure 13.18　A rear-wheel drive power wheelchair.

Control mechanisms

There are different systems available which enable patients to drive power wheelchairs. Most incorporate a joystick which is controlled by either the hand or chin. There are three different electronic set-ups underpinning the way joysticks control the movement of the wheelchair. One type incorporates *microswitches* enabling patients to control the direction but not the speed of the wheelchair with movement of the joystick. Moving the joystick moves the wheelchair but the speed is fixed. Patients nominate between two or three different settings with pre-selected speeds. In contrast, the second type of joystick uses *proportional* control mechanisms where movement of the joystick controls both the direction and speed of movement. A larger movement of the joystick moves the wheelchair faster. A third type of control uses an 'on–off' mechanism. Once forward movement is precipitated, the wheelchair continues to move forwards until a stop switch is activated.

The electronic circuitry of a power wheelchair can be programmed to suit the needs of patients. Some of the features which can be changed include the rate of acceleration and deceleration, turning speed, sensitivity of the joystick to movement, and top speed. Most have two or three pre-set channels which patients select depending on whether they are in- or outside. Switches are required to turn the wheelchair on and off. More sophisticated wheelchairs also require switches to elevate the leg rests, tilt the wheelchair in space, recline the wheelchair and raise the wheelchair. Patients with limited or no hand function require large switches which can be activated with arm or head movement (see Figure 13.19). Often control mechanisms and joysticks need to be modified to enable very weak patients to control them (see Figure 13.20).

Figure 13.19 Large switches can be strategically placed on wheelchairs enabling patients to use gross movements, rather than fine hand movement, to turn switches on and off. In this example, the wheelchair is driven with a hand-control joystick but its different features are turned on and off using a large switch (A).

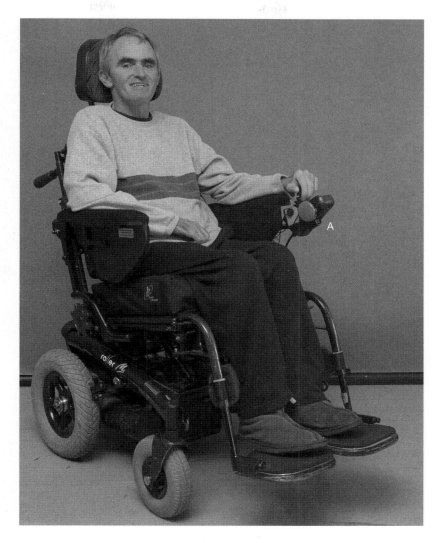

Sitting in vehicles

Sitting in vans, buses, trains or planes is problematic for patients with little trunk control. They can fall from a supported upright position with even small jolts, turns or stops. For this reason chest safety belts are essential. If patients remain in their wheelchairs while travelling, the wheelchair needs to be secured to the vehicle.[16]

Figure 13.20 A typical adaptation to an armrest and hand-control joystick to enable a patient with C4 tetraplegia and small amounts of elbow and shoulder movement to use a hand-control wheelchair. Patients with C4 tetraplegia more commonly use chin-control power wheelchairs.

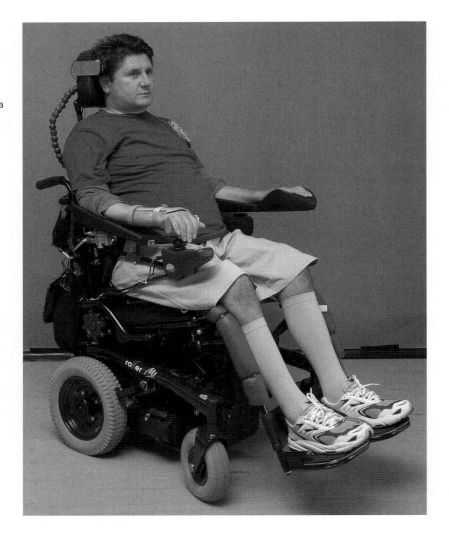

References

1. Zollars JA: Special Seating. An Illustrated Guide. Minneapolis, MN, Otto Bock Orthopedic Industry, 1997.
2. Ham R, Aldersea P, Porter D: Wheelchair Users and Postural Seating: A Clinical Approach. New York, Churchill Livingstone, 1998.
3. Engström B: Ergonomics, Seating and Positioning. Sweden, ETAC, 1993.
4. Conine TA, Hershler C, Daechsel D et al: Pressure ulcer prophylaxis in elderly patients using polyurethane foam or Jay wheelchair cushions. Int J Rehabil Res 1994; 17:123–137.
5. Cullum N, McInnes E, Bell-Syer SEM et al: Support surfaces for pressure ulcer prevention. The Cochrane Database of Systematic Reviews 2004: Issue 3.Art. No.: CD001735. DOI: 10.1002/14651858.CD001735.pub2.
6. Brienza DM, Karg PE, Geyer MJ et al: The relationship between pressure ulcer incidence and buttock–seat cushion interface pressure in at-risk elderly wheelchair users. Arch Phys Med Rehabil 2001; 82:529–533.
7. Stinson MD, Porter-Armstrong A, Eakin P: Seat-interface pressure: a pilot study of the relationship to gender, body mass index, and seating position. Arch Phys Med Rehabil 2003; 84:405–409.

8. Ragan R, Kernozek TW, Bidar M et al: Seat-interface pressures on various thicknesses of foam wheelchair cushions: a finite modeling approach. Arch Phys Med Rehabil 2002; 83:872–875.
9. Geyer MJ, Brienza DM, Karg P et al: A randomized control trial to evaluate pressure-reducing seat cushions for elderly wheelchair users. Adv Skin Wound Care 2001; 14:120–132.
10. Miller GE, Seale JL: The mechanics of terminal lymph flow. J Biomech Eng 1985; 107:376–380.
11. Bolin I, Bodin P, Kreuter M: Sitting position — posture and performance in C5–C6 tetraplegia. Spinal Cord 2000; 38:425–434.
12. Lim R, Sirett R, Conine T et al: Clinical trial of foam cushions in the prevention of decubitis ulcers in elderly patients. J Rehabil Res Dev 1988; 25:19–26.
13. Mayall JK, Desharnais G: Positioning in a Wheelchair: A guide for Professional Caregivers of the Disabled Adult. Thorofare, NJ, SLACK Incorporated, 1995.
14. Cooper RA, Gonzalez J, Lawrence B et al: Performance of selected lightweight wheelchairs on ANSI/RESNA tests. Arch Phys Med Rehabil 1997; 78:1138–1144.
15. Somers MF: Spinal Cord Injury: Functional Rehabilitation, 2nd edn. Upper Saddle River, NJ, Prentice Hall, 2001.
16. Axelson P, Minkel J, Perr A et al: The Powered Wheelchair Training Guide. Minden, NV, PAX Press, 2002.

The way forward

CHAPTER 14
Evidence-based
physiotherapy

275

Evidence-based physiotherapy

The movement towards evidence-based practice has changed physiotherapy. It is no longer acceptable to unquestioningly adopt the beliefs about physiotherapy management of people with spinal cord injury which have been passed down through the years. Instead, we are encouraged to challenge long-held beliefs and to critically appraise the evidence underpinning them.

The desire to base practice on high quality clinical research is both promising and problematic. On the one hand, evidence-based practice has the potential to improve patient outcomes. It also increases job satisfaction for clinicians knowing that what they do each day is clearly effective. On the other hand, research evidence is always limited, both in quantity and quality. This means that we are often faced with clinical scenarios for which there is little or no evidence to guide practice. Transparency about the state of current evidence leads to ambiguity and complexity which is particularly confusing for junior physiotherapists. Junior physiotherapists faced with the day-to-day management of people with spinal cord injury want clear guidance of what to do when. It is difficult to provide this type of guidance in the presence of real uncertainty.

Ideally, most decisions about management would be based on evidence-based clinical practice guidelines. Evidence-based clinical practice guidelines are recommendations for practice based on a transparent assessment of the available evidence including, where possible, randomized controlled trials and systematic reviews (see Table 14.1).[1–3]

Recommendations for clinical practice should take into account patients' priorities and perspectives. Most importantly, there needs to be careful consideration of whether the effects of interventions justify the time, cost and inconvenience associated with providing them. Interventions which are expensive, inconvenient, uncomfortable and time-consuming should only be considered if they make a substantial and clear difference to patients' lives. A balance needs to be achieved between encouraging patients to devote time, money and effort to therapeutic interventions which may have small benefits, and encouraging patients to spend their time participating in the broader aspects of life (e.g. returning to work, participating in family life, and engaging in social, sporting and community activities).

TABLE 14.1 Recommendations within clinical guidelines are rated from A to D according to the level of evidence supporting them

A	consistent level 1 studies
B	consistent level 2 or 3 studies *or* extrapolations from level 1 studies
C	level 4 studies *or* extrapolations from level 2 or 3 studies
D	level 5 evidence *or* troublingly inconsistent or inconclusive studies of any level

where:

Level 1 studies	systematic review (with homogeneity) of randomized controlled trials, or individual randomized controlled trial (with narrow confidence interval)
Level 2 studies	systematic review (with homogeneity) of cohort studies, or individual cohort study (including low quality randomized controlled trial; e.g. <80% follow-up), or 'outcomes' research
Level 3 studies	systematic review (with homogeneity) of case-control studies, or individual case-control study
Level 4 studies	case-series (and poor quality cohort and case-control studies)
Level 5 studies	expert opinion without explicit critical appraisal, or based on physiology, bench research or first principles

After www.cebm.net[109] with permission of the Oxford Centre for Evidence-Based Medicine.

A search of the Cochrane[4] and physiotherapy-specific[5] databases in 2006 retrieved 36 randomized controlled trials,[6–41] three systematic reviews[42–44] and four sets of clinical guidelines[45–48] directly relevant to physiotherapy management of people with spinal cord injury (there are additional trials,[41,49–68] systematic reviews[69–77] and clinical guidelines[78–81] but they are not directly relevant to physiotherapy). Unfortunately, most trials involving patients with spinal cord injury are inconclusive (i.e. statistically underpowered) so few provide high quality evidence about the efficacy of physiotherapy practice. This problem is reflected in clinical guidelines. The few physiotherapy-specific recommendations contained within existing guidelines are generally based on low quality evidence.

Evidence-based practice is not only about treatment effectiveness. The goal-setting process also requires high quality physiotherapy-specific research. Ideally, physiotherapy goals would be based on algorithms which predict the probability of patients with different neurological presentations and attributes mastering different motor tasks, given individual environmental and personal circumstances. Such algorithms can be derived from cohort studies which follow representative samples of patients over time.[46,82–88] The most notable cohort studies use data collected for a large USA-based registry of spinal cord injuries [the American Uniform Data System for Medical Rehabilitation (UDSMR)].[89,90] While the results of these, and similar studies, are helpful for physiotherapists trying to set realistic and attainable goals for patients, most studies rely on global measures of activity limitations[86,91–96] captured in assessments such as the Functional Independence Measure®.[87,88,97,98] These measures primarily reflect the ability to perform a few key motor tasks, but do not provide sufficient or detailed information across the wide range of motor tasks which physiotherapists are responsible for addressing, and which people with spinal cord injury need to master. The widespread use of the Functional Independence Measure® to reflect the mobility of wheelchair-dependent patients is particularly problematic. It has poor sensitivity in this domain and fails to distinguish between those with different levels of wheelchair mobility.[87,99]

No doubt physiotherapy-related research will continue to grow. The increasing number of clinical trials and systematic reviews in the area of spinal cord injuries will make possible the compilation of evidence-based clinical guidelines in the future. Perhaps emerging trials will challenge some aspects of current clinical practice, as is currently happening with contracture management (see Chapter 9). However, there are and always will be difficulties completing randomized controlled trials involving people with spinal cord injury. The most obvious difficulty is the small number of potential participants.[100–103] Less obvious difficulties are the lack of research-trained physiotherapists working in the area of spinal cord injuries and the difficulties attracting financial support to investigate the effectiveness of interventions which have long since become standard practice. Clinical decisions will therefore continue to be made on the basis of lower quality evidence than perhaps hoped for. Sometimes, results of research involving other patient groups will provide the best available estimate of treatment effects. For example, randomized controlled trials indicating the effectiveness of strength training in patients with peripheral neuropathies, multiple sclerosis, stroke or traumatic brain injury may provide the best evidence about the effectiveness of strength training in patients with partial paralysis following spinal cord injury (see Chapter 8).

The challenge for the physiotherapy profession is to critically reflect on what it does and work towards providing high quality evidence to support current practice as well as new and emerging therapies. When new evidence does emerge, the challenge is to respond to the results of clinical trials in a sensible and informed way and to change practice where appropriate.[104]

References

1. Grimmer KA, Bialocerkowski AE, Kumar S et al: Implementing evidence in clinical practice: the 'therapies' dilemma. Physiotherapy 2004; 90:189–194.
2. Handoll HG, Howe TE, Madhok R: The Cochrane Database of Systematic Reviews. Physiotherapy 2002; 88:714–716.
3. Wakefield A: Evidence-based physiotherapy: the case for pragmatic randomised controlled trials. Physiotherapy 2000; 86:394–396.
4. The Cochrane Library, Issue 4. Chichester, Wiley, 2006.
5. Herbert R, Moseley A, Sherrington C: PEDro: a database of randomised controlled trials in physiotherapy. Health Inf Manag 1998; 28:186–188.
6. Beekhuizen KS, Field-Fote EC: Massed practice versus massed practice with stimulation: effects on upper extremity function and cortical plasticity in individuals with incomplete cervical spinal cord injury. Neurorehabil Neural Repair 2005; 19:33–47.
7. Ben M, Harvey L, Denis S et al: Does 12 weeks of regular standing prevent loss of ankle mobility and bone mineral density in people with recent spinal cord injuries? Aust J Physiother 2005; 51:251–256.
8. Cheng PT, Chen CL, Wang CM et al: Effect of neuromuscular electrical stimulation on cough capacity and pulmonary function in patients with acute cervical cord injury. J Rehabil Med 2006; 38:32–36.
9. Crowe J, MacKay-Lyons M, Morris H: A multi-centre, randomized controlled trial of the effectiveness of positioning on quadriplegic shoulder pain. Physiother Can 2000; 52:266–273.
10. Curtis KA, Tyner TM, Zachary L et al: Effect of a standard exercise protocol on shoulder pain in long-term wheelchair users. Spinal Cord 1999; 37:421–429.
11. Diego MA, Field T, Hernandez-Reif M et al: Spinal cord patients benefit from massage therapy. Int J Neurosci 2002; 112:133–142.
12. Davis G, Plyley MJ, Shephard RJ: Gains of cardiorespiratory fitness with arm-crank training in spinally disabled men. Can J Sport Sci 1991; 16:64–72.
13. de Groot PC, Hjeltnes N, Heijboer AC et al: Effect of training intensity on physical capacity, lipid profile and insulin sensitivity in early rehabilitation of spinal cord injured individuals. Spinal Cord 2003; 41:673–679.
14. Derrickson J, Clesia N, Simpson N et al: A comparison of two breathing exercise programs for patients with quadriplegia. Phys Ther 1992; 72:763–769.
15. DiPasquale-Lehnerz P: Orthotic intervention for development of hand function with C-6 quadriplegia. Am J Occup Ther 1994; 48:138–144.
16. Dobkin B, Apple D, Barbeau H et al: Weight-supported treadmill vs over-ground training for walking after acute incomplete SCI. Neurology 2006; 66:484–493.

17. Field-Fote EC, Lindley SD, Sherman AL: Locomotor training approaches for individuals with spinal cord injury: a preliminary report of walking-related outcomes. J Neurol Phys Ther 2005; 29:127–137.

18. Gounden P: Progressive resistive loading on accessory expiratory muscles in tetraplegia. Sth Afr J Physiother 1990; 46:4–12.

19. Harvey L, Simpson D, Pironello D et al: Does three months of nightly splinting reduce the extensibility of the flexor pollicis longus muscle in people with tetraplegia? Physiother Res Int 2007; 12:5–13.

20. Harvey LA, Batty J, Crosbie J et al: A randomized trial assessing the effects of 4 weeks of daily stretching on ankle mobility in patients with spinal cord injuries. Arch Phys Med Rehabil 2000; 81:1340–1347.

21. Harvey LA, Byak AJ, Ostrovskaya M et al: Randomised trial of the effects of four weeks of daily stretch on extensibility of hamstring muscles in people with spinal cord injuries. Aust J Physiother 2003; 49:176–181.

22. Harvey LA, de Jong I, Geohl G et al: Twelve weeks of nightly stretch does not reduce thumb web-space contractures in people with a neurological condition: a randomised controlled trial. Aust J Physiother 2006; 52:251–258.

23. Harvey LA, Smith MB, Davis GM et al: Functional outcomes attained by T9–12 paraplegic patients with the walkabout and the isocentric reciprocal gait orthoses. Arch Phys Med Rehabil 1997; 78:706–711.

24. Hicks AL, Martin KA, Ditor DS et al: Long-term exercise training in persons with spinal cord injury: effects on strength, arm ergometry performance and psychological well-being. Spinal Cord 2003; 41:34–43.

25. Klose KJ, Needham BM, Schmidt D et al: An assessment of the contribution of electromyographic biofeedback as an adjunct therapy in the physical training of spinal cord injured persons. Arch Phys Med Rehabil 1993; 74:453–456.

26. Klose KJ, Schmidt DL, Needham BM et al: Rehabilitation therapy for patients with long-term spinal cord injuries. Arch Phys Med Rehabil 1990; 71:659–662.

27. Kohlmeyer KM, Hill JP, Yarkony GM et al: Electrical stimulation and biofeedback effect on recovery of tenodesis grasp: a controlled study. Arch Phys Med Rehabil 1996; 77:701–706.

28. Latimer AE, Ginis K, Hicks AL: Buffering the effects of stress on well-being among individuals with spinal cord injury: a potential role for exercise. Ther Recreation J 2005; 39:131–138.

29. Liaw MY, Lin MC, Cheng PT et al: Resistive inspiratory muscle training: its effectiveness in patients with acute complete cervical cord injury. Arch Phys Med Rehabil 2000; 81:752–756.

30. Lopes P, Figoni SF, Perkash I: Upper limb exercise effect on tilt tolerance during orthostatic training of patients with spinal cord injury. Arch Phys Med Rehabil 1984; 65:251–253.

31. Loveridge B, Badour M, Dubo H: Ventilatory muscle endurance training in quadriplegia: effects on breathing pattern. Paraplegia 1989; 27:329–339.

32. MacPhee AH, Kirby RL, Coolen AL et al: Wheelchair skills training program: a randomized clinical trial of wheelchair users undergoing initial rehabilitation. Arch Phys Med Rehabil 2004; 85:41–50.

33. Martin Ginis KA, Latimer AE, McKechnie K et al: Using exercise to enhance subjective well-being among people with spinal cord injury: the mediating influences of stress and pain. Rehabil Psychol 2003; 48:157–164.

34. McLean KP, Skinner JS: Effect of body training position on outcomes of an aerobic training study on individuals with quadriplegia. Arch Phys Med Rehabil 1995; 76:139–150.

35. Nash MS, Jacobs PL, Woods JM et al: A comparison of 2 circuit exercise training techniques for eliciting matched metabolic responses in persons with paraplegia. Arch Phys Med Rehabil 2002; 83:201–209.

36. Needham-Shropshire BM, Broton JG, Cameron TL et al: Improved motor function in tetraplegics following neuromuscular stimulation-assisted arm ergometry. J Spinal Cord Med 1997; 20:49–55.

37. Popovic MR, Thrasher TA, Adams ME et al: Functional electrical therapy: retraining grasping in spinal cord injury. Spinal Cord 2006; 44:143–151.

38. Postans NJ, Hasler JP, Granat MH et al: Functional electrical stimulation to augment partial weight-bearing supported treadmill training for patients with acute incomplete spinal cord injury: A pilot study. Arch Phys Med Rehabil 2004; 85:604–610.

39. Zupan A, Savrin R, Erjavec T et al: Effects of respiratory muscle training and electrical stimulation of abdominal muscles on respiratory capabilities in tetraplegic patients. Spinal Cord 1997; 35:540–545.

40. Best KL, Kirby RL, Smith C et al: Wheelchair skills training for community-based manual wheelchair users: a randomized controlled trial. Arch Phys Med Rehabil 2005; 86:2316–2323.

41. Diego MA, Field T, Hernandez-Reif M et al: Spinal cord patients benefit from massage therapy. Int J Neurosci 2002; 112:133–142.

42. Sipski ML, Richards JS: Spinal cord injury rehabilitation: State of the science. Am J Phys Med Rehabil 2006; 85:310–342.

43. Brooks D, O'Brien K, Geddes EL et al: Is inspiratory muscle training effective for individuals with cervical spinal cord injury? A qualitative systematic review. Clin Rehabil 2005; 19:237–246.
44. Stiller K, Huff N: Respiratory muscle training for tetraplegic patients: a literature review. Aust J Physiother 1999; 45:291–299.
45. Eng JJ, Teasell RW, Miller WC et al: Spinal Cord Injury Rehabilitation Evidence. Vancouver, SCIRE, 2006.
46. Consortium for Spinal Cord Medicine: Outcomes following Traumatic Spinal Cord Injury: Clinical Practice Guidelines for Health Care Professionals. Washington, DC, Paralyzed Veterans of America, 1999.
47. Consortium for Spinal Cord Medicine: Preservation of Upper Limb Function Following Spinal Cord Injury: A Clinical Practice Guideline for Health Care Professionals. Washington, DC, Paralyzed Veterans of America, 2005.
48. Consortium for Spinal Cord Medicine: Respiratory Management Following Spinal Cord Injury: A Clinical Practice Guideline for Health Care Professionals. Washington, DC, Paralyzed Veterans of America, 2005.
49. Aydin G, Tomruk S, Keles I et al: Transcutaneous electrical nerve stimulation versus baclofen in spasticity: clinical and electrophysiologic comparison. Am J Phys Med Rehabil 2005; 84:584–592.
50. Baker LL, Rubayi S, Villar F et al: Effect of electrical stimulation waveform on healing of ulcers in human beings with spinal cord injury. Wound Repair Regen 1996; 4:21–28.
51. Baldi JC, Jackson RD, Moraille R et al: Muscle atrophy is prevented in patients with acute spinal cord injury using functional electrical stimulation. Spinal Cord 1998; 36:463–469.
52. Becker DM, Gonzalez M, Gentili A et al: Prevention of deep venous thrombosis in patients with acute spinal cord injuries: use of rotating treatment tables. Neurosurgery 1987; 20:675–677.
53. Bugaresti JM, Tator CH, Szalai JP: Effect of continuous versus intermittent turning on nursing and non-nursing care time for acute spinal cord injuries. Paraplegia 1991; 29:330–342.
54. Daniel A, Manigandan C: Efficacy of leisure intervention groups and their impact on quality of life among people with spinal cord injury. Int J Rehabil Res 2005; 28:43–48.
55. Dinsdale S, Thurber D, Hough E et al: Community based monitoring for spinal man. Can J Public Health 1981; 72:195–198.
56. Dyson-Hudson TA, Shiflett SC, Kirshblum SC et al: Acupuncture and Trager psychophysical integration in the treatment of wheelchair user's shoulder pain in individuals with spinal cord injury. Arch Phys Med Rehabil 2001; 82:1038–1046.
57. Erzurumlu A, Dursun H, Gunduz S et al: Spinal kord yarali hastalarda kronik agri tedavisa. Amitriptilin-karbamazepin kombinasyonu ve elektroakupunktur uygulamasinin etkinlikerinin karsilastirilmasi (The management of chronic pain in spinal cord injured patients. The comparison of effectiveness of amitriptyline and carbamazepine combination and electroacupuncture application) [Turkish]. Eur J Phys Med Rehabil 1996; 7:176–180.
58. Gass EM, Gass GC, Pitetti K: Thermoregulatory responses to exercise and warm water immersion in physically trained men with tetraplegia. Spinal Cord 2002; 40:474–480.
59. Liu XF, Liao ZA, Deng WH et al: Effects of drug injection at eight-liao point combined with bladder function training on bladder dysfunction due to spinal cord injury. Chin J Clin Rehabil 2005; 9:142–143.
60. Merli GJ, Herbison GJ, Ditunno JF et al: Deep vein thrombosis: prophylaxis in acute spinal cord injured patients. Arch Phys Med Rehabil 1988; 69:661–664.
61. Nussbaum EL, Biemann I, Mustard B: Comparison of ultrasound/ultraviolet-C and laser for treatment of pressure ulcers in patients with spinal cord injury. Phys Ther 1994; 74:812–825.
62. Salzberg CA, Cooper-Vastola SA, Perez F et al: The effects of non-thermal pulsed electromagnetic energy on wound healing of pressure ulcers in spinal cord-injured patients: a randomized, double-blind study. Ostomy Wound Manage 1995; 41:42–44, 46, 48 passim.
63. Taly AB, Sivaraman Nair KP, Murali T et al: Efficacy of multiwavelength light therapy in the treatment of pressure ulcers in subjects with disorders of the spinal cord: a randomized double-blind controlled trial. Arch Phys Med Rehabil 2004; 85:1657–1661.
64. Warden SJ, Bennell KL, Matthews B et al: Efficacy of low-intensity pulsed ultrasound in the prevention of osteoporosis following spinal cord injury. Bone 2001; 29:431–436.
65. Wong AM, Leong CP, Su TY et al: Clinical trial of acupuncture for patients with spinal cord injuries. Am J Phys Med Rehabil 2003; 82:21–27.
66. Davis GM, Shephard RJ, Leenen FH: Cardiac effects of short term arm crank training in paraplegics: echocardiographic evidence. Eur J Appl Physiol Occup Physiol 1987; 56:90–96.
67. Griffin JW, Tooms RE, Mendius RA et al: Efficacy of high voltage pulsed current for healing of pressure ulcers in patients with spinal cord injury. Phys Ther 1991; 71:433–442.
68. Webborn N, Price MJ, Castle PC et al: Effects of two cooling strategies on thermoregulatory responses of tetraplegic athletes during repeated intermittent exercise in the heat. J Appl Physiol 2005; 98:2101–2107.
69. Olyaee Manesh A, Flemming K, Cullum NA et al: Electromagnetic therapy for treating pressure ulcers. The Cochrane Database of Systematic Reviews 2006: Issue 2. Art. No.: CD002930. DOI: 10.1002/14651858.CD002930.pub3.

70. Ada L, Foongchomcheay A, Canning C: Supportive devices for preventing and treating subluxation of the shoulder after stroke. The Cochrane Database of Systematic Reviews 2005: Issue 1. Art. No.: CD003863. DOI: 10.1002/14651858.CD003863.pub2.

71. Cullum N, McInnes E, Bell-Syer SEM et al: Support surfaces for pressure ulcer prevention. The Cochrane Database of Systematic Reviews 2004: Issue 3. Art. No.: CD001735. DOI: 10.1002/14651858.CD001735.pub2.

72. Elkins MR, Jones A, van der Schans C: Positive expiratory pressure physiotherapy for airway clearance in people with cystic fibrosis. The Cochrane Database of Systematic Reviews 2006: Issue 2. Art. No.: CD003147. DOI: 10.1002/14651858.CD003147.pub3.

73. Latham N, Anderson C, Bennett D et al: Progressive resistance strength training for physical disability in older people. The Cochrane Database of Systematic Reviews 2003: Issue 2. Art. No.: CD002759. DOI: 10.1002/14651858.CD002759.

74. Moseley AM, Stark A, Cameron ID et al: Treadmill training and body weight support for walking after stroke. The Cochrane Database of Systematic Reviews 2005: Issue 4. Art. No.: CD002840. DOI: 10.1002/14651858. CD002840.pub2.

75. Jones AP, Rowe BH: Bronchopulmonary hygiene physical therapy for chronic obstructive pulmonary disease and bronchiectasis. The Cochrane Database of Systematic Reviews 1998: Issue 4. Art. No.: CD000045. DOI: 10.1002/14651858.CD000045.

76. Saunders DH, Greig CA, Young A et al: Physical fitness training for stroke patients. The Cochrane Database of Systematic Reviews 2004: Issue 1. Art. No.: CD003316. DOI: 10.1002/14651858.CD003316.pub2.

77. White CM, Pritchard J, Turner-Stokes L: Exercise for people with peripheral neuropathy. The Cochrane Database of Systematic Reviews 2004: Issue 4. Art. No.: CD003904. DOI: 10.1002/14651858.CD003904.pub2.

78. Consortium for Spinal Cord Medicine: Acute Management of Autonomic Dysreflexia: Individuals with Spinal Cord Injury Presenting to Health-care Facilities. Washington, DC, Paralyzed Veterans of America, 2001.

79. Consortium for Spinal Cord Medicine: Prevention of Thromboembolism in Spinal Cord Injury. Washington, DC, Paralyzed Veterans of America, 1999.

80. Consortium for Spinal Cord Medicine: Depression Following Spinal Cord Injury: A Clinical Practice Guideline for Primary Care Physicians. Washington, DC, Paralyzed Veterans of America, 1998.

81. McCool FD, Rosen MJ: Nonpharmacologic airway clearance therapies: ACCP evidence-based clinical practice guidelines. Chest 2006; 129:S250–S259.

82. Daverat P, Sibrac MC, Dartigues JF et al: Early prognostic factors for walking in spinal cord injuries. Paraplegia 1988; 26:255–261.

83. Schonherr MC, Groothoff JW, Mulder GA et al: Prediction of functional outcome after spinal cord injury: a task for the rehabilitation team and the patient. Spinal Cord 2000; 38:185–191.

84. Dahlberg A, Kotila M, Kautiainen H et al: Functional independence in persons with spinal cord injury in Helsinki. J Rehabil Med 2003; 35:217–220.

85. Welch RD, Lohley SJ, O'Sullivan SB et al: Functional independence in quadriplegia: critical levels. Arch Phys Med Rehabil 1986; 67:235–240.

86. Yarkony GM, Roth EJ, Heinemann AW et al: Rehabilitation outcomes in C6 tetraplegia. Paraplegia 1988; 26:177–185.

87. Middleton JW, Truman G, Geraghty TJ: Neurological level effect on the discharge functional status of spinal cord injured persons after rehabilitation. Arch Phys Med Rehabil 1998; 79:1428–1432.

88. Beninato M, O'Kane KS, Sullivan PE: Relationship between motor FIM and muscle strength in lower cervical-level spinal cord injuries. Spinal Cord 2004; 42:533–540.

89. Marino RJ, Ditunno JF, Donovan WH et al: Neurological recovery after traumatic spinal cord injury: data from the Model Spinal Cord Injury Systems. Arch Phys Med Rehabil 1999; 80: 1391–1396.

90. Putzke JD, Richards JS, Hicken BL et al: Interference due to pain following spinal cord injury: important predictors and impact on quality of life. Pain 2002; 100:231–242.

91. Catz A, Itzkovich M, Agranov E et al: SCIM — spinal cord independence measure: a new disability scale for patients with spinal cord lesions. Spinal Cord 1997; 35:850–856.

92. Catz A, Itzkovich M, Agranov E et al: The spinal cord independence measure (SCIM): sensitivity to functional changes in subgroups of spinal cord lesion patients. Spinal Cord 2001; 39:97–100.

93. Yarkony GM, Roth EJ, Heinemann AW et al: Spinal cord injury rehabilitation outcome: the impact of age. J Clin Epidemiol 1988; 41:173–177.

94. Yarkony GM, Roth EJ, Heinemann AW et al: Benefits of rehabilitation for traumatic spinal cord injury: Multivariate analysis in 711 patients. Arch Neurol 1987; 44:93–96.

95. Marino RJ, Rider-Foster D, Maissel G et al: Superiority of motor level over single neurological level in categorizing tetraplegia. Paraplegia 1995; 33:510–513.

96. Marino RJ, Goin JE: Development of a short-form Quadriplegia Index of Function Scale. Spinal Cord 1999; 37:289–296.

97. Stineman MG, Marino RJ, Deutsch A et al: A functional strategy for classifying patients after traumatic spinal cord injury. Spinal Cord 1999; 37:717–725.

98. Ota T, Akaboshi K, Nagata M et al: Functional assessment of patients with spinal cord injury: measured by the motor score and the Functional Independence Measure. Spinal Cord 1996; 34:531–535.

99. Middleton JW, Harvey LA, Batty J et al: Five additional mobility and locomotor items to improve responsiveness of the FIM in wheelchair-dependent individuals with spinal cord injury. Spinal Cord 2006; 44:495–504.

100. Samsa GP, Govert J, Matchar DB et al: Use of data from nonrandomized trial designs in evidence reports: An application to treatment of pulmonary disease following spinal cord injury. J Rehabil Res Dev 2002; 39:41–52.

101. Martin Ginis KA, Hicks AL: Exercise research issues in the spinal cord injured population. Exerc Sport Sci Rev 2005; 33:49–53.

102. Jackson AB: Methodological issues in performance of SCI clinical trials. Top Spinal Cord Inj Rehabil 2006; 11:1–11.

103. Cardenas DD, Yilmaz B: Recruitment of spinal cord injury patients to clinical trials: challenges and solutions. Top Spinal Cord Inj Rehabil 2006; 11:12–23.

104. Maher CG, Sherrington C, Elkins M et al: Challenges for evidence-based physical therapy: accessing and interpreting high-quality evidence on therapy. Phys Ther 2004; 84:644–654.

105. Oxford Centre for Evidence-Based Medicine: Levels of evidence and grades of recommendation. http://www.cebm.net/levels_of_evidence.asp; 2001.

Appendix

TABLE A1 Innervation of upper limb muscles

Joint	Movement	Muscle	C3	C4	C5	C6	C7	C8	T1
Scapula	Elevation	Upper trapezius	■	■					
		Levator scapulae	■	■	■				
	Depression	Lower trapezius	■	■					
	Retraction	Middle trapezius	■	■					
		Rhomboids		■	■				
Shoulder	Protraction	Serratus anterior			■	■	■		
	Flexion	Anterior deltoid			■	■			
		Pectoralis major (clavicular head)			■	■			
		Pectoralis major (sternocostal head)					■	■	■
		Coracobrachialis				■	■		
	Extension	Posterior deltoid			■	■			
		Infraspinatus			■	■			
		Teres minor			■	■			
		Teres major			■	■	■		
		Latissimus dorsi				■	■	■	
	Abduction	Middle deltoid			■	■			
		Supraspinatus			■	■			
	Adduction	Pectoralis major (sternocostal head)				■	■	■	■
		Latissimus dorsi				■	■	■	
		Coracobrachialis			■	■	■		

(continued)

TABLE A1 *(continued)*

Joint	Movement	Muscle	C3	C4	C5	C6	C7	C8	T1
	Horizontal abduction	Posterior deltoid			■	■			
	Horizontal adduction	Pectoralis major (clavicular head)			■	■			
		Pectoralis minor					■	■	■
		Anterior deltoid			■	■			
	Medial rotation	Subscapularis			■	■			
		Teres major			■	■	■		
		Latissimus dorsi				■	■	■	
		Anterior deltoid			■	■			
	Lateral rotation	Infraspinatus			■	■			
		Teres minor			■	■			
		Posterior deltoid			■	■			
Elbow	Flexion	Biceps brachii			■	■			
		Brachialis			■	■			
		Brachioradialis			■	■	■		
	Extension	Triceps					■	■	
	Supination	Biceps brachii			■	■			
		Supinator				■	■		
	Pronation	Pronator quadratus						■	■
		Pronator teres				■	■		
Wrist	Flexion	Flexor carpi radialis				■	■		
		Palmaris longus					■	■	■
		Flexor carpi ulnaris					■	■	■
	Extension	Extensor carpi radialis longus			■	■			
		Extensor carpi radialis brevis					■	■	
		Extensor carpi ulnaris					■	■	
	Radial deviation	Extensor carpi radialis longus			■	■			
		Extensor carpi radialis brevis					■	■	
		Flexor carpi radialis				■	■		
	Ulnar deviation	Extensor carpi ulnaris					■	■	
		Flexor carpi ulnaris					■	■	■
Fingers	Flexion (MCP/PIP)	Flexor digitorum superficialis					■	■	■
	Flexion (DIP)	Flexor digitorum profundus					■	■	■
		Dorsal interossei						■	■
		Palmar interossei							■
	Flexion (MCP)	Flexor digiti minimi brevis						■	■
	Extension (MCP/ PIP/DIP)	Extensor digitorum					■	■	
		Extensor indicis					■	■	
		Extensor digiti minimi					■	■	
	Extension (PIP/DIP)	Lumbricals						■	■
	Abduction	Dorsal interossei						■	■
		Abductor digiti minimi						■	■
	Adduction	Palmar interossei							■
	Opposition	Opponens digiti minimi						■	■

(continued)

TABLE A1 *(continued)*

Joint	Movement	Muscle	C3	C4	C5	C6	C7	C8	T1
Thumb	Flexion (IP)	Flexor pollicis longus					■	■	
	Flexion/rotation (MCP)	Flexor pollicis brevis						■	■
	Extension (MCP)	Extensor pollicis brevis					■	■	
	Extension (IP)	Extensor pollicis longus					■	■	
	Abduction	Abductor pollicis longus					■	■	
	Abduction/rotation	Abductor pollicis brevis						■	■
	Adduction/rotation	Adductor pollicis						■	■
	Adduction/flexion (IP)	Palmar interossei						■	■
	Opposition	Opponens pollicis						■	■

The spinal nerve roots which predominantly innervate a muscle are indicated with heavy shading. (Abbreviations: DIP = distal interphalangeal joint; IP = interphalangeal joint; MCP = metacarpophalangeal joint; PIP = proximal interphalangeal joint.) Adapted from Reference 1 with permission of Elsevier.

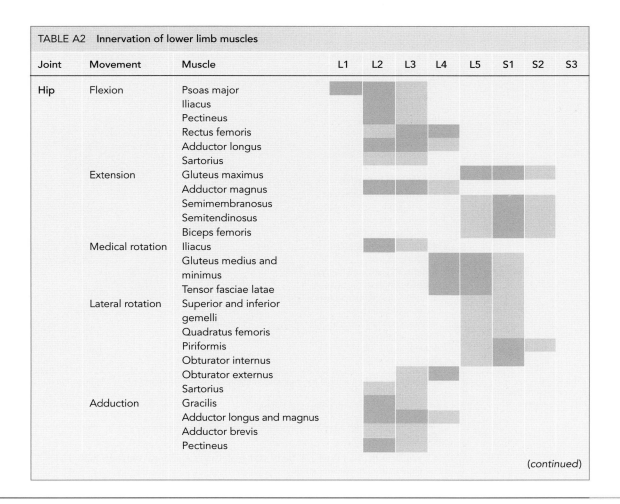

TABLE A2 Innervation of lower limb muscles

Joint	Movement	Muscle	L1	L2	L3	L4	L5	S1	S2	S3
Hip	Flexion	Psoas major	■	■						
		Iliacus		■	■					
		Pectineus		■	■					
		Rectus femoris		■	■	■				
		Adductor longus		■	■	■				
		Sartorius		■	■					
	Extension	Gluteus maximus					■	■	■	
		Adductor magnus		■	■					
		Semimembranosus					■	■	■	
		Semitendinosus					■	■	■	
		Biceps femoris					■	■	■	
	Medical rotation	Iliacus		■	■					
		Gluteus medius and minimus				■	■	■		
		Tensor fasciae latae				■	■	■		
	Lateral rotation	Superior and inferior gemelli					■	■	■	
		Quadratus femoris					■	■		
		Piriformis						■	■	■
		Obturator internus					■	■	■	
		Obturator externus			■	■				
		Sartorius		■	■					
	Adduction	Gracilis		■	■					
		Adductor longus and magnus		■	■	■				
		Adductor brevis		■	■					
		Pectineus		■	■					

(continued)

TABLE A2 (continued)

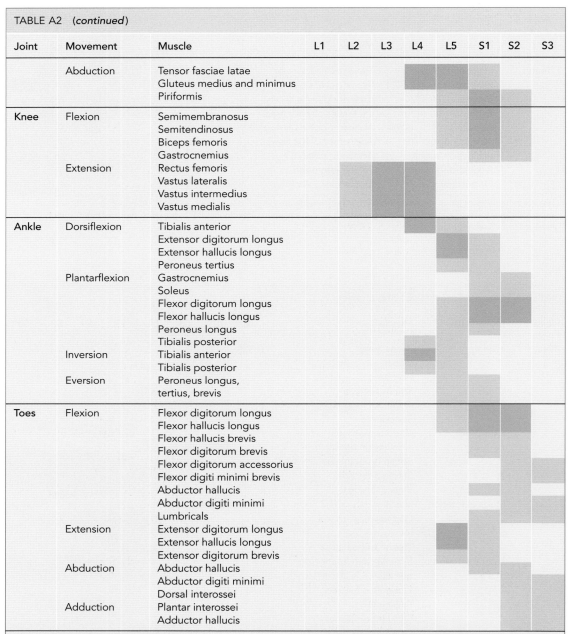

Joint	Movement	Muscle	L1	L2	L3	L4	L5	S1	S2	S3
	Abduction	Tensor fasciae latae				■	■			
		Gluteus medius and minimus					■	■		
		Piriformis						■	■	
Knee	Flexion	Semimembranosus					■	■		
		Semitendinosus						■	■	
		Biceps femoris						■	■	
		Gastrocnemius						■	■	
	Extension	Rectus femoris		■	■	■				
		Vastus lateralis			■	■				
		Vastus intermedius			■	■				
		Vastus medialis			■	■				
Ankle	Dorsiflexion	Tibialis anterior				■				
		Extensor digitorum longus					■	■		
		Extensor hallucis longus					■	■		
		Peroneus tertius					■	■		
	Plantarflexion	Gastrocnemius							■	
		Soleus							■	
		Flexor digitorum longus						■	■	
		Flexor hallucis longus						■	■	
		Peroneus longus						■		
		Tibialis posterior				■	■			
	Inversion	Tibialis anterior				■				
		Tibialis posterior				■	■			
	Eversion	Peroneus longus, tertius, brevis					■	■		
Toes	Flexion	Flexor digitorum longus						■	■	
		Flexor hallucis longus						■	■	
		Flexor hallucis brevis						■	■	
		Flexor digitorum brevis						■	■	
		Flexor digitorum accessorius							■	■
		Flexor digiti minimi brevis							■	■
		Abductor hallucis						■	■	
		Abductor digiti minimi							■	■
		Lumbricals						■	■	
	Extension	Extensor digitorum longus					■	■		
		Extensor hallucis longus					■	■		
		Extensor digitorum brevis						■	■	
	Abduction	Abductor hallucis						■	■	
		Abductor digiti minimi							■	■
		Dorsal interossei							■	■
	Adduction	Plantar interossei							■	■
		Adductor hallucis							■	■

The spinal nerve roots which predominantly innervate a muscle are indicated with heavy shading. Adapted from Reference 1 with permission of Elsevier.

Reference

1. Williams PL, Bannister LH, Berry MM et al: Gray's Anatomy, 38th edn. New York, Churchill Livingstone, 1995.

Index

Page numbers in **bold** refer to tables. Page numbers in *italics* refer to figures.

Notes: as spinal cord injuries are the subject of this book, all entries refer to this, unless otherwise stated.

A

abdominal binders, 217
abdominal distension, 211
abdominal muscle paralysis, 63
aetiology, 3
after-load, 233
aging, 26
air-based cushions, *246*, *247*
American Spinal Injury Association
        (ASIA) assessment, 6–11, 157
    form, *8*
    impairment scale, 10–11
    manual muscle test, 157
    motor level, 7–9, **9**
    neurological level, 9–10
    sensory level, 9, **10**
American Uniform Data System for
        Medical Rehabilitation (UDSMR),
        276
ankle–foot orthoses (AFO), 120–124
    downward slope, *125*
    gait-related activities, 123–124
ankle muscle innervation, **286**
ankle paralysis, walking and, 119–124
    AFO and *see* ankle–foot orthoses
        (AFO)
    dorsiflexor muscle paralysis, *119*,
        119–120
    plantarflexor muscle paralysis, 120,
        120, *121*
anterior cervical cord syndrome, 11
anterior horn cells, 6, 12
anti-tip bars, 83, 90, 263, *265*
arm ergometers, 234, *235*
arm rests, 266–267
arm troughs, *198*
arterio-venous oxygen difference, 233–234
ASIA classification *see* American Spinal
        Injury Association (ASIA)
        assessment
aspiration, 211
assisted cough, *213–214*, 213–215
associative stage, training tasks, 138

atelectasis, 208–209
autonomic dysreflexia, 17–18
autonomic pathways, 6, *7*
autonomous stage, training tasks, 138

B

backrests, 256–259
    height, 258
    inclination, 259
    sling type, 250, *257*
    width, 256–258
back wheels, wheelchairs, *253–254*, *255*,
        260–263
balance, *148*, 148–149
Barthel Index, **37**
bed mattresses, 23–24
bed mobility, 57–76
bicep muscles, 73, 94
bi-level positive airway pressure support,
        218–219
bladder function, 18, 19
blood pressure, 17–18
blood volume, 233
body weight, lift and transfer, 45
Borg exertion scale, 229, **230**
bowel function, 18, 19
braces, *14*
brakes, 263
Brown-Sequard lesion, 11
bulbocavernosus reflex, 15

C

C1–C3 tetraplegia
    hand function, 93–94
    independence attained, **43**, 43–44
    mobilization, 44
    ventilation, 219–221
    wheelchair mobility, 44, *44*, 79
C4 tetraplegia
    contractures, 185

C4 tetraplegia (*continued*)
  hand function, 93–94
  independence attained, **43**, 44
  respiratory function, 205
  wheelchair mobility, 79
C5 tetraplegia
  contractures, 185
  hand function, 94, *95*
  independence attained, **43**, 44–45
  respiratory function, 205
  wheelchair mobility, 79
C6 tetraplegia
  contractures, 185
  hand function, 94–96, *97*
  independence attained, **43**, 45
  respiratory function, 205
  transfer and mobility strategies, 57
    rolling, 60, **60**
    unsupported sitting, 58, *58*, *59*
    vertical lift, 64–65, **66**, **67**, **68**
    wheel chair mobility, 79
C7 tetraplegia
  hand function, 94–96
  independence attained, **43**, 45
  respiratory function, 205
  wheel chair mobility, 79
C8 tetraplegia
  hand function, 97–98
  independence attained, **43**, 45
  respiratory function, 205
  wheel chair mobility, 79
Canadian Occupational Performance
  Measure (COPM), **38**
Capabilities of Upper Extremity
  Instruments (CUE), **39**
cardiac output, **231**, 231–233
cardiovascular fitness, 227
  assessment, 228–231
    field exercise tests, 230, **230**
    peak oxygen consumption tests,
     228–229, 231
    submaximal exercise tests, 229,
     230
  training *see* cardiovascular fitness
    training
  see also exercise
cardiovascular fitness training, 227–237
  exercise in the community, 237
  exercise prescription, 234–237
  importance, 227
  principles, 228
  responses, 231–234
  see also exercise
catheterization, 19
cauda equina lesions, 12
central cord lesion, 11
central pattern generators, 150–151

chin-controlled wheelchairs, 44
classification *see* American Spinal Injury
  Association (ASIA) assessment
Clinical Outcomes Variable Scale
  (COVS), **37**
cognitive stage, training tasks, 138
Common Object Test (COT), **39**
comorbid brain injury, 25
complete lesions
  goal planning/setting, **43**, 43–46
  paraplegia *see* paraplegia
  tetraplegia *see* tetraplegia
  see also specific lesion level
complex regional pain syndrome, 200
continuous positive airway pressure
  (CPAP), 218
contractility (cardiac), 232
contracture management, 277
contractures, *177*, 177–189, *178*, 185
  anticipation, 185–188
  assessment, 178–179
  causes, 177
  differentiation, 179
  effects of, 177–178
  goal planning, 178
  predisposing factors, 185–188
  prevention, 93–94, 100, 185–188
  spasticity, 188
  treatment, 179–185
    non-stretch-based modalities, 189
    prioritizing, 188–189
    stretch and passive movements *see*
     stretch and passive movements
  see also specific types/locations
conus, 12
corticospinal tracts, 5
cough, assisted, *213–214*, 213–215
Craig Handicap and Reporting Technique
  (CHART), **37**
cross section (spinal cord), *5*
'crouch' gait, 120
cuneate tract, 6
cutlery, adapted, *96*
cycle ergometer, 236

D

deep tendon reflex, spinal shock, 15
deep vein thrombosis, 15–16
definitions, 3–4
deltoid muscles, 197
depression, 24–25
dermatomes, 9
diaphragm
  function, 43
  innervation level, **206**

diaphragmatic pacing, 220
dorsiflexion, ankle–foot orthoses, 124
dorsiflexor muscle paralysis, *119,*
        119–120
double metal upright AFO, 122–123,
        124

E

ectopic ossification, 21
elbow collapse, 64–65, *68*
elbow muscles
    flexors
        contracture, *178*
        stretches, *186*
    innervation, **284**
    pronator, stretches, *187*
elderly
    exercise prescription, 236–237
    spinal cord injuries and, 25
electrical stimulation
    assisted cough, 214
    exercise, 236
    hand function, 104–105
    motor task training, 146–148
    muscle fatigue, 128
    partially paralysed muscles, 170
    voluntary strength, 170
    walking and standing, 128
electromyographic (EMG) feedback, 169
endurance (muscle), 164
environmental factors, 243–271
    see also wheelchair(s)
epidemiology, 3, *4*
evidence-based physiotherapy, 275–277,
        276
exercise
    adherence to, 235
    community-based, 237
    prescription, 234–237
        elderly, 236–237
        electrical stimulation and, 236
        frail, 236–237
        intensity, 234
        thermoregulation and, 237
        type, selection, 234–236
    recreational, 236
    spinal cord injuries and responses to,
        231, 231–234
        arterio-venous oxygen difference,
            233–234
        cardiac output, 231–233
    testing, 228–231
        see also cardiovascular fitness
expiratory flow rates, 209–210
external drainage sheaths, 19

F

family, psychological well-being and, 25
field exercise tests, 230, **230**
finger muscles
    extensor, 103
    flexor, 189
    innervation, **284**
fitness-training programmes, 228
Five Additional Mobility and Locomotor
        Items (5-AML), **40**
flexor-hinge splints, 103–104, *104*
foam-based cushions, *246,* 248
folding wheelchair frames, 250, *251*
footplates, *251,* 263–266, *265*
forced expirations, 209
friends, psychological well-being and, 25
'frog breathing,' 220–221
'frog' position, *182*
front castors, wheelchairs, 259–260, *260*
Functional Independence Measure
        (FIM®), **37,** 276
functional residual capacity, 209
Functional Standing Test (FST), **39**

G

gait-related activities, 123–124
    assessment tools, **39**
gait training, 143, 151
gel-based cushions, *246,* 247–248
glossopharyngeal breathing, 220–221
goal planning/setting, 35, 40–46, 276
    benefits, 40–41
    complete lesions, **43,** 43–46
        see also specific lesion levels
    contracture management, 178
    guidelines, 41–42, **42**
gracile tract, 6
grade-aids, 263, *264*
Grasp and Release Test (GRT), **39–40**

H

hamstring muscles
    excessive extensibility, 189
    paralysis, 126
    unsupported sitting, 59, *59*
hand function, 93–105
    C4 (and above) tetraplegia, 93–94
    C5 tetraplegia, 94, *95, 96*
    C6 tetraplegia, 94–96, *97*
    C7 tetraplegia, 94–96
    C8 tetraplegia, 97–98
    electrical stimulation, 104–105

hand function (*continued*)
  feeding equipment, *96*
  reconstructive surgery, 104–105
  therapy principles, 93–98
  see also splints/splinting
hand-held myometers, 159, 162, *162*
hanger angle, 266
headrests, 267
heart rate, **231**, 231–232
heterotopic ossification, 21
hinged solid plastic AFO, 122, *123*
hip extension, 113, *113*
hip flexion contracture, *177*
hip guidance orthosis, 115, *116*
hip–knee–ankle–foot orthoses, 115–119,
    118
  types, 115–117, *116, 117*
  walking using, 117–118, *118*
hip muscles
  abductor paralysis, 128
  extensor paralysis, 127–128
  flexor paralysis, 126–127
  innervation, **285–286**
hip paralysis, walking and, 126–128
  hip extensor paralysis, 127–128
  hip flexor paralysis, 126–127
hip stretches, *182–183, 188*
hybrid exercise, 236

I

impairment(s), 13–21
  activity restrictions, links, 46
  assessment, 40, 46–47
    ASIA scale, 10–11
    physiotherapy, 40
    see also specific tests/measures
  autonomic dysreflexia, 17–18
  bladder dysfunction, 18, 19
  bowel dysfunction, 18, 19
  cardiovascular, 227
  contractures *see* contractures
  DVT and pulmonary embolism, 15–16
  heterotopic ossification, 21
  management, 135–242
    cardiovascular fitness *see*
      cardiovascular fitness training
    contracture management *see*
      contractures
    motor task training *see* motor task
      training
    pain *see* pain management
    respiratory *see* respiratory
      management
    strength training *see* strength training

osteoporosis, 21
paralytic ileus, 15, 211
physiotherapy identification of, 46–47
postural hypotension, 18
sexual dysfunction, 18, 19–21, *20*
spasticity *see* spasticity
spinal shock, 13, 15
vertebral, 13
incomplete lesions
  goals, 46
  neurological loss patterns, 11
  standing and walking, 107, 118–128
    ankle paralysis *see* ankle paralysis,
      walking and
    hip paralysis *see* hip paralysis,
      walking and
    knee paralysis *see* knee paralysis,
      walking and
independence, 42, **43**
indwelling catheter, 19
innervation levels, 41, **42**
inspiratory muscle training, 217
intermittent catheterization, 19
intermittent positive pressure breathing,
  219
International Classification of
  Functioning, Disability and
  Health (ICF), 35, *36*, 36–48
interphalangeal (IP) joints
  flexion, 94, *94, 101*
  sustained stretches, *184*
  tenodesis grip, 100, *101, 102*
intrathoracic positive pressures, 209
invasive mechanical ventilation,
  219–220
ischial tuberosities
  air-based cushions, 247
  foam-based cushions, 248
  gel-based cushions, 247, *247*
  pressure relief, 23
  seat rake, 256
isokinetic dynamometers, 162–163

J

joint angle, 178
joysticks, 268, *269, 270*
jumping gait pattern, 111, **112**

K

Katz Index of ADL, **38**
kerbs *see* wheelchair mobility
kidney failure, 19

knee–ankle–foot orthoses (bilateral),
110–115, *111*
   sitting to standing, 113–115, **114**
   walking with, 111–115, **112**, *113*
knee extension, unsupported sitting, 58
   unsupported sitting, *59*
knee hyper-extension, 126, *127*
knee muscle innervation, **286**
knee paralysis, walking and, 124–126
   hamstring paralysis, 126
   quadriceps paralysis, 124–126
knee splints, 126
knowledge of performance, 146

L

lateral key grip, 98–99
lateral trunk support, *257*
latissimus dorsi muscle, 45
leg rests, 263–266, 265, *266*
life expectancy, 26
long-term ventilation, 220
lower limb innervation, **285–286**
lower limb paralysis
   standing and walking, 107–128
   strength training, 155
   transfers and mobility, 57–76
      influencing factors (mobility), 74–76
      lying to long sitting, 61–63, **61–63**, *64*
      rolling, **60**, 60–61
      sitting unsupported, 57–60, *58*, *59*
      transfers, 68–74
      transfer strategies, **69–70**, **71–72**, *73*
      vertical lift, 64–66, **65**, **66**, *67*, *68*
      vertical transfers, 74, **75–76**
lower motor neurons, 6
   lesions, 12
lumbar paraplegia, **43**, 46
lumbosacral paraplegia, **43**, 46, 107–108
lungs
   compliance, 208, 210
   mechanical inflation, 214
   pulmonary embolism, 15–16
   secretions, 210
      suctioning, 215–216
   see also respiratory function
lying to long sitting
   lower limb paralysis, 61–63, **61–63**, *64*
   tricep muscle paralysis, 63

M

male fertility, 20
manual muscle test, 157–158, **158**

manual wheelchairs
   arm rests, 266–267
   back wheels, 260–263
   brakes, 263
   footplates, *251*, 263–266, *266*
   front castors, 259–260, *260*
   headrests, 267
   leg rests, 263–266, 265, *266*
   pushrims, 261, *261*, *262*
   seat depth, *252*, 254–255
   seat rake, *252*, *253*, 256
   seat-to-floor height, 250–254, *252*, *253*
   seat width, 255
   side guards, *258*
   spoke guards, *262*, 263
   wheel camber, *252*, 263
   see also backrests; wheelchair cushions
marital status, 25
mattresses, 23–24
mechanical in-exsufflator, 214, *216*
medial-linkage orthosis, 117, *117*
metacarpophalangeal (MCP) joints
   hyper-extension, 94, *94*, 100
   sustained stretches, *184*
mid-drive wheelchairs, 267, *268*
minitracheostomies, 216
mobility
   bed mobility and transfers, 57–76
      see also transfers; *specific
         strategies/techniques*
   muscle strength and, 155, *156*
      see also strength training
   tasks, 74–76
   wheelchairs *see* wheelchair mobility
   see also sitting; standing; walking
Modified Ashworth Scale, 16, **16**
Modified Benzel Classification, **39**
Modified Functional Reach Test
   (mFRT), **40**
'modified' one repetition maximum,
   159
motor control, 137–138
motor imagery, 169
motor learning, 137–138
   see also motor task training
motor neurons, 4, 6, 12
motor pathways, 4, *5*, 6
   assessment, 7–9, *9*
   motor control, 137–138
   motor learning, 137–138
'Motor Relearning Approach,' 137
motor schema theory, 137–138
motor task analysis, 57–133
   hand function *see* hand function
   realistic framework for, 47
   standing *see* standing

motor task analysis (*continued*)
 transfers *see* transfers
 walking *see* walking
 wheelchair mobility *see* wheelchair
  mobility
 see also motor task training; *specific tasks*
motor task training, 137–151
 control, 137–138
 electrical stimulation, 146–148
 goals, 146
 learning, 137–138
 methods, 145–148
  demonstration, 145
  feedback, 145–148
  instructions, 145
  'similar but simpler' approaches,
   139–140, 139–143, *141–142*
 motivation maintenance, 144
 novel, learning of, 137
 practice, importance of, 139–145
  outside formal therapy sessions,
   143–145
  training booklets, 144, *144*
 principles, 138–149
 progression, 143
 stages, 138
 treadmill training, 149–151
movement restrictions, 13
muscle endurance, 156
muscle fatigue, 128
 respiratory muscles *see* respiratory
  muscles
muscle shortening, 180
muscle strength
 assessment *see* strength assessment
 training/improvement *see* strength
  training
 transfers/mobilty and, 155, *156*
myometers, hand-held, 159, 162, *162*
myositis ossificans, 21

N

Needs Assessment Checklist (NAC), **38**
nerve roots, 4, *5*
neurological assessment *see* American
  Spinal Injury Association (ASIA)
  assessment
neurological losses, 11
neuromuscular weakness, respiration, 213
neuropathic pain, 193, **194**, 195
nociceptive pain, 193, **194**, 196–200
 back, 196
 complex regional pain syndromes, 200
 management
  analgesics, 196

 electrical stimulation, 197
 immobilization, 196
 lifestyle interventions, 200
 physical supports, 197, *198*
 physiotherapy interventions, 196
 surgery, 196
 neck, 196
 overuse limb pain, 199–200
 shoulder *see* shoulder pain
non-invasive negative ventilation, 220
non-invasive positive airway pressure
  support, 217–219
non-invasive ventilation, 219

O

one repetition maximum (1RM) test,
  158–159, *159–161*
orthoses *see specific types*
osteoporosis, 21
overhead suspension, 149, *150*
overuse syndromes, 199–200

P

pain
 assessment, 194–195, **195**
  intensity measures, 194
 chronic
  back/neck, 196
  overuse syndromes, 199–200
  psychosocial factors, 200–201
 classification, 193, **194**
 management *see* pain management
 neuropathic, 193, **194**, 195
 nociceptive *see* nociceptive pain
 see also specific regions
pain management, 193–201
 neuropathic pain, 195
 nociceptive pain, 196–200
 psychosocial factors, 200–201
 respiratory, 211
 see also specific methods
palmar bands, 97
palmar tenodesis grip, *98*
paradoxical breathing, 210
parallel bars, *109*, 164, *166*
paralytic ileus, 15, 211
paraplegia
 definition, 3
 goal planning/setting, 46
 life expectancy, 26
 standing and walking, 107
 transfer and mobility strategies

lying to long sitting, 61, **61–63,** 63, *64*
  vertical lift, 64, **65**
  wheelchair mobility, 79
  see also specific lesion levels
parasympathetic nerves, 6
ParaWalker, 115, *116*
partially paralysed muscles
  electrical stimulation, 170
  motor tasks, 155
  strength training, 166–170, *167–168,*
    169
passive joint range of motion, 178–179
passive movements, 184–185
  animal studies, 179–180
  clinical trials, 180–181
passive tenodesis grip, 99
peak flow cough, 209
peak oxygen consumption tests,
    228–229, 231
percussion, 215
The Physical Activity Recall Assessment
    for People with Spinal Cord Injury
    (PARA-SCI), **38**
physiotherapy, 35–48
  activity limitations, 36–40
    assessment tools, 36–37, **37–40**
  evidence-based, 275–277
  goals, 35, 40–46
    benefits, 40–41
    complete lesions, **43,** 43–46
    guidelines, 41–42, **42**
    incomplete lesions, 46
    significance, 41
    see also goal planning/setting
  impairment
    assessment, 40
    identification, 46–47
  multi-disciplinary team, 48
  outcome measurements, 47–48
  participation restrictions, 36–40, **37–40**
    assessment tools, 36–37
  purpose, 35
  recommendations, 275, **276**
  respiratory management, 213
  treatment identification, 47
  see also specific techniques
pincer tenodesis grip, *98,* 98–99
plantarflexor muscles
  paralysis, 120, *120, 121*
  stretches for, *182, 186*
plastic solid AFO, 121–122, *122*
pneumatic front castors, 259
position changes, pressure sore
    prevention, 23
positioning, respiratory management,
    216–217
posterior leaf spring AFO, 121, *122*

postural adjustments, balance, 148
postural hypotension, 18
power wheelchairs, 80, 267–268, *268*
  circuitry variations, 268
  control mechanisms, 268
  joysticks, *270*
pressure-relieving equipment, 23–24
pressure ulcers, 22–24
  causes, 22
  early signs, 22
  education, 23
  prevention, 22–24
  treatment, 24
prevalence, 3, *4*
prognosis, 12
progressive resistance training, 163–166,
    165, 166
  general well-being, 171
  muscle power and endurance,
    164–166
  specificity, 164
prolonged bedrest, respiratory
    complications, 211
psychological well-being, 24–25
psychosocial factors, chronic pain,
    200–201
pulmonary compliance, 208
  secretions, 210
pulmonary embolism, 15–16
PULSES, **37**
pushrims, 261, *261, 262*

Q

quadricep muscle paralysis, 124–126
quadriplegia *see* tetraplegia
Quadriplegic Index of Function (QIF), **38**
Quebec User Evaluation of Satisfaction
    with Assistive Technology
    (QUEST), **40**

R

range of motion, 178–179
rear-wheel drive wheelchairs, 267, *268*
reciprocating gait orthosis, 116, *116*
reflux voiding, 19
residual volume, 210
respiratory complications
  C1 tetraplegia, 205
  C2 tetraplegia, 205
  C3 tetraplegia, 205
  immediate post-injury, 210–212
  muscle weakness, 206–210, *207,*
    208, 211

respiratory function, 205
    assessment, 212–213
    expiratory flow rates, 209–210
    functional residual capacity, 209
    lesion level effects, **206**
    pulmonary compliance and, 208, 210
    residual volume, 210
    rib cage compliance and, 208
    rib cage distortion, 210
    tidal volume, 206–209, *207*, **207**
    total lung capacity, 206–209, *207*, **207**
    vital capacity, 206–209, *207*, **207**
respiratory management, 205–221
    assessment of function, 212–213
    positioning, 216–217
    treatment options, 213–219
        assisted cough, 213–215, *214–215*
        bi-level positive airway pressure,
            218–219
        continuous positive airway pressure,
            218
        intermittent positive pressure
            breathing, 219
        muscle training, 217
        non-invasive positive airway
            pressure, 217–218
        non-invasive ventilation, 219
        percussion, vibration, shaking, 215
        positioning, 216–217
        suctioning, 215–216
    ventilation in C1–C3 tetraplegia,
        219–221
respiratory muscles
    fatigue, 206–210, **207**, *207*, *208*, 211
    innervation levels, **206**
rib cage
    compliance, 208
    distortion, 210
    expansion, 208
rigid frame wheelchairs, 250, *251*
rolling, **60**, 60–61

S

sacral paraplegia, **43**, 46
sacral pressure ulcers, 24
sacral sparing, 11
scales, motor task training, *147*
scapula muscle innervation, **283**
seat depth, *252*, 254–255
seat rake, *252*, *253*, 256
seat-to-floor height, 250–254, *252*
seat width, 255
secretions, lung, 210, 215–216
sensory pathways, *5*, 6
    assessment, 9, **10**

serial casts, 181
sexual function, 18, 19–21, *20*
sexuality, 20
SF-36® Health Survey, **38**
shaking (chest), 215
shoulder
    muscle innervation, **283–284**
    pain *see* shoulder pain
    stretches, *181*, *187*
    support, 197, *198*
    weight bearing, 146, *147*
shoulder adductor stretches, *187*
shoulder extensor stretches, *181*
shoulder pain, 196–199
    soft tissue trauma, physical handling,
        198–199
    subluxation, 197–198
Sickness Impact Profile (SIP-136), **38**
side guards, 255, *258*
'similar but simpler' approach, *139–140*,
        139–143, *141–142*
sitting
    lying to long sitting
        lower limb paralysis, 61–63, **61–63**,
            64
        tricep muscle paralysis, 63
    to standing, knee–ankle–foot orthoses,
        113–115, **114**
    unsupported, 57–60, *58*
    in vehicles, 269
6 m Walk Test, **39**
skin management, 22–24
    see also pressure ulcers
sleep apnoea, 218
slideboards, 73, *73*
    strength training and, 167, *168*
sliding tilt tables, strength training, 167,
        169, *169*
sling backrests, 250, *257*
slings, strength training and, 167, *167*
SMART, goal setting, 41
solid front castors, 259
spasticity, 16–17, 76
    classification, 16, **16**
    contractures, 188
    management, 17
    neurophysiology, 16–17
Spinal Cord Independence Measures
        (SCIM), **37**
The Spinal Cord Injury Functional
        Ambulation Inventory (SCI-FA),
        39
spinal orthosis, 13, *14*
spinal pathways, 4–6, *5*
spinal shock, 13, 15
spinothalamic tracts, *5*, 6
splints/splinting

hand function and
  C4 (and above) tetraplegia, 94, *94*
  C5 tetraplegia, 95, *96*
  C6 tetraplegia, 97, *97*
  flexor-hinge splints, 103–104, *104*
  tenodesis grip promotion, 99–103,
    100, 101, 102
  wrist splints, *100*
  knee splints, 126
spoke guards, *262, 263*
spotter training strap, 81, *83*
stairs *see* wheelchair mobility
standing
  duration, 110
  electrical stimulation, 128
  lower limb paralysis, 107–128
  therapeutic, 108–110
    equipment, 108, *109*
  see also walking
standing frame, *109*
strength assessment, 157–163
  hand-held myometers, 159, 162, *162*
  isokinetic dynamometers, 162–163
  manual muscle test, 157–158, **158**
  one repetition maximum (1RM) test,
    158–159, *159–161*
  wheel devices, *168*
strengthening exercises, subluxation, 197
strength training, 155–171, 277
  agonist, antagonist muscle imbalances,
    170
  complications, 170–171
  electrical stimulation *see* electrical
    stimulation
  flickers of movement, 169
  general well-being, 171
  injury avoidance, 170–171
  neurally intact muscles, 163–166
  partially paralysed muscles, 166–170,
    167–168, 169
  progressive resistance *see* progressive
    resistance training
  see also strength assessment; *specific
    methods/devices*
stretch and passive movements, 179–185
  animal studies, 179–180
  clinical trials, 180–181
  contracture prevention, *186, 187, 188*
  sustained stretch *see* sustained stretches
stroke volume, **231**, 232–233
subluxation, 197–198
submaximal exercise tests, 229, **230**
suctioning (airway), 215–216
suicide, 25
supraspinatus muscles
  overuse, 200
  subluxation prevention, 197

sustained stretches, 181–184
  elbow flexor muscles, *186*
  elbow pronator muscles, *187*
  hamstring muscles, *182*
  hip
    adductor muscles, *182, 188*
    extensor muscles, *183*
    internal rotator muscles, *182, 183*
  interphalangeal joints of finger, *184*
  metacarpophalangeal joints of fingers,
    184
  plantarflexor muscles, *182, 186*
  shoulder adductor muscles, *187*
  shoulder extensor muscles, *181*
  soleus muscles, *183*
swing through pattern, 111, **112**
sympathetic nerves, 6

T

T1 paraplegia, independence attained, 46
'Task-oriented Approach,' 137
10 m Walk Test, **39**
ten repetition maximum, 163, 167
tendon transfers, 105
tenodesis grip, *98*, 98–104
  motor task training, 142
  splinting and taping, 99–103
    duration of wear, 102
tetraplegia
  definition, 3
  goal planning/setting, **43**, 43–45
  hand function *see* hand function
  life expectancy, 26
  shoulder pain, 196–199
  standing and walking, 107
  see also specific lesion levels
Tetraplegic Hand Activity Questionnaire
  (THAQ), **39**
thermoregulation, 237
thoracic paraplegia
  independence attained, **43**, 46
  lying to long sitting transfer, *64*
  respiratory function, 206
  'similar but simpler' approach, 142, *143*
  standing and, 107
  strength training, 155, 156
  transfer strategies, 57
    muscle strength and, 155, *156*
  walking and, 107, 110–118
    bilateral knee–ankle–foot orthosis,
      110–115, *111*, **112**, *113*
    hip–ankle–foot orthosis, 115–119,
      116, 117, 118
    see also specific orthoses
  wheelchairs, appropriate, *258*

thumb
  adductor contracture, *178*
  extensor muscles, 103
  flexor muscles, excessive extensibility, 189
  muscle innervation, **284**
  tenodesis grip promotion, 100, 102, *102*
thumb loop, 102, *103*
tidal volume, 206–209, **207**
'tilt-in-space', 267
tilt table, *109*, 167, 169, *169*
Timed Motor Test (TMT), **40**
Timed Up and Go, **39**
toe-off AFO, 122, *123*
toes, muscle innervation, **286**
total lung capacity, 206–209, **207**
transfers, 57–76, 68–74
  bicep muscles, 73
  definition, 68
  leg position, 68
  lower limb paralysis, 57–76
  muscle strength and, 155, *156*
    see also strength training
  rotary strategy, **69–70**, 71
  strategies, 68
  translatory strategy, 71, **71–72**
  tricep muscle paralysis, 74
  wheelchair, 73, *73*, 74, **75–76**
  see also specific tasks/strategies
traumatic brain injury comorbidity, 25
treadmill training, 149–151
tricep paralysis
  lying to long sitting, 63
  transfers, 74
  vertical lift, 64–65
Tufts Assessment of Motor Performance
    (TAMP), **38**
12-minute wheelchair propulsion test,
    230, **230**

U

upper limb(s)
  functional assessment, **39–40**
  muscle innervation, **283–285**
  strength, 155
upper motor neurons, 4, 6
  lesions, 12

V

Valutazione Funzionale Meilolesi (VFM),
    38
venous return, 232
verbal encouragement, 146
verbal feedback, 146
vertebrae, 4, *5*

vertebral column, 4, *5*
  damage, 13
  instability, 13
  orthoses, 13, *14*
    see also specific types
vertical lift, 23
  lower limb paralysis, 64–66, **65, 66, 67,**
    68
  tricep muscle paralysis, 64–65
vertical transfers, lower limb paralysis, 74
vibration (chest), 215
vital capacity, 206–209, **207**
VO$_{2\,max}$, 229
VO$_{2peak}$ test, 228–229, 231
voluntary strength, electrical stimulation,
    170

W

walking, 107–128
  electrical stimulation, 128
  lower limb paralysis, 107–128
  orthoses
    ankle–foot orthoses *see* ankle–foot
      orthoses (AFO)
    hip–knee–ankle–foot *see*
      hip–knee–ankle–foot orthoses
    knee–ankle–foot orthoses *see*
      knee–ankle–foot orthoses
      (bilateral)
  partial lower limb paralysis, 118–128
  thoracic paraplegia, 110–118
  see also standing
Walking Index for Spinal Cord Injury
    (WISCI), **39**
The Walking Mobility Scale, **39**
walk tests, **39**
wheel camber, *252*, 263
wheelchair(s)
  back wheels, *253–254*, *255*, 260–263
  frame types, 250, *251*
  front castors and back wheels, distance
    between, 259
  manual *see* manual wheelchairs
  powered *see* power wheelchairs
  seating, 24, 245–270
    backrest *see* backrests
    cushions *see* wheelchair cushions
    manual wheelchairs, 249–267
    power wheelchairs, 267–268
    seat, 250–256
    sitting in vehicles, 269
  set-up, 249–250
  'tippiness', 259
  transfer to, 73, *73*, 74, **75–76**
  see also wheelchair mobility

Wheelchair Circuit Test (WCT), **40**
wheelchair cushions, 24, 245–249, *246*
  assessment, 246
  cost, 249
  maintenance, 248
  posture, 248–249
  prescriptions, 246, 249
  stability, 248–249
  weight, 249
wheelchair mobility, 79–92
  assessment tools, **40**
  assistance, 90–92
  corners, 80, *81*
  kerbs
    ascending, 88, *88, 89*
    ascending forwards, 90
    descending backwards, 85, *86*
    descending forwards, 85, *87*
  manual chairs, 80–90
  power chairs, 80
  stairs
    ascending, 90, *91*

    descending backwards, 85, *86*, 90, *90*
    descending forwards, 85, *87*
    wheelstands *see* wheelstands
Wheelchair Skills Test (WST), **40**
'wheelie' *see* wheelstands
wheelstands, 80–85
  ease, 84–85
  grassy slopes, 88–90, *89*
  maintaining, 84
  moving onto, 83
  tilt required, *82*
wrist extensor contracture, *178*
wrist muscle innervation, **284**
wrist pain, 199
wrist splints, *100*

Z

zones of partial preservation, 11